Test

Ch. 1

Ch. 2.

Ch. 3 - diag. equip., rt, left hemi chart p.56
    not: rt/left /Clem's

    Localiz.
    See p. 60

Ch. 4. not: memory

A Survey
of Adult Aphasia

A SURVEY
OF ADULT APHASIA

G. ALBYN DAVIS

University of Massachusetts

PRENTICE-HALL, INC. *Englewood Cliffs, N.J. 07632*

Library of Congress Cataloging in Publication Data

DAVIS, G. ALBYN,   (date)
    A survey of adult aphasia.

    Bibliography: p.
    Includes index.
    1. Aphasia. I. Title.
RC425.D38 1983   616.85′52   82-13169
ISBN 0-13-878207-5

Editorial/production supervision by Marion Osterberg
Cover design by Ray Lundgren
Manufacturing buyer: Ron Chapman

Printed in the United States of America

10   9   8   7

ISBN 0-13-878207-5

Prentice-Hall International, Inc., *London*
Prentice-Hall of Australia Pty. Limited, *Sydney*
Editora Prentice-Hall do Brazil, LTDA, *Rio de Janeiro*
Prentice-Hall Canada Inc., *Toronto*
Prentice-Hall of India Private Limited, *New Delhi*
Prentice-Hall of Japan, Inc., *Tokyo*
Prentice-Hall of Southeast Asia Pte. Ltd., *Singapore*
Whitehall Books Limited, *Wellington, New Zealand*

Contents

Preface

Within the rehabilitation team for neurologically-impaired patients, the speech-language pathologist is the expert on communication processes, impairments of these processes, and treatment of these impairments. This expertise enables the clinician to identify and differentiate the specific abilities and disabilities that relate to language function, to plan and carry out various treatment procedures in a way that is relevant to each patient, and to assess recovery of different communicative functions. Physicians and families of patients turn to the speech-language clinician for answers to their questions about the nature of aphasia and its recovery.

A Survey of Adult Aphasia is a comprehensive presentation of literature and prevailing ideas. The book begins with definitions of the disorder, related disorders, and symptoms and syndromes of aphasia. The next few chapters provide background for a thorough understanding of aphasia and of how investigators go about developing this understanding. Direct presentation of the clinical process begins with Chapter 6; and from there the reader is taken through the principles and methods of diagnosis and assessment, the intricacies of recovery, and the principles and procedures of language rehabilitation. I have attempted a balanced approach in that most of the concepts coming out of basic and applied research are covered. However, my own point of view about the logic underlying prevailing concepts and about the coherency of the clinical process shapes the organization, terminology, and explanation found in this book. While I have tried to present an overview and analysis which would be of interest to the experienced clinician and academician, my main purpose is to provide the graduate student in speech-language pathology with an introduction to varied aspects of aphasiology.

Basic research, diagnosis, and treatment are glued together by a single chain of thought: in order to treat a patient's deficit appropriately, we should identify the appropriate deficit; and in order to identify deficits, we should know what to look for as determined by basic research. Theory, research, and clinical practice are related intimately. A coherent clinical process which is to help the aphasic person is out of reach in the face of false dichotomies like the clinician-researcher distinction. Unfortunately, this dichotomy is false in concept but not in how activity and self-concepts are divided among professionals. Presently clinicians tend to have their own set of terms and definitions, while many researchers have their own concepts which are divided further because of different backgrounds in neurology, psychology, and linguistics. I have made a few attempts to sort through all of this in a way that hopefully will make it a little easier to travel the different corridors of aphasiology.

My motivation for this endeavor came not only from my enjoyment of aphasic people and treatment activity but also from my respect for students in speech-language pathology and their requests for adequate preparation. This preparation includes a comprehensive understanding of the disorder which contributes to clinical thinking and procedures. A fully functioning clinician should be familiar with information that often is discarded as being clinically irrelevant. We do read the research literature which is filled with varied logic, concepts, and terms; and we do attend conferences where we listen to neurolinguists and psycholinguists. The clinician should be prepared to engage in the kind of thinking required to interpret research, diagnostic test results, and improvements made by patients. The clinician should have confidence that he or she possesses a comprehensive foundation in clinical aphasiology.

I have refrained from presenting new terms to pile onto old terms for the same ideas; however, I have attempted in some areas to select what appear to me to be the most useful and valid existing terms rather than give equal weight to all of them. There is a heightened sensitivity to use of the term *aphasia*. I have chosen to employ this word generically rather than use *dysphasia*, a term which denotes degrees of impairment while aphasia is suggestive of total loss of language to some clinicians. The British tend to use dysphasia instead of aphasia. I have no quarrel with the conceptual distinction implied by the two terms. The reader simply should be aware that I use aphasia to refer to all variations of the disorder. Also, there are objections to use of *aphasic* as a noun instead of as the adjective that it is, as in "aphasic patient" or "aphasic subject." I use aphasic as a noun frequently, as many other writers have done, and I appeal to the natural forces of language use as a partial justification. Furthermore, it is often easier to write "aphasic" instead of "aphasic person."

I was able to complete this project largely because of the support and patience so generously given by my parents, George and Mary Jane, and the rest of my family. Motivating encouragement was plentiful from my friends, colleagues, and students. A special thank you is for Daniel Beasley, department chairman. Numerous people read portions of the book and made important editorial contributions. They include Gary Barnes, Carol Blossom, Jane Canale, Paula Cheslik, Amy Fleisher, Audrey Holland, Joel Kahane, Jay Rosenbek, Hillary Soloff, and Terry Wertz. Many students reviewed chapters, too many to cite here; but I appreciate all of you. I do want to acknowledge Ann Haire, Pat Larkins, Pete Marincovich, and Karen Shamel for their assistance. I could not thank anyone without the reliability, professionalism, and good humor of typists

Shirley Rias, Patricia Harris, Marcia Elam, and Donna Douglas. I would not know how to learn about aphasia without my mentors Audrey Holland, Joann Fokes, Richard Dean, Danny Moates, and Jon Eisenson. What they have taught me was developed further because of opportunities provided by a grant from the U.S. Veterans Administration. Finally, I reserve special admiration and a thank you for the aphasic people I have known at Ohio University, the Pittsburgh VA Medical Center, and Memphis State University.

G. Albyn Davis

A Survey
of Adult Aphasia

1 Definition, Symptoms, and Syndromes

Aphasia is a communication disorder that usually appears suddenly, often without warning. Some patients will think of an idea and say, "I know what it is but I just can't think of the word." Wulf (1979) called her own aphasia a "weird disorder," because, in spite of her impaired speaking, much of her ability to perceive, think, and remember remained intact. A person with aphasia can hear speech clearly but has difficulty understanding it. Newspaper print is sharply visible but does not make sense. Furthermore, aphasia is manifested as different language disorders. One patient struggles to say one word at a time. Another talks effortlessly and profusely, using many strange words that no one recognizes.

For over a century, aphasia has been an important clue to understanding the elusive relationship between the mind and the brain. Linguists, psychologists, and neurologists have converged on this disorder; and since 1950 their investigations have combined under the headings of psycholinguistics, neuropsychology, and neurolinguistics. The human tragedy of brain injury was magnified by World War II, and psychologists and speech-language pathologists created several new programs for rehabilitating the victims of aphasia.

During the 1970s, clinical aphasiology emerged as a circumscribed area of investigation within the speech-language pathology profession. This specialty simply embraces what has been learned in several fields, mixes in its own discoveries about aphasia, and directs this information toward rehabilitation of the aphasic person.

A DEFINITION OF APHASIA

Accurate identification of aphasia is the first step in delivering effective treatment. It is defined as *an acquired impairment of language processes underlying receptive and expressive modalities and caused by damage to areas of the brain which are primarily responsible for the language function.* A corollary to this definition is that aphasia by itself leaves distinctly non-verbal processes of reasoning and memory relatively intact.

Definitional problems arise because "aphasia" has been used to refer to a wider variety of impairments of language which are caused by brain damage or are suspected to be caused by brain damage. However, language impairment is the primary characteristic of aphasia, while language impairment may be a secondary

1

characteristic of multifaceted disorders such as psychosis or dementia. Investigators such as Wertz (1978) have preferred not to use aphasia to label the language problems of generalized mental deficits (dementia), while Benson (1979a), on the other hand, wrote of the "aphasia of Alzheimer dementia." There are several reasons for defining aphasia in a way that restricts it to language impairment as the primary disorder: (1) the linguistic symptomatology of aphasia differs qualitatively from language in psychosis and dementia, (2) neuropsychological conditions for promoting recovery separate aphasia from generalized disorders, and (3) it is the circumscribed language disorder which traditionally has been treated by speech-language pathologists.

An Acquired Disorder

"Aphasia" has been used for certain infrequent language disorders in children which are not necessarily the same as adult aphasia. They have been defined as congenital or developmental disorders caused by brain damage (Eisenson, 1972) or without concrete evidence of neuropathology (Stark, 1980). These childhood aphasias have generally been investigated independently from the aphasias of adulthood, but the definition of aphasia can be consistent with language disorders which can occur with children. A child can suffer circumscribed brain damage from trauma and even from a rare stroke. Dennis (1980c) identified aphasia with expressive language disorders caused by brain damage occurring "after language has developed but before it is fully mastered" (p. 45). We can be most confident that an aphasia in children is basically the same disorder as aphasia in adults when it occurs after at least most language development has been completed normally in the preschool years. By that time, the language function in childhood is more like the function impaired in adulthood.

Etiology

Areas of the brain which are primarily responsible for the language function are located in the left half of the brain for most people. Neuropathologies capable of singling out these areas include disruption of blood supply to the brain (stroke), abnormal growth of brain tissue (tumor), and head injury (trauma). Also, a small part of the brain may be damaged necessarily during life-saving surgery, for example, to remove a tumor. For any of these causes, the resulting pathologically altered brain tissue is referred to in general as a *lesion*. About 80 percent of the adult aphasia caseload in speech clinics of hospitals is the result of stroke (Davis and Holland, 1981). Stroke is associated often with the arteriosclerotic processes of normal aging; and so the average age of the clinical population with aphasia is around fifty-five to fifty-seven years.

Contrasted with neurological diseases that proceed insidiously over a period of months, most causes of aphasia operate in a brief time frame. The common characterization of the onset of aphasia as sudden offers a useful contrast to other neurogenic disorders; yet it is an oversimplification of what actually occurs. The symptoms of aphasia seem to appear in an instant; but in many cases they take seconds, minutes, and sometimes hours to evolve to maximum impairment. Also, symptoms of aphasia may arise gradually from a slow-growing tumor. The time characteristics of onset is one of the many clues used by the neurologist to infer the exact nature of the neuropathology.

A Language Disorder

The third major component of the definition of aphasia is that it is an impairment of language processing. This impairment reduces a person's ability to derive meaning from language that is heard or read and reduces the ability to express ideas with language, especially in speaking and writing. In terms of impact, the common denominator is social in that the disorder reduces a person's ability to receive and send messages in conversations. Though patients continue to communicate feelings and ideas, impairments in the use of language limit the range and subtlety of messages conveyed. It also may affect the ability to follow the dialogue in a television program, reduce the inclination to answer the telephone, and prohibit simply jotting down a grocery list.

A Disorder of Symbolization. A symbol is any sign, verbal or nonverbal, that is invented by people to stand for something else. A symbol can be quite arbitrary in that it can bear no physical relationship to what it stands for and, therefore, can be used for communication only when two or more people share a knowledge of its meaning. The term symbolization refers to the mental processes of comprehending symbols and of retrieving them from memory for expression. Aural-oral language is a comprehensive symbol system, with rules of semantics, syntax, and phonology designed to represent a full range of concepts.

Finkelnburg, in an 1870 lecture, described cases of aphasia in which not only the aural-oral verbal symbol function was disrupted but also the use of other symbols was impaired (cited in Duffy and Liles, 1979). A pious Catholic woman could not initiate the sign of the cross; a violinist continued to be able to play by ear but could not read musical notation. The composer Ravel, whose aphasia was described by Alajouanine (1948), recognized musical pieces and an untuned piano quite easily but had difficulty reading music, naming musical notes, and finding the location of particular notes on the keyboard of his piano. In his classic introduction to speech and language disorders, Van Riper (1972) defined aphasia as "the general term used for disorders of symbolization." Head (1920) defined aphasia as a disruption of

"symbolic thinking and expression"; Wepman and Van Pelt (1955) considered it to be a disorder of the symbolic processes or symbolic formation.

This attention to symbols expands our consideration of behaviors impaired in aphasia beyond the more frequent attention given to verbal language. The tendency to concentrate on verbal language in research, assessment, and treatment is related to its being the primary vehicle of communication for most people and its being the most significant concern of most patients. The intricacies of structure in verbal language are of great interest to researchers attempting to discover relationships among language, mind, and the brain. Yet, when we think of language and its disorders, we should keep in mind the nonverbal symbol systems such as American Sign Language for the deaf and American Indian Sign Language. Aphasic impairment of gestural language of the deaf, for example, has been described to a limited extent (Kimura, 1976). Moreover, several studies have indicated that the concept of symbol disorder extends even beyond the formal verbal and nonverbal languages to the ability of verbal language users to understand and produce nonlinguistic symbols such as pantomime (Duffy and Duffy, 1981). It is this attention to pantomime which has enhanced the perspective that aphasia is a disorder of symbolization.

The symbol deficit in aphasia, however, does not apply to all symbols. Wapner and Gardner (1981) found that aphasics perform as well as normals in recognizing correct drawings of objects, in choosing the traffic sign which goes with a pictured context, and in choosing the best object for displaying a trademark. In fact, certain brain-damaged persons without aphasia are confused by incorrect object drawings, traffic signs, and trademarks; and they have a much greater difficulty recognizing the proper use of mathematical signs or the dollar sign (see Chapter 6). Wapner and

Gardner concluded that symbolization cannot be viewed as a "unitary" category of behavior. People with aphasia still show their clearest deficit with respect to purely linguistic symbols.

A Central Disorder.   Aphasia is an impairment of a level of cognition that corresponds to a functional level of the nervous system. Comprehension of language is the culmination of a process that begins with receiving an acoustic signal at the ear and ends with relating a version of the signal to its meaning in the brain. Expression of language begins with an idea which is translated into a linguistic form in the brain, which is then translated into a complex combination of neural impulses directing the movement of muscles for speech. In psychological terms, aphasia is a disturbance somewhere *between* thinking of an idea to convey and directing the tongue, lips, and vocal folds to make rapid and coordinated movements that produce words. Levels of function in expression were acknowledged decades ago by physicians who inferred their existence from damage to different levels of the nervous system (Kussmaul, 1877).

Joseph Wepman, a pioneer of clinical aphasiology, defined aphasia and related disorders with respect to functional levels shown in Figure 1–1 (Wepman, Jones, Bock, et al., 1960). Different levels of function are related to input and output transmission and to processes that integrate input and output at these levels. Different nonaphasic disorders of input transmission can arise from damage to individual sensory modalities at levels of reception (reflex), perception, and recognition (conceptual). Different nonaphasic disorders of output transmission can arise from damage to individual motor systems at levels from the brain to the nerves carrying impulses to the muscles. Aphasia is represented as an impairment of complex functions which are "between" input and output transmission

and which involve processes shared by the individual transmission channels. Wepman, et al. (1960) added that deficits could occur at different points within the integration process: " . . . in the arousal of a meaningful state, in the semantic process of word selection, or in the syntactic process" (p. 328). Brookshire (1978b) reinforced this view of aphasia as a disturbance to a central "processor" of verbal information.

The centrality of aphasia is illustrated with word-retrieval deficit, a basic characteristic of this disorder. This deficit is observed when a patient is asked to name common objects. Caramazza and Berndt (1978) attributed aphasic object-naming problems to failure of a "central stage" between object recognition and motor planning for word production. This stage, in which the mental representation of the object is matched with a corresponding word, is independent of the sensory modalities through which the object may be presented. Goodglass, Barton, and Kaplan (1968) presented objects to aphasics by either sight, sound, feel, or smell. Naming impairment was the same no matter which sensory channel was used to present the idea. Similar results were obtained by Spreen, Benton, and Van Allen (1966).

A   Multimodality   Disorder.   If the mental processes of symbolization are shared by the different modalities, then an impairment of this central function should be observed in the use of language with any modality. Indeed, aphasia is manifested in each of the modalities with comprehension deficits in listening and reading and with expressive deficits in speaking and writing (Basso, Taborelli, and Vignolo, 1978; Duffy and Ulrich, 1976; Schuell and Jenkins, 1961b; Smith, 1971). Early investigators, however, tended to differentiate aphasias based on impairment of either input or output modalities. One type of aphasia was referred

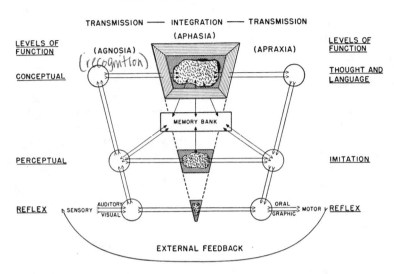

<——— CENTRAL NERVOUS SYSTEM ———>

Figure 1-1. Functional levels correspond to levels of the nervous system presented in Chapter 2. Aphasia is a central impairment of integration. Other communicative disorders result from impairment of other levels in the system. *(Reprinted by permission of the author and the American Speech-Language-Hearing Association from Wepman, J. M., et al., Studies in aphasia: Background and theoretical formulations. Journal of Speech and Hearing Disorders, 25, 323–332, 1960)*

to as motor or expressive aphasia, with disturbance of speech production and good auditory comprehension. Another type was referred to as sensory or receptive aphasia, with severe disturbance of auditory comprehension and fluent speech production. Weisenburg and McBride (1935) softened this modality-focused orientation by suggesting that deficits may be "predominantly" expressive or receptive. Now, aphasia is commonly viewed as a multimodality disorder. Current classifications of different aphasias are based on criteria other than degrees of impairment among modalities.

Even though characterizing an aphasia as receptive or expressive is somewhat misleading, degree of impairment often differs among modalities. Comprehensive tests enable the clinician to compare modalities as to the degree of deficit. Comparisons have been made with large groups of patients who have been given these tests (Porch, 1967; Schuell, Jenkins, and Jimenez-Pabon, 1964). Results indicate that (1) expressive modalities usually are more impaired than receptive modalities, (2) reading is usually more impaired than auditory comprehension, and (3) writing is usually more impaired than speech. Smith (1971) found that writing is generally the most severely impaired modality. Exceptions to this pattern often indicate that the aphasic patient possesses an additional modality-specific disorder.

A Disorder of Propositional Language. This feature of the language deficit has been described for over a century. It characterizes the apparent contradiction in patients who, on the one hand, do not verbalize for conversation or who struggle to answer a question with even a single word and, on the other hand, who fluently count to ten or readily remark "I can't say that" or quickly curse when frustrated. The most severely impaired patients may say only recurring, stereotypical utterances such as "Where's my hat" as a reply to anything. In aphasia the propositional/volitional use of language is impaired and the nonpropositional/nonvolitional use of language is preserved to a greater degree. Propositional utterances were defined by Eisenson (1973) as calling for "a creative formulation of words with specific and appropriate regard to the situation," as opposed to certain nonpropositional forms which "come 'ready made' or preformulated for the speaker" (p. 7).

Even when a patient is unable to converse at all, it may be possible, sometimes with a little urging from the clinician, for him or her to produce nonpropositional language forms. These forms include *automized sequences* such as counting, reciting the alphabet, or saying the days of the week in order; *memorized sequences* such as a prayer or song; *recurrent social speech* as "I'm fine" or "How are you?"; and *emotional speech* such as any words, often profanity, which occur only as part of an emotional outburst. These forms are not used for intentional communication.

A Disorder of Communication. Although aphasia is referred to as a disorder of language function and as a disorder of communication, language function and communication are not equivalent phenomena. Communication is a process of interaction between at least two people where the goal of each participant is the exchange of messages. Language is one tool that a person uses to send messages to a receiver, and language is one source of information used by the receiver to comprehend a message. Portions of messages are exchanged with motion of a hand, a shift of gaze, or a smile. What is said and understood depends on situational con-

texts in which verbal and nonverbal channels are used. For example, giving directions to a destination which is in view of the sender and receiver will be different from directions given when the destination is a few miles away. The amount of information shared by participants in a conversation contributes to the extent of communication achieved. Aphasia affects the use of language to convey messages; other means of conveying messages remain relatively intact, and the situational context and the listener continue to contribute to the communicative exchange.

RELATED DISORDERS

Several disorders are related to aphasia because they are caused by damage to the nervous system and may interfere with communication. It is important to identify these disorders because they may accompany aphasia, may be confused with aphasia, and definitely require different approaches for rehabilitation. Though Wepman's model of functional levels in Figure 1–1 does not specify the intricacy of processes involved in the language function, it does specify levels of processing input and output which are related to language processes. Most of the disorders discussed here are related to levels of either input or output processing suggested by this model.

Receptive Transmission

There are several disorders of single sensory modalities which occur at the functional levels of reception and recognition of stimuli. These disorders may coexist with aphasia for two reasons: either a patient has had at least two medical conditions producing at least two different disorders, or the damage producing aphasia extended to an area of the brain responsible for a particular sensory function.

Sensory Disorders. Reduction of sensory sensitivity can occur with damage to the receptors, to their pathways to the brain, and to the regions where sensations arrive at the brain. Reductions of auditory and visual acuity are common by age seventy. Peripheral hearing loss due to deterioration of the inner ear is called *presbycusis,* and gradual loss of near-distance vision with age is called *presbyopia.* Speech discrimination can be reduced with damage to auditory pathways and the auditory-receiving areas of the brain. Vision can be impaired in selected portions of the visual field depending on location of damage to the visual system. Half-field deficits, from damage to one half of the brain, are common with aphasia. Called *homonymous hemianopsia* (or hemianopia), the patient cannot see the right or left of center depending on which half of the brain was damaged. With damage to the left brain, the patient cannot see to the right of center. Brain damage can diminish sensation for touch, temperature, and pain; this sensory impairment is called *hemianesthesia* when one side of the brain is affected.

Disorders of Recognition. At a higher level of input processing (the conceptual level of transmission in Figure 1–1), focal damage of the brain may result in impaired recognition of auditory stimuli while hearing is preserved. This is called **auditory agnosia,** a term which has been used inconsistently with respect to whether recognition of nonverbal or verbal stimuli or both is deficient. Hecaen and Albert (1978) defined auditory agnosia as impaired recognition of nonverbal (environmental) sounds, and cases have been reported with this modality-specific deficit without a language comprehension problem. Cases of auditory agnosia for speech, also called *pure word deafness,* without deficits in other language modalities are rare and are usually accompanied by mild word-retrieval difficulties. The presence of this type of auditory agnosia is sometimes considered in certain cases of aphasia with a pronounced auditory comprehension deficit. Agnosia for both nonverbal and verbal sounds while other modalities remain relatively intact has also been reported. The varieties of auditory agnosia were reviewed by Ulrich (1978).

Visual agnosia is rare in pure form, but it can appear with aphasia and be hidden by the language disorder. It is an impairment in the recognition of nonverbal stimuli in the absence of a loss of visual reception. Several types of visual agnosia have been identified (Hecaen and Albert, 1978; Williams, 1979). *Visual object agnosia* is of special interest, since it can be confused with the object-naming deficit of aphasia. The two disorders can appear together or separately. With visual object agnosia the patient can see the object but cannot name it, demonstrate its function, or remember having seen it before. This failure to name an object on visual confrontation may appear to be an aphasic symptom; but when it is due to agnosia, the patient can use the name in conversation and can retrieve the name when stimulated through other modalities, as when touching the object. *Color agnosia* involves preserved color discrimination but an inability to identify all colors of the same hue. Verbal manifestations of this disorder, in absence of aphasia, include failures to point to colors on command, to name colors, and to retrieve the name of the color or color-specific objects such as a tomato or grass. Agnosia for faces, called *prosopagnosia,* is the inability to recognize previously known people, including very familiar people and people just met.

Just as the auditory modality can be affected with respect to verbal recognition, the visual modality can be impaired at the level of recognition of graphic verbal stimuli without impaired visual reception and without a deficit in the general language function. Though this isolated deficit, which is very uncommon, has been referred to as agnosic alexia, it is not clear as to whether it should be considered to be comparable to auditory agnosia for speech. This modality-specific reading deficit more often has been called *pure word blindness, alexia without agraphia,* or *pure alexia.* It is usually discussed as a syndrome which can be accompanied by color agnosia and which occurs without aphasia. The deficit is found only with visual linguistic material; recognition of numbers remains intact. Reading-related skills through other modalities, such as oral spelling or recognition of letters presented through the sense of touch, also remain unimpaired. The patient with pure alexia, strangely, can write but cannot read what he has just written.

Tactile agnosia, also called *astereognosis,* is the inability to recognize an object through the sense of touch. It can occur in the absence of hemianesthesia and is confirmed when objects can be recognized when seen. The neurologist asks the patient to close his eyes when being tested for tactile agnosia.

Expressive Transmission

Modality-specific impairments of motoric functions, especially of the speech mechanism, can occur which are analogous to the disorders of reception and recognition within isolated input modalities. The speech-language pathologist is most concerned with disorders affecting output mechanisms used for communication such as the movement of body parts used for speaking, writing, and gesturing.

Motor Disorders. Muscle movement is innervated by fibers which connect the motor area of the brain's surface to the specific muscles of the body. These connectors consist of multiple systems and levels. Damage to different locations between the brain's surface and these muscles produces a variety of impairments including weakness, paralysis, rigidity, and incoordination. Neuromotor impair-

ment of the speech musculature is called **dysarthria.** The term dysarthria represents a variety of speech disorders depending on location of damage to the nervous system (Darley, Aronson, and Brown, 1975; Rosenbek and LaPointe, 1978). They involve impairments of respiration, phonation, resonance, and articulation, each contributing to deficient speech production. Dysarthric speech has been described as consisting of distorted speech sounds, slurring, excessive nasal emission, and breathiness. These and other symptoms occur in different patterns depending on the site of lesion.

Similarly, there are motor disorders with muscle weakness affecting the extremities. *Hemiplegia* is the weakness or paralysis of one side of the body and may accompany aphasia. This term may be restricted to complete paralysis, while *hemiparesis* is used to denote varying degrees of weakness on one side. Designations of right or left hemiplegia refer to the side of paralysis instead of the side of the brain that was damaged (see Chapter 2).

Common problems directly related to hemiplegia include lack of sensation on the paralyzed side, difficulty with balance and muscle control, pain of the extremities, especially the shoulder, and fluid retention (edema) in the tissues of the affected hand and wrist or foot and ankle. The patient has reduced physical endurance and fatigues easily. As a result, the patient has reduced independence in basic self-care activities such as locomotion, eating, dressing, and bathing. Some patients must learn transfers between the wheelchair and a bed, another chair, a bathtub, and an automobile. A sling is needed for arm support and elevation in order to keep the arm and hand in a functional and safe position, lessen the fluid retention, and relieve pain that may come from excessive pulling on the shoulder (Sister Kenny Institute, 1977). Paralysis and its impact on the activities of daily living are treated by physical and occupational therapists.

Most victims of brain injury experience

some degree of motor deficit at onset, and frequently at that time both upper and lower limbs are affected. For some, muscle function is recovered quickly and completely. For others, functional impairment remains on either side, depending on the site of the brain damage. In the aphasic, the lower extremity is usually less impaired and improves more quickly than the upper extremity, because arm and hand movement are controlled by an area of the brain which is located closer to speech areas than the area controlling leg and foot movement. Those with aphasia usually have hemiplegia on the right side.

Disorders of Motor Planning. At a higher level of motor function, other areas of the brain's surface are responsible for programming the intricate interactions of muscle movements in order that they may perform certain functions. The volitional control of movements for the purpose of speaking can be disrupted without muscle weakness, and this is called **apraxia of speech** (Johns and LaPointe, 1976; Rosenbek, 1978). Because the area of the brain which is responsible for speech programming is located near the areas responsible for the language function, apraxia of speech sometimes accompanies aphasia, thereby compounding the individual's expressive communication problem. Without muscle weakness, the verbal apraxic patient has no difficulty using the lips, tongue, and pharynx for nonspeaking purposes such as chewing and swallowing food. Even in the volitional movement of these muscles for other purposes, the patient with this disorder may have no difficulty. However, when intending to put these muscles in gear for speaking, the patient shows visible signs of awkwardness in the selection and sequencing of movements. It is as if the articulators veer off into directions not intended by the speaker, who occasionally may reach for his tongue like a parent scolding a wayward child.

A disturbance in the volitional move-ment of the jaw, lips, and tongue for nonspeaking purposes, called *oral apraxia* (oral nonverbal apraxia, bucco-facial apraxia), may or may not occur with apraxia of speech. Oral apraxia is observed when the patient is unable to protrude his tongue or whistle on command. Mateer has concluded that impaired nonverbal oral movement at different levels of complexity is characteristic of persons with aphasia (Mateer, 1978).

Disorders of limb movement can occur without neuromuscular weakness or rigidity. These disorders are called *limb apraxia, ideomotor apraxia,* and *ideational apraxia* and represent an inability to carry out common acts on command, without muscle weakness, while maintaining an ability to perform these acts spontaneously. The patient may not be able to strike a match and light a candle on command but will be able to do it when the electricity goes out in an emergency (Williams, 1979). It is risky to suggest a stable definition for each of these disorders, since definitions vary among different authors. One set of definitions follows the distinctions among these three apraxias originally outlined by Liepmann in 1900 and equates limb apraxia with ideomotor apraxia (Brookshire, 1978b). Another set follows Liepmann fairly closely but distinguishes between limb and ideomotor apraxia (Hecaen and Albert, 1978). Another set focuses on ideomotor apraxia and does not include the others (Williams, 1979). Williams (1979) added that the distinction between ideomotor and ideational apraxia " . . . has been seen by many authors to be more confusing than helpful" (p. 90).

Generalized Disorders

In contrast to aphasia and to the modality-specific disorders just described, a reduction of all mental functions can occur due to diffuse brain damage or multifocal lesions (see Chapter 6). The symptoms of diffuse brain damage can be revealed through the use of language with extremes of a continuum in which, at one end, a patient is facile using language per se (performing well on most tests of language function) and, at the other end, a patient may be unable to talk at all. When the patient can use language, deficits are revealed which are not usually found in cases of aphasia; these deficits include disorientation as to time and place, poor memory for events, faulty judgment, and generally reduced intellectual function. Terms for these disorders include *acute* or *chronic brain syndrome* (also, organic brain syndrome), and the symptomatology of these disorders is referred to collectively as *dementia*. Certain investigators in the field of speech-language pathology have chosen to refer to these disorders as generalized intellectual impairment (Halpern, Darley, and Brown, 1973; Wertz, 1978).

SYMPTOMS OF APHASIA

The specific deviations of language behavior in aphasia are varied; and a great deal of research has been devoted to identifying, sorting, and labeling these behaviors. A *symptom* is a deviation from normal function which indicates the presence of a disorder. A catalogue of aphasic symptoms can enhance the clinician's sensitivity to nuances of aphasic behavior. One aphasic patient will exhibit only a few of these symptoms, and another patient will exhibit a different combination of symptoms. Also, a patient's language behavior will consist of some of these characteristics soon after onset of aphasia; and, as recovery occurs, these early characteristics will lessen or disappear gradually and others will take their place. Therefore, an awareness of these possibilities enables the clinician to differentiate aphasic behavior from other disorders, differentiate among types of aphasia, and monitor the stages of recovery in each patient. Furthermore, regularly occurring types of symptoms provide clues to the basis for the patient's

deficit, enabling the clinician to plan treatment strategies which are most appropriate for the individual's problems.

Spoken Language

Inadequate or inappropriate use of language through speech is the most readily observed and thoroughly classified collection of symptoms in aphasia. There are symptoms of omission in which linguistic units cannot be retrieved or are partially omitted, and symptoms of commission in which incorrect elements are selected unintentionally.

Anomia, for example, is a general term for almost any condition in which an aphasic person has difficulty finding a word. Anomia is an inappropriate term for retrieved words that are articulated poorly. It is reflected in symptoms of omission when an intended word cannot be produced and in symptoms of commission when mistakes in word selection are made. Also, a patient may take an inefficient path toward accurate word finding by pausing before producing the word or by self-correcting after producing an unintended word. Anomia is a broad category for *negative symptoms* which arise from a malfunctioning language mechanism. Aphasic people also exhibit certain *positive symptoms* which arise from language mechanisms that remain unimpaired. A positive symptom is *circumlocution* in which, upon failure to retrieve a word, a patient talks around the intended word, giving definitions, descriptions, or even sound effects. The circumlocuting patient might say, "I wear it right here" (pointing to his wrist) "and I tell time with it."

Many symptoms of aphasia are identified with reference to levels of analysis used by linguists to describe normal language. These levels include the phoneme, the morpheme, and grammar. This approach not only makes the aphasic deviation from the norm more apparent but also lends some precision to the identification of different symptoms. As Lesser (1978) put it, "The linguistically-oriented student of aphasia would not be satisfied with a statement such as 'This patient has difficulty in repetition' or 'This patient has reading problems' but would wish to analyze the difficulties in terms of the structures and systemic features which are disrupted or retained" (p. 23).

Paraphasias. A paraphasia is a symptom of commission in that it is an incorrect word substituted for an intended or targeted word. It is the product of a breakdown at a stage of the word-retrieval process and, as such, is a dominant symptom within the more general category of anomia. Paraphasias are produced *unintentionally* and are found primarily with patients whose speech is uttered *fluently.* In contrast, circumlocutions are produced intentionally, while also being produced fluently. Goodglass and Kaplan (1972) noted that "the distorted pronunciation of patients with poor articulation does *not* come under this heading" (p. 8).

The major types of paraphasia are the phonemic, verbal, and neologistic. They are identified in terms of the linguistic relationship between the spoken incorrect word and the target word. Knowing the patient's intended word is not always possible when paraphasias are produced in extended speech or conversation. However, situational and linguistic context may assist in the identification of target words occasionally. Types of paraphasia are revealed best when the patient is asked to name an object or to repeat or read aloud a particular word or sentence.

The first general category is substitutions which are related in sound structure to the intended word. **Phonemic paraphasias,** also called *literal paraphasias,* involve the substitution, addition, or rearrangement of speech sounds so that the error can be identified as sounding like the target. Goodglass and Kaplan (1972) used the criterion that more than half of the in-

tended word is preserved. The different definitions of phonemic paraphasia leave it unclear as to whether these errors should be restricted to dictionary words such as saying "pike" instead of *pipe* (Goodglass and Kaplan, 1972) or should be restricted to nondictionary words such as saying "kipe" instead of *pipe* (Lesser, 1978) or should encompass dictionary and nondictionary words (Lecours and Vanier-Clement, 1976). These varied definitions point toward a subtle ambiguity in this category of symptoms. In addition, phoneme substitution in phonemic paraphasia is a different phenomenon from the substitutions in apraxia of speech (see Chapter 5).

The second major category of paraphasias is the **verbal paraphasias,** which are identified based on whether there is a semantic relationship between the error and the intended word. Verbal paraphasias are dictionary words or words from the patient's language. A *semantic verbal paraphasia* (or, simply, semantic paraphasia) is a word substitution which bears a relationship in meaning to the intended word. Buckingham and Rekart (1979) provided several examples of these paraphasias which are identified from the contexts of extended speech: "Well, my wife..." instead of *husband;* "...way down in the north..." instead of *south;* and "I can see you talking that way..." instead of *hear you.* Neurolinguists have been fascinated by the possibility that semantic paraphasias might provide clues as to how words are organized in permanent memory (Whitaker, 1970; Rinnert and Whitaker, 1973). Also, these errors can be considered to reflect difficulties at a deeper level of the word-retrieval process than the phonemic level mentioned earlier. With many phonemic paraphasias, it can be surmised that the correct word was retrieved but was put together poorly; while with verbal paraphasias it can be surmised that the patient was unable at a particular moment to retrieve the correct word. Dictionary words for which no semantic relationship can be determined in comparison with the target word are called *unrelated verbal paraphasias* (or random paraphasias). A patient may look at a fork and confidently call it a "doorkey." She may talk about the "turnips" in her laundry.

The third major category of paraphasias is the **neologism.** A neologism is a fluently spoken word form which cannot be identified as having come from the patient's language or, unless coincidentally, from any other language. Like the unrelated verbal paraphasia, it bears no phonemic or semantic similarity to the target word. It sometimes has been described as an invented word, a characterization which inappropriately attributes intentionality to the patient. Like all paraphasias, these strange words appear unintentionally. In his hospital room, the patient might ask someone to turn on the "pinwad" or request a "ferbish" to quench his thirst. A patient might even call a comb a "planker" and then insist, "p-l-a-n-k-e-r!"

There has been some overlap between phonemic paraphasia and neologism in the classification of nondictionary words. Examples of neologisms given by Eisenson (1973), such as saying "spork" as a combination of *spoon* and *fork,* were considered by Lecours and Vanier-Clement (1976) to be a special class of phonemic paraphasias which they called *phonemic telescopages.* It has been suggested that neologisms may be simply a severe result of the breakdown which produces phonemic paraphasias, the neologism representing a modification in sound structure of more than 50 percent of the target (Buckingham and Kertesz, 1976). This is plausible, since a neologism certainly is not extracted from the patient's permanent storage of language in long-term memory. Also, phonemic paraphasia and unrelated verbal paraphasia can come close together, as when a patient says "pickle tacks" instead of *tackle box.*

Some authors refer to anomia, verbal paraphasias, and circumlocution as independent categories of symptoms. Verbal paraphasias and circumlocution are conceptualized here as examples of a more general category of symptoms called anomia.

Agrammatism. This is a category of symptoms designating inadequacies of sentence production. It is characterized by omissions and sometimes is called *motor agrammatism.* The earliest mention of this symptom was by Kussmaul (1877), who described "agrammatismus" as affecting three prerequisites for sentence production: an "unbroken flow of words"; use of articles, verb auxiliaries, and prepositions; and arrangement of words in a certain order. Agrammatism, as the term is commonly used, refers to attempts at sentence formulation in which the muscle is present but the skeleton is missing. Content words, such as nouns and main verbs, are produced; but the function words, such as articles, verb auxiliaries, and prepositions, are omitted. Other grammatical details are dropped out as well, such as bound morphemes used for pluralization, tense, and subject-verb agreement. Utterances sound like a telegram, a manner of speaking sometimes called telegraphic speech or "telegramese" (Gardner, 1974b). Utterances are described as nonfluent, with hesitant and often labored word production; frequently agrammatism is accompanied by apraxia of speech. Functors and bound morphemes also are omitted when the patient is repeating and reading aloud. This symptom has been investigated extensively by Goodglass (1976) and his colleagues (see Chapter 5). Zurif (1980) has investigated the possibility that patients with agrammatic speech may have difficulties processing functors in comprehension as well.

Agrammatism varies in degree based on the number of omissions of grammatical support units and on the number of content words retrieved. Hesitant initiation and pauses reflecting the conscious planning of utterances always appear to some degree. In its most severe form, one content word is produced with much effort; and in its mildest form, a lengthy and sometimes complete sentence is produced, but the hesitancy and pauses are still there. The listener must usually be patient and wait while a complete utterance is being formulated. These differences are illustrated with three possible descriptions of a picnic scene with parents preparing food on a table and children playing in the background: (1) "Uh, boy . . . and, uh, girl . . . That's all"; (2) "Mother, father . . . making dogs . . . hot dogs; a boy, no two boys . . . and baseball . . . running and hot"; (3) "It's a mother and . . . a father fixing hot dogs . . . a picnic; I have two sons like this . . . boys playing baseball . . . they are playing baseball." In these examples, the utterances increase in length from (1) to (3); phrases are longer, functors are added, and complete sentences appear in (3). All utterances relate to the scene in some way; but the first utterance especially is ambiguous because of its meagerness and, therefore, is not very communicative. These examples could represent differences in severity among different agrammatic patients or differences in stages of recovery by one patient.

Telegramese has been called motor agrammatism in order to contrast it with another symptom called *sensory agrammatism*. Also called paragrammatism, the sensory form occurs primarily in fluent and complete utterances; it is a symptom of commission in that mistakes are made in the use of grammatical elements instead of their simply being omitted. Sensory agrammatism has received little attention from researchers, possibly because it is difficult to detect in rapidly flowing speech which is often filled with paraphasias. It is one characteristic of jargon.

Jargon. Almost the opposite of telegramese in many respects, jargon is lengthy, fluently articulated utterance which makes little or no sense to the listener. It is replete with verbal paraphasias and neologisms and is referred to informally as jibberish or word salad. While agrammatism is a reduction in number of words, jargon can seem to be an excess of words. While the words in motor agrammatism are generally on target, the speaker's reference with jargon is usually indeterminable. While agrammatic speech is hesitant and often articulated awkwardly, jargon is initiated quickly and spoken smoothly. In addition, while the awkward articulatory formulations accompanying agrammatism may result in sound substitutions, jargon may include fluently produced phonemic paraphasias which might also be recorded as sound substitutions. This latter contrast lies in the means to an apparently similar end-product. Jargon has been characterized broadly as incomprehensible, incoherent, and lacking in meaning, a "disappearance of that very quality which gives signification to speech" (Alajouanine, 1956, p. 22). There is a tendency to start talking before another speaker has relinquished his turn in conversation or to continue talking indefinitely. This tendency for excessive speech is called *press for speech*.

Jargon has been classified as being of at least two types depending on the proportion of verbal paraphasias (dictionary words) or neologisms in the patient's utterances. A heavy concentration of neologisms is called *neologistic jargon,* while a higher proportion of semantic and unrelated verbal paraphasias is called *semantic jargon.* With reference to English, Goodglass and Kaplan (1972) distinguished between extended neologistic jargon and extended English jargon. Though these terms may characterize the expression of different patients, they also may represent stages of recovery, namely, from neologistic to semantic forms (Kertesz and Benson, 1970). Other types have been proposed, including undifferentiated jargon (Alajouanine, 1956) and phonemic jargon (Buckingham and

Kertesz, 1976). Undifferentiated jargon is the repetitive fluent production of one or two phonemes; this was considered by Buckingham and Kertesz not to be true jargon, but, rather, a type of stereotypic utterance found in global or very severe aphasia. Phonemic jargon is a stream of varied speech sounds of which almost nothing is recognizable.

Several examples of semantic jargon have appeared in the literature (Brown, 1981b). The following example was presented by Kinsbourne and Warrington (1963); the patient had been asked to describe his job as a draftsman:

> "My job was . . . original . . . him . . . concerned with . . . particulars . . . of . . . so that I could tell him exactly what to take, and, where to . . . take it from . . . so that I could get away to the . . . gestures for the conditions of one side . . . which would give me particular items or discussion according to that. I should have then convolve to the complete asculation . . . which would give me particulars to tendon, but I am not . . . not . . . available throwing back particulars until they were given to me." (p. 32)

This example consists mostly of dictionary or English words. The neologisms include "convolve" and "asculation." It illustrates a tendency for semantic jargon to maintain the syntactic component of language while the semantic component is elusive.

Verbal Stereotypes.   Except for a complete inability to say anything, the most severe expressive impairment is the exclusive use of stereotypic utterances or what Alajouanine (1956) called verbal stereotypy. These forms are produced involuntarily. The patient is generally aware of the language disorder but is not aware of the nature of this particular symptom. A verbal stereotype is a very restricted form of expression as it is used repeatedly by a patient, as if it were the only language form available. A common manifestation

is the use of "yes" and "no" as the only verbalization. It may be a bland "I think so"; or it may be a word such as "shit." Ask a patient his name, and he will reply "shit."

Alajouanine (1956) described two types of permanent verbal stereotypes, which are established at the onset of aphasia and persist for several months "without apparent modification of their structure" (p. 5). The first type consists of *nondictionary verbal forms:* either one syllable repeated several times, called iterative stereotypy; or an unrecognizable word form, called jargonized (or neologistic) stereotypy. An example of iterative stereotypes would be "dee-dee-dee." The neologistic stereotype was observed by the nineteenth-century neurologist Hughlings Jackson during a boyhood experience (Critchley, 1960):

> When quite a child on a seaside holiday, he lodged at a house where the landlady—as he discovered to his wonderment and awe—could say nothing but "watty." This unlikely disyllable was articulated with such a range of cadence that it could express a variety of emotions. Her laugh was merry and ringing, and when anything amused her she would say: "Watty, watty, watty." (p. 8)

The common feature of the nondictionary forms is that they are not composed of legitimate words or, as Alajouanine put it, are devoid of meaning. The second type of permanent verbal stereotype consists of *dictionary words.* These may be either single words such as "yes" or "no" or a single recurring sentence. The recurring phrase or sentence received special attention from Alajouanine, since there has been some question as to the origin of these utterances.

Aphasiologists have thought that the particular verbal stereotype may have been on the patient's mind or even spoken by the patient just prior to or at the time of onset of aphasia. Alajouanine described several examples from the literature. A railway signalman suffered a stroke while on the job, and his recurring utterance was "Come on to me." Another patient was injured in a fight and could utter only "I want protection." Another patient, injured in a fight at a tavern, uttered "on the booze" all the time. A young lady "of dubious morals" suffered a hemorrhage and subsequently would say only "Not tonight, I am too tired." An issue was whether these were the last utterances just prior to these injuries or represented the situation at the time of injury. They may simply have come from the patient's way of life.

Written Language

Aphasic writing usually exhibits patterns which are similar to the speaking impairment (Goodglass and Hunter, 1970). The writing component of aphasia is called *agraphia* or *dysgraphia*. Terminology for writing deficits corresponds to the terms used for deficits in speech. Graphic word-retrieval errors are called *paragraphias,* with graphemic paragraphia corresponding to phonemic paraphasia, and so on. Terms such as *jargonagraphia* are found in the literature (Lecours and Rouillon, 1976). Writing skill, including sentence structure and spelling, varies widely within the normal population depending on educational, vocational, and cultural experience. Some people are not interested in writing much more than their name. These factors are considered in the diagnosis and treatment of writing disturbance in aphasia. Furthermore, patients with hemiplegia, usually on the right side, may be initially unwilling to try writing with the inexperienced left hand. Linguistic symptoms can be masked by right-handed muscle weakness and by left-handed awkwardness.

Hemiplegia contributes to making writing a more limited channel of communication than speech in most cases of aphasia. Also, writing and reading involve a different code, a graphemic code, which is learned after the more facile phonemic code of aural-oral language. Theories of writing suggest that it entails generating a mental phonemic code which is translated into a graphemic code, a process called transcoding (Weigl and Fradis, 1977). Some patients have a pronounced inability to write to dictation which requires transcoding the auditory-phonemic code into the visual-graphemic code. Because writing is more severely impaired than speech, examination of writing is valuable for detection of mild aphasia (Keenan, 1971).

Auditory Comprehension

Deriving meaning from an utterance is a private event, occurring in the mind. The symptomatology of comprehension deficit, therefore, comes from behaviors through which the observer can only infer the nature of the impairment. They include a quizzical look, an irrelevant response to a question, or failure to follow an instruction correctly. Some people with aphasia have such serious problems with comprehension that they appear not to be attending to a speaker, as if they are deaf. Other patients are quite adept at masking their comprehension deficits by appearing to be paying careful attention and by using standard phrases such as "Oh yes, I think so" or "That's good." This ruse fails when a patient who is asked "Where do you live?" replies "That's good." Mild comprehension problems are reflected in delayed responses or requests for repetition.

Comprehension deficit is one aspect of aphasia for which the diagnostic skills of the speech-language pathologist can be quite informative for the family and hospital staff. The clinician presents carefully selected language stimuli to the patient without helpful clues from facial expression or the environment and requires simple unequivocal responses from the patient to indicate whether the stimuli were comprehended. In this way, the clinician can avoid the overestimates or underestimates of a patient's comprehension ability which can often be made by observing conversation in natural settings.

A few preliminary attempts have been made to specify the hidden events of impaired auditory comprehension. Schuell dealt with this problem to some extent. "Partial auditory imperception" was a term that she used for impaired processing at a level prior to attaching meaning to the auditory signal (Schuell, et al., 1964). This modality-specific deficit pertains to perception of the signal and is similar to auditory agnosia for speech or pure word deafness. A similar disruption, called "intermittent auditory imperception," is a random fading in and out of comprehension which can occur in some cases of aphasia (Marshall, Jefferies, Rau, et al., 1978). Brookshire (1974, 1978b) has inferred several possible auditory processing deficits in aphasia. These include slow rise time (missing the initial portion of messages), noise buildup (missing the later portion of messages), retention deficit (failure to hold certain amount of input in short-term memory), and intermittent auditory imperception. The existence of these private deficits has not been verified by repeated and varied experimentation.

Differences in comprehension deficits among cases of aphasia are sometimes based on whether the patient can repeat auditory stimuli. Ability to repeat is considered to be evidence that the patient can perceive the auditory stimulus. Therefore, Benson (1979a) distinguished between perceptual deficit (patients who cannot comprehend and cannot repeat) and semantic deficit (patients who cannot comprehend but can repeat). However, there are aphasic patients who can comprehend an utterance which they cannot repeat, rendering repetition a weak test of perception.

The most common delineation of comprehension deficits is made with respect to the kind of stimuli with which a patient has the most difficulty or has isolated difficulty. An aphasic patient may be said to be deficient in comprehending isolated words, sentences, or paragraphs. A patient may have a pronounced problem comprehending phrases or sentences which contain a preposition; may be able to comprehend short utterances but not long ones or complex ones; or may have a problem in answering questions or a problem in following instructions. Without a valid and complete model of the mental operations of comprehension, we continue to define this deficit according to what can be observed directly.

Mild comprehension deficits can be especially tricky to detect, and a valuable investigative tool for the clinician includes simply asking the patient to describe the problem. Butler wrote of his aphasia: "... difficulties in conversation arise mainly from my seemingly frequent inability to understand adequately the main point of a discussion or the implication of a remark" (Sies and Butler, 1963, p. 265).

Reading

Moss (1972) and Dahlberg (Dahlberg and Jaffe, 1977), in describing their initial experiences with stroke, mentioned reading more than auditory comprehension, perhaps because they were alone at the time of onset and for periods thereafter. Moss recalled "trying to read the headlines of the *Chicago Tribune* but they didn't make any sense to me at all" (p. 4). Wulf (1979) wondered: "What in the world was I to do with anything as big and cumbersome as a newspaper? And all those words! An article was tackled only to find that all the words were a complete jumble of letters signifying nothing!" (p. 59). One patient told Rolnick and Hoops (1969), "Sometimes in the paper if it's real long sentences I have trouble. I have to go over and over to see what it means." He continued, "When there is little print I have trouble if it's real small'' (p. 52). Published material has some compensations for aphasic people, however; as another patient remarked, ''The only thing I look at is pictures and try to get some idea what it has to be'' (Rolnick and Hoops, 1969, p. 52).

The reading deficit in aphasia has been called *alexia, dyslexia,* or, more specifically, *acquired dyslexia.* A problem with referring to aphasic reading in this way is that these terms are used to label the relatively uncommon pure alexia noted previously in this chapter. In order to distinguish between pure alexia and reading deficit in aphasia, various types of deficit have been proposed. Marshall and Newcombe (1973), for example, described *visual dyslexia,* involving visual perception of letters (graphemes), *surface dyslexia,* involving the transcoding of graphemes into the auditory (phonemic) code, and *deep dyslexia,* involving semantic interpretation. This classification becomes confusing because impaired grapheme-to-phoneme conversion has been used to explain the semantic errors of deep dyslexia (see Chapter 5). Warrington (cited in LaPointe and Horner, 1979) distinguished between *peripheral dyslexias* and *central dyslexias.* Her central dyslexias included surface and deep dyslexias. Reading deficits have simply become an area of active research from which unresolved differences of definition have arisen.

The dyslexias are observed in two ways, either during silent reading for comprehension or during reading aloud. In tests of silent reading for comprehension, the patient is asked to select a word that goes with a picture. Surface dyslexia is revealed when the patient has a pronounced difficulty in selecting from words that sound alike. Deep dyslexia is inferred from errors concentrated in choosing from words that are similar semantically. Many studies of acquired dyslexia have focused on reading aloud. When a patient is asked to read words aloud, the dyslexias are inferred from the patient's incorrect verbalizations

which are called *paralexias.* Saying a word that sounds like the tested word is indicative of surface dyslexia, and saying a word that is similar in meaning is indicative of deep dyslexia.

Perseveration

Perseveration is a common symptom of brain damage which is not unique to a particular location of injury and, therefore, not unique to language behavior. Disruption of a basic neural function, shifting from one neural network to another, may be responsible for this symptom (Luria, 1974). Its appearance in the language behavior of aphasic persons was analyzed by Buckingham, Whitaker, and Whitaker (1979) who defined perseveration as ''the recurrence, out of context and in the absence of the original stimulus, of some behavioral act'' (p. 329). The patient appears to be stuck in a behavior pattern. The repeated response occurs involuntarily and often when the patient is fatigued or frustrated with a task. Eisenson (1973) considered it to be a clinical signal that a task is too difficult for the patient. An example would be when a patient is asked to name a series of pictures; one picture is named correctly as ''steak,'' the next one of a cup is called ''steak,'' and the next one of a fork is called ''steak.'' The patient often recognizes these incorrect productions, shaking his or her head in frustration.

Awareness and Self-Correction

Aphasic patients differ in level of awareness of their language disorder. Lack of awareness of symptoms is referred to by neurologists as *anosognosia.* Anosognosia for language deficit accompanies some language symptoms more than others, and it is almost invariably a companion of jargon. Of course, when a patient does not identify a problem, he or she does not attempt to correct it. Yet aphasic persons, who are aware of their problem and recognize specific errors when they occur, frequently attempt to improve their language behavior on their own. Wepman (1958) considered this positive symptom to be a favorable sign for recovery.

SYNDROMES

For over a century, people with aphasia have been recognized as displaying different combinations of symptoms, and these combinations have been related to specific sites of brain damage. Many investigators over the years have described the same symptom patterns and yet have used different labeling systems. As Benson (1979a) noted, "the resulting aphasic syndromes represent one of the most confusing aspects of the complex topic of language disturbance" (p. 57). Not only does the mere quantity of classification schemes create confusion, but also speech-language clinicians often have difficulty finding clear examples of these categories in their caseloads.

Overview of Syndrome Classification

The multitude of classification systems arose from three traditions: from modification of the traditional distinction between sensory and motor aphasias (Weisenburg, 1934; Weisenburg and McBride, 1935; Goldstein, 1948); from attempts to make the aphasias fit into certain linguistic concepts (Jakobson, 1971; Wepman and Jones, 1961, 1964); and from different approaches to analyzing aphasic behavior (Luria, 1964, 1966; Howes, 1964, 1967; Goodglass, Quadfasel, and Timberlake, 1964). The notion that the aphasias can be divided into two major categories has been a regular theme: for instance, Jakobson's similarity and contiguity disorders, Howe's Type A and Type B aphasias, and fluent and nonfluent categories of aphasic speech. Others have

stayed away from a simple dichotomy. Head (1921, 1926) applied linguistic terminology by describing nominal, semantic, verbal, and syntactical language deficits. Luria derived sensory, amnestic-acoustic, semantic, efferent motor, afferent motor, and dynamic aphasias from his neuropsychological conceptualizations of brain function. Wepman and Jones identified syntactic, semantic, and pragmatic aphasias in addition to jargon and global aphasias. Schuell did not differentiate among aphasias but developed a classification system incorporating related disorders which may accompany aphasia (Schuell, et al., 1964). Because the varied classification systems represent the same disorders, several authors have presented charts which suggest comparisons among the many systems (Benson, 1979a; Green, 1969b; Kertesz, 1976, 1979).

In addition to the bewilderment caused by the number of labels for one type of aphasia, some clinicians have been frustrated at being unable to find cases which match the textbook descriptions of syndromes. Schuell's view that aphasia varies only in degree and not in kind has been appealing, and Smith (1971, 1972, 1977) was skeptical about the validity of traditional classification. Benson (1979a) suggested that clinicians may have been too demanding of the syndrome definitions possibly resulting from a misunderstanding as to the medical use of the term syndrome. He defined *syndrome* as "a group of findings, signs and/or symptoms which occur together in a given disease process with sufficient frequency to suggest the presence of that disease process..." (p. 57). He added:

Unfortunately, many individuals discussing aphasia consider an aphasic syndrome to be a fixed group of language findings and that each finding must invariably be present if a specific disorder is to be diagnosed. An exact syndrome is just as rare in aphasia as in any other medical disorder and many investigators interpret this variability negatively, implying that the syndromes of aphasia have little validity. In one sense this is true; the individual components of the syndrome are not firm and fixed. . . . In a broader sense, however, there is a strong tendency for the features of aphasia to bunch together into a few comparatively consistent clusters. . . . (p. 57)

Discernible syndromes of aphasia are suggestive of the presence of brain damage in a particular location of the brain. Yet often a stroke, tumor, or trauma do not attack a particular area but, rather, damage more than one of these specialized locations or somewhere between. This is why syndromes frequently are not clearly evident in the clinical population.

The Basic Dichotomy

In spite of individual differences in the details of symptom patterns, aphasic patients can be divided broadly into two distinct groups. The division is based on patterns of verbal output and is referred to as *fluent aphasia* and *nonfluent aphasia*. Aphasias corresponding to these general characteristics result from damage to either the anterior region of the brain in cases of nonfluent aphasia or the posterior regions of the brain in cases of fluent aphasia (see Figure 2–1). Therefore, some investigators use the terms *posterior* and *anterior aphasias*. The neoclassical division based on fluency has been substantiated empirically as descriptive of aphasic symptom patterns (Kerschensteiner, Poeck, and Brunner, 1972; Kreindler, Mihailescu, and Fradis, 1980; Wagenaar, Snow, and Prins, 1975) and as correlated with sites of brain lesion (Benson, 1967; Yarnell, Monroe, and Sobel, 1976; Mazzocchi and Vignolo, 1979).

The nonfluent-fluent distinction has been made according to at least ten parameters of verbal expression (Benson, 1967; Kerschensteiner, et al., 1972). These parameters include word selection, verbal paraphasias, grammatical com-

pleteness, perseveration, and several factors more directly tied to fluency such as phrase length, effort, rate of speaking, pauses, articulation, and prosody. Nonfluent aphasias tend to consist of word selection dominated by nouns, relatively few verbal paraphasias, incomplete grammar, frequent perseverations, short phrases usually less than four words, marked effort, a slow rate of speaking, many pauses, sometimes awkward articulation, and minimal prosody. The dominant symptom of nonfluent aphasias is agrammatism. In contrast, fluent aphasias tend to consist of a variety of word classes including functors, frequent verbal paraphasias, completeness of grammar, few perseverations, phrase length of more than four words, minimal effort, normal or sometimes faster rate of speaking, absence of noticeable pausing, smooth articulation, and varied intonation which appears to be near-normal. Depending on the type of fluent aphasia, dominant symptoms include circumlocution, paraphasias of all types, and jargon.

One symptom difficult to include in one of these divisions is nonpropositional verbal stereotypes, which may be a short phrase produced perseveratively and fluently. Patients with nonfluent aphasia and apraxia of speech may be able to produce only fluent stereotypic utterances in conversation. These patients are sometimes misdiagnosed as having fluent aphasia.

The Syndromes of Aphasia

When damage occurs to a certain functional area of the brain leaving other areas unscathed, a certain form of aphasia is the result. When the damage is not so discrete, the resultant pattern of aphasia can be thought of as a mixture or overlap of syndromes. The discrete syndromes are presented here as prototypes which illustrate the variability of disorders included under the label "aphasia." The best substantiated classification of aphasias was developed by Harold Goodglass, Norman Geschwind, and their colleagues in Boston (Geschwind, 1970, 1979; Goodglass and Kaplan, 1972). This neoclassical system fits well within the nonfluent (anterior) —fluent (posterior) dichotomy. Most current investigations of differences in aphasic deficits utilize the Boston classification system for identifying different groups of subjects.

Nonfluent Aphasias. The aphasias with limited verbal expression are Broca's aphasia, global aphasia, and transcortical motor aphasia.

Broca's aphasia, named after the French physician who discovered the site of speech in the brain, consists of relatively good auditory comprehension and of agrammatism as the dominant feature of verbal expression. Speech has all the characteristics of nonfluent aphasia. Historically, this symptom pattern has been referred to as motor aphasia or expressive aphasia because of the difference between receptive and expressive functions. The awkwardness of articulation found with Broca's aphasia represents a combination of two disorders, namely, Broca's aphasia and apraxia of speech. Agrammatism is a central language component, and apraxia is a motor speech component. Much research has been done to determine whether the central syntactic deficit seeps into auditory comprehension. The patient with Broca's aphasia often communicates successfully for two reasons. One, the few words produced usually represent a portion of the patient's message. Two, the listener may guess the rest of the message by asking yes/no questions, and the patient's good functional comprehension often enables him or her to answer the listener appropriately.

Global aphasia is a severe depression of language function in all modalities. Though these patients can be alert and aware of their surroundings, they do not comprehend language very well and have no functional speech. They convey feelings and simple wishes through facial, vocal, and manual gesture. Speech may appear at a nonpropositional level. For example, serial speech such as counting to ten may be possible with assistance from the clinician. Verbal stereotypes are common productions.

Transcortical motor aphasia is a rare syndrome. In conversation, this patient is similar to one with Broca's aphasia with good auditory comprehension and nonfluent, agrammatic verbal expression. The transcortical patient may tend more to possess "a stumbling, repetitive, even stuttering spontaneous output" (Benson, 1979a, p. 84). These patients may use a distinct body movement as a prompt for initiating speech. However, the cardinal feature of this syndrome is a startling ability to repeat fluently to a degree that would not be expected from observing spontaneous speech. The patient may struggle and stammer when answering a question, and then be able to repeat a fifteen-word sentence without missing a beat.

Fluent Aphasias. This category includes a more diverse group of syndromes which differ widely in overall severity of communicative impairment. The fluent aphasias are Wernicke's aphasia, conduction aphasia, anomic aphasia, and transcortical sensory aphasia.

Wernicke's aphasia has been known by many other names, such as sensory aphasia, receptive aphasia, and jargon aphasia. Carl Wernicke was a nineteenth-century German physician who, at the age of twenty-six, published a paper in which this syndrome was identified (Eggert, 1977). The patient's outward appearance is not usually tarnished by hemiparesis, and so the fluent jargon surprises the unfamiliar observer. The patient's continued muddled talking without the slightest evidence of concern is even more baffling. Basically, Wernicke's aphasia consists of poor language comprehension, jargon of different forms, and an anosognosia for the speech symptom. The jargon may be semantic or neologistic. The patient cannot repeat, and attempts often bear no relationship to the stimulus. Communicating with Wernicke's patients is a challenging project, since they comprehend poorly and use speech which eludes interpretation. Sparks (1978) described them as having a poor "therapeutic set," because they do not perceive the intent of tasks presented to them.

Conduction aphasia is characterized mainly by an impairment of repetition that is disproportionately severe relative to the adequacy of auditory comprehension and spontaneous speech. Comprehension is quite good, and conversational speech is communicative. Verbal expression is hampered occasionally by word finding delays and phonemic paraphasias. In spite of auditory comprehension which appears normal, the patient with conduction aphasia struggles to repeat. Verbal output in repetition deteriorates as the stimulus becomes longer and less familiar. With short, familiar phrases, the repetition may contain one phonemic paraphasia. However, as stimuli increase in difficulty, the phonemic paraphasias increase until output is reduced to random neologistic forms. Nothing like it occurs in the patients' conversational speech. Theoretical arguments have arisen as to whether conduction aphasia represents a deficient short-term memory, accounting for the repetition problem, or a deficient phonological selection component of the production system, accounting for the paraphasias.

Anomic aphasia consists of good auditory language comprehension and fluent, grammatically coherent utterances weakened in communicative power by a word retrieval deficit. Utterances are vacuous, with indefinite nouns and pronouns filling in for substantive words. A twenty-seven-year-old patient was asked to explain how to drive a car:

When you get into the car, close your door. Put your feet on those two things on the floor. So, all I have to do is pull . . . I have to put my . . . I'm just gonna do it the way I'm thinking of right now. You just put your thing which I know of which I cannot say right now but I can make a picture of it . . . you put it in . . . on your . . . inside the thing that turns the car on. You put your foot on the thing that makes the, uh, stuff come on. It's called the, uh . . .

Specific ideas are not conveyed by this empty speech, but communication with an anomic patient is possible within a situational context or with knowledge of the topic so that the ambiguity can be partly resolved. This patient can convey specific ideas inefficiently with circumlocutions. Realizing that needed words are missing, the patient expresses frustration and reminds the listener that the idea is known but the word is unavailable. When naming objects, the anomic patient retrieves some names quickly or, with other objects, engages in long delays and circumlocutions. Anomic aphasia is seen by some researchers as one end of a continuum of possible symptom patterns, with Wernicke's aphasia at the other end. Goodglass and Kaplan (1972) noted that there are cases at every point along the continuum. Variations occur according to level of auditory comprehension, level of awareness of expressive deficit, and use of paraphasias. Paraphasias are infrequent in anomic aphasia.

In a sense, **transcortical sensory aphasia** is to Wernicke's aphasia what transcortical motor aphasia is to Broca's aphasia. This rare patient possesses features of Wernicke's aphasia but also possesses a remarkable ability to repeat. Echolalia, where the patient repeats a question instead of answering it, is a prominent feature of this syndrome. It is as if the mechanism of speech production has been separated from intentions and meanings generated in the rest of the brain. For this reason, transcortical sensory aphasia was equated with "isolation of the speech area" by Goodglass and Kaplan (1972). However, Benson (1979a) and Kertesz (1979) considered isolation syndrome to be a separate disorder characterized by Benson as a "mixed transcortical aphasia."

The Caseload. Benson (1979a) concluded that "only about half of the cases of aphasia seen routinely in a clinical practice can clearly be placed into one or another of the syndromes and even this figure is dependent on some degree of diagnostic flexibility" (p. 136). Reasons for this low yield of clear syndromes include the presence of multiple or extensive lesions and lesions often superimposed upon a brain already impaired by previous lesions or aging processes. Benson added: "In view of the many potential complicating factors, however, it is not at all surprising that pure examples of the aphasic syndromes are not common, and in fact it is remarkable that the recognizable syndromes shine through as often as they do" (p. 137). While Darley (1982) emphasized the commonalities among patients, division into syndromes turns our attention to the differences. Therefore, the syndromes are considered here to represent prototypes of the different directions in which aphasia varies. The multiplicity of disorders in aphasia is an important fact requiring some flexibility in the administration of language treatment. One implication is that some patients can repeat and others cannot, resulting in differences in what can be done in treatment.

When syndromes are identifiable, some are found in the clinic more frequently than others. Benson (1979a) and Kertesz (1979) identified their cases in somewhat different ways but still reported proportions of syndromes which were similar. Both found that 85 to 90 percent of the caseload is made up of Broca's, global, Wernicke's, conduction, and anomic aphasias. The remaining small amount includes the transcortical aphasias and modality-specific disorders such as pure word deafness, alexia with agraphia, and alexia without agraphia. Benson reported the distribution of 263 cases with an unequivocal diagnosis of syndromes and 181 cases with a less definite identification of syndromes. Of the unequivocal diagnoses, 65 percent were somewhat evenly distributed among Broca's, Wernicke's, and anomic aphasia. Broca's aphasia was 26 percent of all aphasias in Benson's study, while anomic aphasia comprised 29 percent in Kertesz's study. Global and conduction aphasia were around 10 percent each of the total caseload in Benson's report. When the less certain diagnoses were considered, the proportion of global aphasias jumped to 31 percent while the other aphasias dropped in representation.

CLINICAL SETTINGS

The many settings in which a patient may receive speech-language treatment vary widely in terms of advantages and disadvantages for the clinician in providing services. The aphasic may be treated as an *in-patient,* a temporary or permanent resident of an institution, or as an *out-patient,* a visitor to a hospital or clinic in order to receive treatment. This represents a variation, not only in the setting of treatment, but also in patients' living environments to which the clinician directs generalization of clinical activity. The amount and types of assessment and treatment may depend on time and facilities dictated by the setting. Many of the prominent writers on clinical aphasiology have shared their experiences from a Veterans Administration Hospital or Medical Center. We are only beginning to become aware of the special circumstances for treatment dictated by home health care and nursing home environments.

The *acute care hospital* is where the patient can be seen by the clinician soon after onset. However, the length of stay in these hospitals is brief, only long enough to take care of medical problems so that the patient is well enough to go home or to another setting designed for long-term care and rehabilitation. The stroke patient may not stay in an acute care facility longer than thirty days, the time it takes for most aphasic patients to present a clear pattern of impaired and spared functions. The importance to the patient of clinical services in this setting includes reassurance felt with early awareness that there is a professional who understands and can help with initial adjustments to the communication disorder.

There are several advantages to providing speech-language treatment in the hospital setting. The availability of medical charts, physicians, nurses, and rehabilitation professionals such as physical therapists and social workers provides immediate and easy access to information for differential diagnosis and prognosis and to consultation and coordination of services. Through in-service programs and informal contact, there is a convenient opportunity to familiarize these personnel with the goals and methods of clinical aphasiology. The in-patient also is readily available for observation and treatment. One potential frustration in the acute care setting is that the clinician may not be able to carry out a vision of the patient's language treatment. However, referrals and sharing this vision with the next clinician can be of immense value to the patient.

Rehabilitation centers frequently provide in-patient and out-patient services, and are concerned with the rehabilitation of chronic cases for an extended period of time. They may be associated with an acute care hospital or combined with an acute care facility as in Veterans Administration Medical Centers, or they may be an independent facility. Services include speech-language treatment, phys-

ical therapy, occupational therapy, recreational therapy, and psychiatry. Requirements for admission may include the need for at least two of these services, which reduces the possibility that fluent aphasias are seen in this setting. Anomic, conduction, and many Wernicke's aphasics will not have the additional paralysis requiring physical and occupational therapies.

A big advantage of rehabilitation centers is the opportunity to carry out a long-term and varied treatment program for aphasia. This program can be coordinated with physical and occupational therapies, and daily living environments provided in occupational therapy may be made available for communication practice. Access to medical information and other professionals is similar to that found in acute care hospitals. One problem is the often busy schedule of patients who receive several therapies in a day; the speech-language clinician may see a tired patient, especially in the afternoon.

Five percent of the United States population over age sixty-five resides in an institution such as a *nursing home* (Lubinski, 1981b). A nursing home provides residential care which includes a room, meals, laundry, and personal care such as help with dressing, bathing, and toileting. The level of care varies widely; and Medicare and Medicaid have established two categories of nursing homes. A skilled nursing facility (SNF) provides a level of care similar to hospital care with twenty-four-hour nursing services. Regular medical supervision and rehabilitation services are provided. An intermediate care facility (ICF) provides regular nursing service but not twenty-four-hour service. Most ICF homes have rehabilitation programs, but personal care and social services are emphasized. Chapey, Lubinski, Chapey, et al. (1979) found that only 3 percent of respondents in a survey of nursing homes offered full-time speech-language pathology services, and part-time services were available in 27 percent of these homes.

The nursing home combines the advantage of ready access to medical information, medical assistance, and rehabilitation personnel, with the advantages of treatment being conducted in the patient's place of residence. The clinician has a convenient opportunity to observe, understand, and manipulate the patient's environment outside of direct, individual treatment. Of course, the clinician must enlist the cooperation of nursing home personnel and deal with the patient's adjustment to this living environment. Residents recently moved into a nursing home may be experiencing stages of reaction to loss of a loved one, external objects, security, and the sense of self derived from familiar surroundings and companions (Tanner, 1980). The resident may be angry or depressed. Furthermore, the nursing home may present what Lubinski (1981b) called a "communication-impaired environment," defined as "a setting in which there are few opportunities available for successful, meaningful communication" (p. 352).

Many persons confined to home require regular medical and rehabilitative services, which are provided by a *home health care agency*. Home health care may be administered by different levels of local government, visiting nurse associations (VNA), or hospital-based agencies. They provide nursing, physical, occupational, and speech-language services. A survey by Lubinski and Chapey (1980) showed that most agencies employed one or two part-time speech-language clinicians. Most clinicians had an average weekly caseload of between one and five patients, and as many as fifty communicative impaired patients were assisted by one agency. Most of the clinician's caseload consisted of aphasia or apraxia of speech. Most of their time was spent in treatment, and time spent in diagnosis equaled the time spent traveling.

One advantage of home-based services is the naturalness of the communicative context, and the availability of family for participation in the treatment program (Lubinski, 1981b). Problems with home health care which were found in the survey included the distance and traveling between patients, parking difficulties, and weather inconveniences.

The final setting considered here is *community* or *university clinics*. The community clinic may be supported by private donations (United Way), third party payments (private insurance, Medicare, Medicaid), and fees. These clinics service a wide variety of speech, language, and hearing impairments of children and adults. Clients are served as out-patients, and so the aphasics are generally in better health and from more supportive home environments than many seen in hospital and nursing home settings. The clinicians in these settings may not have the extent of specialized experience with aphasia found in the other settings because of the variety of caseload or their status as trainees in a university clinic. One difficulty of these settings is the lack of immediate availability of medical information and medical support. Medical records must be requested from a variety of sources, and this information may be received in a variety of forms, including a cursory letter or hastily photocopied handwritten progress notes. The clinician, therefore, must establish a clear understanding with potential sources of information.

Though the settings may be the same as those just described, the mechanism for delivering services is different with *private practice*. The number of private practitioners increased dramatically in the 1970s. In a survey of these clinicians, the largest proportion of their cases included hearing impairment and aphasia (Chapey, Chwat, Gurland, et al., 1981). Services are provided in the clinician's own offices, at the patient's home, or in a hospital through contractual arrangement with the hospital. Payment is provided by medical insurance, Medicare, Medicaid, and direct client payment.

THE CLINICIAN'S ROLE

The clinician's primary roles in aphasia rehabilitation include differential diagnosis and assessment, treatment, education and counseling of patients and their families, and administration according to the requirements of each setting. Diagnosis and assessment (Chapters 6, 7, 8, 9) are carried out for purposes of selecting the caseload, planning treatment, predicting and measuring recovery, and advising family and hospital staff concerning communicative strategies. Treatment (Chapters 10, 11, 12) consists of a variety of activities designed to improve specific impaired language functions and to enhance overall communication effectiveness. Efforts are directed toward guiding the patient to becoming the best possible communicator as independent from the clinician as possible. The sudden communication disorder also requires adjustments in familial, occupational, and social roles by the patient and family; and the clinician can facilitate these adjustments. Clients may request a variety of information about aphasia, some of which may have been given by a physician during a time when shock and disbelief prevented understanding and acceptance of this information. The rehabilitation process is lubricated by interaction with other professions involved in treating the aphasic patient. The speech-language clinician obtains referrals and broadens the rehabilitation effort by educating others on clinical aphasiology and by consulting relative to the goals of other professionals. This places a demand on the clinician to possess familiarity with a range of information that extends beyond the specifics of language assessment and treatment. Some of this information is contained in the chapters which follow.

2 Neurological Structure and Etiology

The physician generally identifies the presence of speech or language difficulties and refers the patient to a speech-language pathologist for assessment and possible treatment. Neurologists such as Rubens (1977c) and Stein (1981) have advocated for clear communication between themselves and the speech-language pathologist. The clinician can feel at ease in a hospital setting by understanding the etiological bases of aphasia and the relationships between symptoms and brain structures. The clinician is often in a situation where an understanding of basic neurology should be drawn upon to answer questions from the patient, the family, and certain hospital staff. The information in Chapters 2 and 3 is the foundation for differential diagnosis and for making certain predictions about recovery.

This chapter provides an elementary introduction to the neuroanatomical structures involved in language processing. Levels of the nervous system are related primarily to simple and general behaviors such as alertness, expression of emotion, and receiving sensory inputs and generating motor responses. Humans share these levels of behavior with other animals. Higher-level functions largely unique to human beings will be the emphasis of Chapter 3.

FUNCTIONAL LEVELS IN THE CENTRAL NERVOUS SYSTEM

Most of the human nervous system consists of the central nervous system (housed within the vertebral column and skull) and the peripheral nervous system (between these structures and the sensory or motor endorgans). Of these divisions, this chapter focuses on the central nervous system (CNS). Dysarthrias, apraxia of speech, and the aphasias can be traced to damage of different levels within the CNS. Certain dysarthrias result from damage to the peripheral nervous system. Gross anatomy of the human brain is shown in the upper drawings of Figure 2–1. Three major structures of the CNS are shown: the cerebrum, brain stem (midbrain, pons, and medulla), and cerebellum. The convoluted lateral surface of the cerebrum, called the cerebral cortex, is shown for the left half of this structure; it is essentially duplicated on the other side. These halves are referred to as the left and right *cerebral hemispheres,* and are connected by a band of commissural fibers, the largest of which is

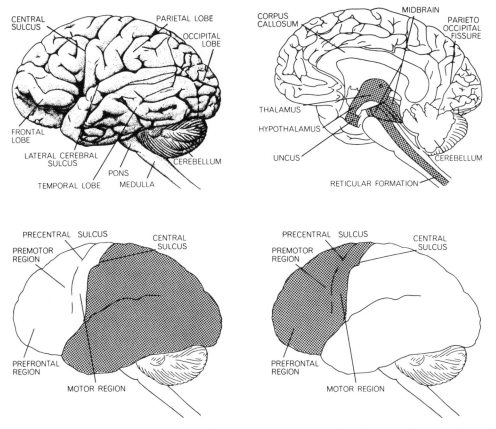

Figure 2-1. Gross anatomy of the brain is depicted in the upper left (lateral view) and upper right (medial view). The shaded regions represent Luria's three functional levels or "blocks": reticular formation, posterior cortex, and anterior cortex. *(Reprinted by permission from Luria, A. R., The functional organization of the brain. Scientific American, 222(3), 66–78, 1970. Copyright © 1970 by Scientific American, Inc. All rights reserved.)*

the corpus callosum. The medial surface of the right hemisphere is shown in the upper right of Figure 2–1, as if the hemispheres of the cerebrum had been pulled apart.

Functional levels of brain structure can be introduced in a broad sense with reference to three levels described by A. R. Luria (1970a) and represented in Figure 2–1. These levels apply to the left and right cerebral hemispheres. The first structural level is the reticular formation within the brain stem. The second structural level is the posterior portion of the cerebral hemispheres, and the third is the anterior portion of the cerebral hemispheres.

In a sense, the cerebrum must be turned on in order to be engaged in a majority of complex mental activities, including the processing of language. Through the brain stem, the reticular formation is plugged into the base of the cerebral mass and is responsible for wakefulness and alertness. The reticular formation is a network of small nerve cells with short interconnections. This network is projected diffusely to all regions of the cortex, forming what is known as the reticular activating system (RAS). The reticular formation receives input from sensory pathways on their way to the cerebral cortex, so that any visual, auditory, or tactile sensation can activate the cortex as a whole as well as proceed to a specific sensory receiving area in the cortex. In effect, the RAS alerts the entire cortex to be prepared for specific information to be analyzed.

The other two levels, according to Luria, are the higher cortical functions. The second level, related to posterior cortex, involves the reception, analysis, integration, and storage of information. The sensory inputs of each modality arrive at different locations within the posterior cortex, where they are analyzed and integrated. The third level, related to the anterior cortex, involves the initiation and coordination of purposeful or goal-directed behavior; it is responsible for willful action. The motor region (Figure 2–1) sends impulses directly to the muscles of the body. The premotor region contains the plans for organizing these impulses to

carry out particular functions. In a simplistic way of looking at these levels, the posterior cortex is responsible for handling stimuli and the anterior cortex generates a purposeful response. This broad division corresponds to the anterior and posterior sites of lesion which produce nonfluent and fluent aphasias.

THE CEREBRUM

Characterizing the incredible information capacity of the human brain, Sagan (1977) suggested that it contains ten trillion bits of information in the form of its neuron connections (synapses). The structure of this marvelous computer is depicted grossly in Figure 2–2. The cortex and internal structures, such as the thalamus, consist of compact collections of neuron networks. These components are commonly referred

Figure 2-2. Frontal (coronal) section of the cerebrum shows location of the layer of cortex and certain interior structures. *(From Willard R. Zemlin,* SPEECH AND HEARING SCIENCE: *Anatomy and Physiology,* © *1968, pp. 466, 469. Reprinted by permission of Prentice-Hall, Inc., Englewood Cliffs, N.J.)*

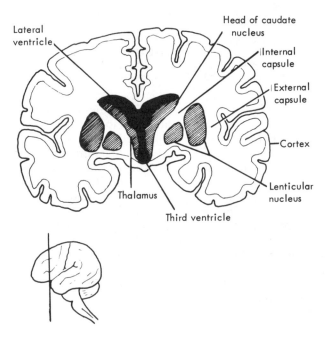

to as gray matter. White matter, such as the internal capsule, consists of axonal fiber tracts traversing to and from the cortex, thalamus, and similar structures. This figure will be referred to again in later pages, but for now let us turn to the most important part of brain structure in the study of language function.

Cerebral Cortex

The surface of the brain is protected by three structural features: the bony skull, membranous tissue covering the cortex, and a cushion of cerebrospinal fluid which is channeled within and around the surface of the brain.

Three membranes cover the cortex and collectively are called *meninges*. The uppermost layer, the *dura mater,* is a dense, durable tissue. The middle layer is the *arachnoid;* and the innermost layer is the *pia mater,* which makes direct contact with the surface of the brain, covering the cortex like cellophane within the ridges of the convoluted surface. A space between the arachnoid and the pia mater, called the subarachnoid space, contains tiny blood vessels and cerebrospinal fluid.

The cortex consists of six layers of over ten billion densely packed nerve cells with varied thickness, from fifty to one hundred cells (1.5 mm to 4.5 mm). This represents

approximately 50 percent of the neurons in the cerebrum and about 40 percent of its weight. The folding which creates the convoluted brain surface permits 2 to $2^{1}/_{2}$ square feet of cortex to be compacted into a small space.

The topography of each cerebral hemisphere provides reference points for defining functional regions of the cortex. The wormy-looking ridges are called *gyri,* and the grooves are generally called *sulci.* Certain larger grooves may be called fissures, but authors vary as to which groove is to be called a sulcus or a fissure. Figure 2–3 shows common terminology used to label these landmarks on the lateral and medial surfaces of the left hemisphere. Some of these landmarks are boundaries for the four major functional regions of each hemisphere. Like the boundaries of American states, some boundaries of these regions are marked by clear terrain features and others are somewhat arbitrary.

Frontal Lobe. The anterior brain, or frontal lobe, is bounded posteriorly by the *central sulcus* and inferiorly by the lateral cerebral fissure or *Sylvian fissure.* The central sulcus has also been called the fissure of Rolando. The *precentral gyrus* is responsible for sending impulses to the muscles, and damage to this gyrus in one hemi-

Figure 2-3. Lateral and medial views of the cerebral cortex show landmarks important for localization of speech and language functions (see Chapter 3).

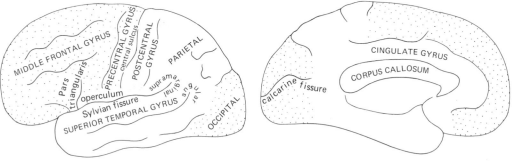

(a) Lateral view

(b) Medial view

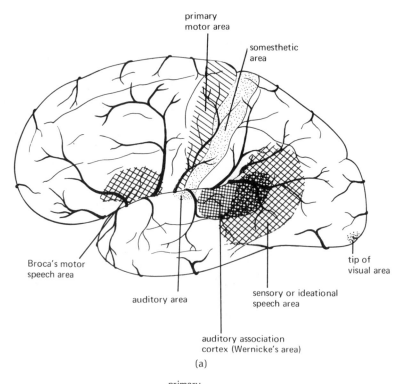

primary
motor area

somesthetic
area

Broca's motor
speech area

tip of
visual area

auditory area

sensory or ideational
speech area

auditory association
cortex (Wernicke's area)

(a)

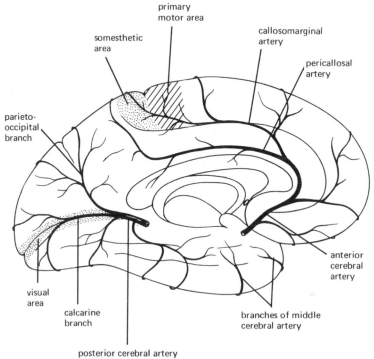

primary
motor area

somesthetic
area

callosomarginal
artery

pericallosal
artery

parieto-
occipital
branch

anterior
cerebral
artery

visual
area

calcarine
branch

branches of middle
cerebral artery

posterior cerebral artery

(b)

Figure 2-4

sphere results in hemiplegia. Functionally, it is referred to as the motor strip or *primary motor area* (see Figure 2-4). Parts of the body are controlled from different locations in the precentral gyrus. Leg movement is directed from the medial portion of this gyrus, while the arm is directed by the superior lateral portion. Moving further down the motor strip, the muscles used for articulation and phonation are directed from the lower half of the lateral portion. The relative proximity of representation for the arm and hand to the oral area is why people with speech impairments tend to retain lower-limb movement better than upper-limb movement.

Important landmarks of the frontal lobe include the inferior frontal gyrus (also called the third frontal convolution) and the operculum. The inferior frontal gyrus contains a premotor zone called *Broca's area*, which is bounded anteriorly by the pars triangularis. It programs the oral and phonatory mechanisms for the movements of speech (see Figure 2-4). At this level of function, the cerebral hemispheres differ from each other; Broca's area is usually in the left hemisphere. A lesion in Broca's area produces apraxia of speech, and this area is prominent in the site of damage resulting in Broca's aphasia.

Parietal Lobe. The parietal lobe is one of three posterior functional regions which receive sensory information. It is bounded anteriorly by the central sulcus, posteriorly by a somewhat arbitrary boundary at the occipital lobe, and inferiorly by the Sylvian fissure and part of the temporal lobe. The *postcentral gyrus* is the sensory counterpart to the motor strip, and it is referred to as the sensory strip or *primary somesthetic area*. Hemianesthesia results

from damage to this area. Representation of body parts corresponds to the location of representation in the motor strip. Though the motor and sensory gyri are side by side, they are not connected directly. Neural communication between these gyri is accomplished via the thalamus.

The region posterior to the precentral gyrus is responsible for tactile recognition and visuospatial orientation. Damage to either hemisphere may result in *astereognosis* (see Chapter 1) or in *constructional apraxia*, causing difficulties in copying geometric forms and drawing from memory. With right parietal lobe damage only the left half of the drawing may be defective, indicative of a general *neglect of the left side* (see Table 3-3). Right hemisphere damage in this region is also responsible for *three-dimensional spatial disorientation* and *dressing apraxia*, an inability to clothe oneself properly. Left parietal lobe lesions, on the other hand, are responsible for *ideomotor/ideational apraxia, right-left disorientation, finger agnosia* (failure to recognize names of individual figures), and *acalculia* (reduction of mathematical skills).

Temporal Lobe. Looking like the thumb of a fist, the temporal lobe is situated inferiorly to the Sylvian fissure and parietal lobe and anteriorly to the occipital lobe. The *primary auditory area* is located on the superior temporal gyrus, where it serves as the lower wall of the Sylvian fissure beneath the parietal lobe. This area, hidden from view in Figure 2-3a, is called *Heschl's gyrus* (also called transverse temporal gyrus). The interpretation of auditory language input in the left hemisphere is handled posteriorly to Heschl's gyrus in a region called *Wernicke's area*. The relationship between Wernicke's area

Figure 2-4. Distribution of the three cerebral arteries to the (a) lateral and (b) medial surfaces of the brain are shown relative to functional areas for speech and language (also see Figure 3-1). The lateral view primarily depicts the middle cerebral artery. (*Reprinted by permission from Barr, M. L., The Human Nervous System. Hagerstown, Md.: Harper & Row, 1974*)

and the primary auditory area is shown in Figure 2-4. The lesion producing Wernicke's aphasia includes this left hemisphere region. Most cases of *agnosia* for environmental sounds have been found to have bilateral temporal lobe lesions, while a lesion in the left Heschl's gyrus is likely to cause *pure word deafness.*

Two other landmarks which are located in the temporal and parietal lobes will be prominent in later discussions of language function. The *supramarginal gyrus* wraps around the posterior portion of the Sylvian fissure, and the *angular gyrus* joins the superior temporal gyrus with the middle temporal gyrus posteriorly.

Occipital Lobe.   The occipital lobe is posterior to the parietal and temporal lobes. A critical feature of this region is the *calcarine fissure,* which is largely on the medial surface (Figure 2-3b). The *primary visual area* for the reception of visual input lays within the banks of the calcarine fissure. Damage to this area in either hemisphere produces homonymous hemianopsia; and, when the lesion is in the left hemisphere and includes the posterior corpus callosum (called the splenium), *alexia without agraphia* and *color agnosia* are the result. *Visual object agnosia* usually occurs after bilateral damage in the occipitotemporal boundary, but it can occur with a unilateral lesion which produces aphasia; *prosopagnosia* occurs after bilateral or right hemisphere damage in this region.

Other Cortical Regions.   There are two additional areas of the cortex. One cannot be seen in Figure 2-3a but can be viewed in the coronal view of Figure 2-2. This area, called the *insula,* can be revealed by prying the frontoparietal lobes and the temporal lobe apart at the Sylvian fissure. This cortical wall is deep to the Sylvian fissure and is continuous with the inferior frontoparietal cortex and the superior temporal cortex. The other area is the *cingulate gyrus,* which, shown in Figure 2-3b, is located on the medial surface of each

hemisphere and is part of the limbic system. The limbic system is responsible for the emotional component of behavior.

Contralateral Connections.   One crucial aspect of brain structure has implications for the functional relationship between the primary motor and sensory areas of the cortex and the endorgans to which they are connected. These cortical areas functionally possess *contralateral connections* with their respective endorgans. That is, the motor strip of the left hemisphere controls the right side of the body and the right hemisphere controls the left side. Similarly, the left sensory strip primarily receives input from the right side, and vice versa. The left primary auditory cortex hears primarily from the right ear, and the right auditory cortex hears primarily from the left ear. This contralateral relationship is not quite the same regarding vision. In this case, the left primary visual cortex sees the right field of vision and the right visual cortex sees the left visual field.

Blood Supply to the Cortex

Because most cases of aphasia are caused by stroke, it is essential to understand the structure of blood flow to the brain. Different patterns of symptoms and different expectations for recovery are related to the location of damage in this arterial system. This system supplies brain tissue with critical nutrients such as oxygen and glucose. Cortical blood supply can be viewed with respect to three structural levels: the vascular system on the surface of the cortex, the origin of this system at the base of the brain, and the arteries in the neck leading up to the base of the brain.

Three cerebral arteries cover the surface of each hemisphere. These are shown in Figure 2-4 for the left hemisphere, and their relationship to the primary motor and sensory areas is noted. The *anterior cerebral artery* is distributed mostly throughout the medial surface of the cortex, extending posteriorly into the parietal lobe (Figure 2–4b). The *middle cerebral artery* (MCA) has a main vessel within the Sylvian fissure and branches to most of the lateral cortex (Figure 2–4a). The MCA supplies the motor and sensory areas involved in speech, audition, and language function. The specific location of a stroke within the MCA is designated usually with reference to the direction of flow from the Sylvian fissure and to the lobe supplied. Branches are identified as upper-division (superior) and lower-division (inferior) and as frontal, parietal, or temporal. The auditory area, for example, is supplied by an inferior temporal branch of this artery. Other designations may be with reference to the central sulcus (Rolandic fissure) and are called pre-Rolandic or post-Rolandic branches. The *posterior cerebral artery* covers the medial surface of the occipital lobe and the base of the temporal lobe. It can be seen in the lateral view reaching around the posterior portion of the left hemisphere. It supplies the primary visual area on the banks of the calcarine.

The three cerebral arteries originate from a circular arterial system at the base of the brain, anterior to the brain stem. This system is called the *Circle of Willis,* consisting of small communicating arteries between the origins of each cerebral artery. From the Circle of Willis, the cerebral arteries proceed upward to their respective hemispheres.

The Circle of Willis is supplied on both sides by arteries in the neck. In the lower neck, the left and right *common carotid arteries* divide at the level of the larynx and become the internal and external carotid arteries on each side of the larynx and spinal column. Only the left and right *internal carotid arteries* proceed to the Circle of Willis. At the Circle of Willis, each internal carotid artery is continuous with its respective middle cerebral artery; and, therefore, the internal carotid supplies the lateral and anterior regions of the brain via its direct connection with the MCA and its indirect connection with the anterior cerebral artery. Another pair of arteries runs upward continuously through the neck, posterior to the carotids. These are the left and right *vertebral arteries,* which travel in openings in the vertebra of the spinal column and enter the base of the skull in the lower portion of the brain stem. The arteries are joined, becoming the *basilar artery* which carries blood to the posterior of the Circle of Willis. The proximity of the basilar artery to the posterior cerebral arteries makes it a supplier of the occipital lobe.

White Fiber Tracts

Three categories of axonal fiber tracts connect different parts of the brain with each other. The cerebral hemispheres are connected by the *commissural fibers.* They include a small bundle of fibers connecting the temporal lobes called the anterior commissure as well as a large bundle called the *corpus callosum* (Figures 2–1 and 2–3). The second category is the *projection fibers,* which connect the cortex with subcortical levels of the nervous system. Sensory (afferent) impulses travel to the cortex and motor (efferent) impulses travel from the cortex by way of the projection fibers. They tend to converge at the center of the brain. They are funneled between the thalamus and corpus striatum as a band of fibers called the *internal capsule* (Figure 2–2). The third category is the *association fibers,* which connect one area of cortex to another within a hemisphere. These tracts, traversing beneath the cortex, permit sensory areas to communicate with each other and also permit sensory areas to communicate with motor areas. They also are referred to as association fasciculi; and the superior longitudinal fasciculus, also called the *arcuate fasciculus,* connects the auditory language area with the motor language area. Association fibers make possible the complex integration of varied information within the cerebral cortex.

Interior Structures
of the Cerebrum

When the brain is sliced open to afford a view of its core (Figure 2-2), three structures are prominent. Two of these are gray matter, masses of nerve cell nuclei; and the other is a system of cavities. These structures are contained in each hemisphere.

The cavities are nearly in the absolute center of the cerebrum and include the *lateral ventricles* and the *third ventricle* (Figure 2-2). The roof of the lateral ventricle is formed by the corpus callosum. Because the mind is a nonmaterial thing, these three cavities were believed a few centuries ago to be the site of mental activity. Actually, the ventricular structures are part of a continuous system of tunnels and spaces throughout the central nervous system, and a clear *cerebrospinal fluid* (CSF) flows through these spaces to provide a cushion for the central nervous system. CSF is produced in the ventricles. The ventricles possess a characteristic size and

shape which become important reference points in certain radiological techniques for the identification and location of brain lesions. A deep space-occupying lesion, such as a tumor, might compress the ventricles.

On each side of the third ventricle and beneath each lateral ventricle is a mass of nerve cells called the *thalamus* (Figures 2-1, 2-2, and 2-5). It is a way station for sensory transmissions scurrying to the cortex and for some motor impulses on their way downward, a kind of "traffic cop" for simultaneous inputs, directing them to their appropriate places in the cortex. The thalamus is composed of different nuclei, such as the medial geniculate nucleus for hearing and the lateral geniculate nucleus for ' vision. The subthalamus contains motor nuclei interconnecting the motor area of the cortex to other structures within the cerebrum, the cerebellum, and the brain stem. The anterior portion is part of the limbic system and, therefore, is involved in emotional response to sensory experience. The thalamus, especially a

Figure 2-5. Transverse section of the cerebrum shows location of certain interior structures. *(From Willard R. Zemlin, SPEECH AND HEARING SCIENCE: Anatomy and Physiology, © 1968, pp. 466, 469. Reprinted by permission of Prentice-Hall, Englewood Cliffs, N.J.)*

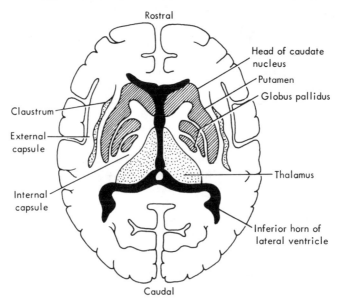

posterior portion called the pulvinar, may have a role in language behavior (see Chapter 3). The posterior cerebral artery supplies the thalamus.

The *corpus striatum* is a complex arrangement of gray masses situated between the cortex and the thalamus. Its several parts are the caudate nucleus, the lenticular nucleus which includes the putamen and globus pallidus, the claustrum, and the amygdaloid nucleus (Figure 2–5). The anterior corpus striatum, including the caudate nucleus, is nourished from a branch of the anterior cerebral artery. The middle cerebral artery supplies the putamen and globus pallidus. The corpus striatum is a major way station for motor neurons. *Basal ganglia* is a term sometimes used for this structure; but, according to Barr (1974), it usually refers to the corpus striatum, subthalamus, and substantia nigra in the brain stem.

Glial Cells

Neuroglia provide structural support for neurons throughout the cerebrum. They are found between nerve cells and axonal fibers but are not involved directly in the transmission of neural impulses. Two types of glial cells, astrocytes and oligodendrocytes, have their own additional uses. Astrocytes assist in the metabolic reactions of neurons, and oligodendrocytes are responsible for the formation of myelin sheaths which cover the axons of the central nervous system. Certain types of malignant tumors grow out of these cells.

PRINCIPAL CAUSES OF APHASIA

Cerebrovascular Accident (Stroke)

A cerebrovascular accident (CVA) is a disruption of blood flow to the brain. There are two general types of stroke, distinguished roughly on the basis of whether too little or too much blood is being supplied to brain tissue. An *ischemic* stroke involves a reduction or cessation of blood flow caused by occlusion of an artery supplying the brain. A *hemorrhagic* stroke is a bursting artery that causes blood to escape onto areas of the brain's surface or into brain tissue. Cerebrovascular disease has been the third most common cause of death over age forty-five in the United States. Ischemic strokes are the most common of the two varieties, with varied incidence figures indicating that they comprise around 75 percent of all CVAs, while hemorrhages are responsible for the remaining 25 percent.

Ischemia. Aphasia results from occlusion of the middle cerebral artery (MCA) or the internal carotid artery because of its continuation with the MCA. The deprivation of blood flow causes an area of brain cells to die (necrose). This tissue, called an *infarct,* softens, is liquified, and then is removed naturally, leaving a cavity on the brain's surface. Astrocytes (glial cells) form a rim of scar tissue around the cavity. Ischemia refers to the occlusion (cause), and infarction refers to the damaged tissue (effect).

Two aspects of recent infarction have important clinical implications. First, upon occurrence of the stroke there is a swelling of necrotic tissue and surrounding gray matter. This edema or excess of tissue fluid reaches a maximum in a few days and may produce a corresponding increase in the neurological deficit. The edema and related deficit may take one or two additional weeks to subside. Compounding this physiological reaction to the infarction is a general reduction of blood flow in both cerebral hemispheres following an infarction in one hemisphere. This reduction of blood flow was found to disappear in the unimpaired hemisphere within two or three weeks after onset (Meyer, Shinohara, Kanda, et al., 1970). Therefore, localized edema and generalized reduction of blood flow are likely to produce a more severe clinical deficit than that which remains after three weeks. The clinician should wait for this period to pass in order to observe the deficit attributable to the infarction itself.

The two types of ischemic stroke, thrombosis and embolism, produce similar clinical characteristics but differ generally in characteristics of history, precipitating causes, and onset.

Thrombosis is the most common cause of focal infarction. It is typically associated with arteriosclerotic disease and consists of sclerotic plaque from the vessel wall at the site of occlusion. There is a higher incidence of thrombosis among people with diabetes mellitus and hypertension. The process of thrombus formation may take minutes or weeks to produce the occlusion. Therefore, though clinical signs may appear suddenly, subsequently they may gradually increase in severity over minutes, hours, or even days. This *stroke-in-evolution* may proceed in a step-wise fashion. The reaching of maximum deficit is referred to as "completed stroke."

A frequent warning signal of impending thrombosis is the *transient ischemic attack,* or TIA. TIAs are temporary disruptions of blood supply that produce specific neurological signs. They are experienced as sudden, transient blurring or loss of vision, weakness (motor) or numbness (sensory) of one side, difficulty with speech, vertigo, diplopia, or any combination of these. They warn that a process of plaque formation, which could lead to a thrombotic stroke, is underway. TIAs usually come to an end in less than an hour but are defined as being completed within twenty-four hours. Not all cases of stroke are preceded by these transient episodes. However, if a person heeds these signals and visits a physician, thrombosis can be delayed or avoided through anticoagulant medication. Common anticoagulants are coumarin agents and heparin. Physicians are careful in prescribing these medications, since the risk of a hemorrhage is great with

hypertensive patients. Surgery to clear the carotid artery (carotid endarterectomy) may be performed as a preventive measure.

An **embolism** is a clot that originates in another part of the circulatory system and then travels through the system to block an artery supplying the brain. The most common source of embolic material is the heart. Therefore, medical history is likely to include arteriosclerotic or rheumatic heart disease. Because the clot was formed elsewhere, clinical onset of embolism differs from that of thrombosis. The development of maximum neurological deficit takes less time, usually seconds or minutes. Stroke-in-evolution is much less frequent with an embolism. There are usually no warning signs such as TIAs, though they may occur when the origin of the embolus is in the arteries of the neck.

The speech-language clinician's first contact with the victim of an ischemic CVA may be in the patient's hospital room during the first few days after admission. The patient may be kept resting in bed with the feet slightly elevated for a few days in order to avoid rapid lowering of blood pressure, especially during stroke-in-evolution. Patients with swallowing problems (dysphagia) are maintained on intravenous fluids. Within twenty-four to forty-eight hours after completion of the stroke, certain physical exercises are begun three or four times per day to prevent development of muscle contractures, and self-care activities are instituted to promote psychological as well as physical well-being. Anticoagulant medication may be administered during stroke-in-evolution and continued indefinitely after the stroke is completed to prevent a recurrent episode.

Hemorrhage. A hemorrhage occurs when a vessel wall breaks and floods the surrounding tissue with blood. The accumulation of blood (hematoma) acts as a rapidly expanding mass which displaces and compresses adjacent structures. Depending on its location, the hematoma can compress arteries and cranial nerves. Hemorrhages are usually associated with hypertension, ruptured aneurysm, or arteriovenous malformation. The several types of hemorrhage are classified according to their location, some occurring in the surface areas surrounding the brain and others occurring deep within the brain. Some of these are associated with trauma rather than vascular impairment. Intracerebral and subarachnoid hemorrhages are associated with vascular disturbance.

An **intracerebral hemorrhage** invades tissue within the brain. Located where sensory-motor projection fibers converge in a small place, these hemorrhages can be devastating. Size and location of the hematoma determine its clinical manifestations. Severe headache is a prominent early clinical symptom, usually preceding development of focal neurological signs. Other signs include nausea and vomiting. About half the cases lose consciousness within minutes to hours after onset. The clinical manifestations of hemorrhage occur suddenly, without warning, and often during activity. Because of the central location of intracerebral hemorrhage, symptoms usually include hemiplegia (motor disturbance) and hemianesthesia (sensory disturbance) of the opposite side of the body. Development of symptoms may progress rapidly over a period of minutes. Medical treatment of intracerebral hemorrhage includes medication to reduce edema, such as steroids or glycerol, and surgical evacuation of the hematoma, especially in the cerebellum.

Subarachnoid hemorrhage occurs within the tissue that covers the surface of the brain and is usually caused by a ruptured aneurysm at the base of the brain. It may also be caused by trauma. An *aneurysm* is a dilated blood vessel that can vary from the size of a pea to that of an orange (Chusid, 1979). This stretches and weakens the vessel wall, and rupture produces an excruciating headache, nausea, and vomiting. Surgical treatment of an accessible aneurysm may prevent rupture, and procedures include "trapping" the aneurysm by applying clips on both sides, clipping the neck of the bulging sac, or packing muscle around the aneurysm. Plastics have been sprayed on the aneurysm and surrounding vessels to prevent rupture.

Risk and Survival. Certain risk factors increase the likelihood of suffering a stroke. The most important to consider are hypertension, TIAs, and cardiac disease. According to Sahs, Hartman, and Aronson (1976), "hypertension is not only a major cause of nonembolic cerebral infarction but also the most important treatable risk factor for this condition" (p. 24). TIAs commonly herald cerebral thrombosis. There is a 23 percent chance of suffering an ischemic stroke during the first year after onset of TIAs, with a 5 percent risk in each of subsequent years. This is more than ten times the rate of expected stroke incidence in a general population of the same age and sex. Embolic stroke is commonly associated with cardiac disease. Advances in the treatment of cardiac diseases have changed the incidence of stroke associated with these disorders. Other potential risk factors include smoking, obesity, and oral contraceptives.

Roughly 50 percent of all stroke cases survive after the first thirty days (Sahs, et al., 1976). Cases due to infarction, the most common cause of stroke, have the best chance of survival, about 60 percent after the first thirty days. Intracerebral hemorrhage has the worst survival rate, at 20 percent. Fifty percent of cases with subarachnoid hemorrhage will survive after thirty days. Therefore, the predominance of cases caused by infarction in the speech pathologist's caseload is due, not only to its higher incidence among causes of stroke, but also to the better chances of living to benefit from long-term rehabilitation.

Tumor

A tumor (neoplasm) is a spontaneous new growth of tissue which serves no useful purpose. Benign tumors are not recurrent and tend to apply mild pressure to adjacent tissue. Malignant tumors not only apply pressure but also invade and destroy surrounding tissue. They grow worse and become resistant to treatment. Tumors within the brain infiltrate widely before destroying a specific location of brain tissue, and early symptoms of these neoplasms usually are very general reductions of function.

Types of Brain Tumor. Tumors are identified with respect to their tissue origin. For example, they may arise from the glial cells that reside among nerve cells in the brain (glioblastoma, astrocytoma, oligodendroglioma), the meninges that cover the brain's surface (meningioma), or the nerve sheath surrounding nerve fibers (schwannoma, neurofibroma). However, location of the tumor is usually more crucial than tissue origin in the neurologist's evaluation of symptoms. Tumors may be classified broadly as either intraaxial, originating from glial cells within the brain, or as extraaxial, originating in the skull, meninges, or cranial nerves.

Glioblastoma multiforme, also known as malignant glioma or *astrocytoma grades 3–4,* is the most common primary brain tumor in adults. Peak incidence is between forty-five and fifty-five years of age. It may originate anywhere in the cerebral hemispheres, with the frontal and temporal lobes being the most frequent sites. The glioma is an infiltrative, rapidly growing mass that is likely to invade both sides of the brain through their connecting pathway. Weiss (1978) reported median survival to be approximately $5^{1}/_{2}$ months, with 20 percent surviving one year and less than 10 percent surviving two years. Chusid (1979) suggested that average survival from glioblastoma is about one year.

Weiss (1978) commented that though neurosurgeons may report "gross total removal of the tumor," it will always recur, usually in months. Radiation therapy or chemotherapy have not been shown to be effective for this type of tumor.

Astrocytomas grades 1–2 (low-grade astrocytoma) and *oligodendrogliomas* in adults are much less common than glioblastoma multiforme but have a more favorable prognosis. These tumors usually expand slowly, and in some cases symptoms such as seizures may appear years before the tumor is discovered. They may remain benign histologically, but over the course of months or years they may assume the terminal characteristics and prognosis of the glioblastoma. Though length of survival following surgery has been given at a median of three to five years (Weiss, 1978) or an average of five to six years (Chusid, 1979), Weiss noted that prognosis is "notoriously uncertain" (p. 222). According to Weiss, the treatment of choice is craniotomy (opening of the skull) followed by the most extensive surgical resection of brain tissue that is possible. Complete removal is seldom accomplished. However, repeated craniotomy and resection can be beneficial when the tumor is in an accessible location such as the anterior regions of the brain. Postoperative radiation therapy may slow down or arrest tumor growth.

Finally, a *meningioma* is a benign tumor that arises from the tissues covering the brain (arachnoid cells). It is the second most common primary brain tumor in adults. Its peak incidence in adulthood is in the thirties and forties, and unlike other brain tumors it occurs more frequently in women than men. Fifty percent occur over the lateral surfaces of the brain, and 40 percent occur at the base of the brain. Meningiomas grow slowly and generally do not invade the cerebral cortex. Complete surgical removal is often possible. This makes prognosis generally favorable, with prolonged survival being a frequent outcome after surgery. Recurrence is possible in a small proportion of cases.

Pathophysiological Mechanisms. The mechanisms that produce symptoms are the same with most types of tumor. The primary mechanism is increased intracranial pressure from the neoplasm, which may obstruct circulation, and from edema in surrounding tissue. This produces headache as one of the earliest symptoms, which is precipitated or intensified by activities such as stooping, straining, or exercising. Nausea and vomiting are common. Sensory impairments and dulling of mental function may occur; and if the tumor is allowed to enlarge, such symptoms may evolve to stupor and coma. The presence of focal neurological signs depends on location of the tumor and may include loss of vision and hearing if there is pressure on the optic and acoustic cranial nerves. As the tumor grows, it may cause loss of speech.

Trauma

Traumatic damage to brain tissue is of two broad types. A *contusion* is when the membranous covering of the brain's surface remains intact but the underlying cortex is bruised. A contusion directly below the site of impact is called a coup lesion; damage to the side of the brain directly opposite the site of impact can also occur, and this is called a contracoup lesion. Blows to the back of the head produce coup and contracoup lesions because the impact causes the brain to move forward, making contact with the forehead of the skull. The other general type of lesion is *laceration,* in which there is a tearing of the surface of the brain. Contusions and lacerations are commonly found beneath skull fractures and around penetrating wounds caused by sharp objects or missiles.

Head injuries are frequently classified as either closed or open, depending on degree of injury to the skull. *Closed* injuries are those in which there is no injury to the skull or in which the skull injury is limited to an undisplaced fracture. Also called nonpenetrating injuries, they can produce mild or severe loss of consciousness, and the less-than-severe forms usually simply bruise the brain. Closed-head injury often produces diffuse effects, and obvious deficits may disappear in a few weeks. *Open* or penetrating head injuries can produce extensive contusions and lacerations of brain tissue.

The most consistent result of head trauma is altered consciousness. Assessment of level of consciousness provides an important index of severity of brain damage and a means of monitoring improvement of brain function after recent injury. Reduction of consciousness has been viewed on a continuum from drowsiness (also called lethargy or obtundation), stupor, light coma, and deep coma. The Glasgow Scale was first reported by Teasdale and Jennett in 1974 as an assessment of altered consciousness. This assessment involves independent observation of eye opening, motor response, and verbal performance (Jennett and Teasdale, 1981). The patient's responsiveness is rated on a scale for each of these features, and a "coma score" is computed. Jennett and Teasdale noted that the Glasgow Scale provides an objective and reliable means of specifying level of consciousness, which has been subject to inconsistent definition and labeling.

Another indicator of severity of impairment is the duration of post-traumatic amnesia (PTA). PTA continues after the patient is judged to have regained consciousness, usually when he begins to speak. "The end of PTA is when the patient begins to lay down conscious memory of on-going events—when he remembers today what happened yesterday and does not begin each day with a blank mind" (Jennett and Teasdale, 1981, p. 89). Jennett and Teasdale added that " . . . the interval from injury to the end of PTA is about four times longer than the interval until he first speaks (unless there has been a specific factor delaying the return of speech)'' (p. 90).

Penetrating open-head injuries have been studied in detail since World War II; they can produce fairly definitive and chronic aphasias. Closed-head trauma, on the other hand, has more ambiguous effects on behavior, and has been receiving an increasing amount of attention in the literature (see Levin, 1981). While several investigators have observed symptoms of aphasia after this injury (Heilman, Safran, and Geschwind, 1971; Levin, Grossman, and Kelly, 1976; Thomsen, 1975), general memory deficits have been observed as well (Thomsen, 1975; Groher, 1977). Hematomas, in many cases, are diffuse and bilateral. Closed-head trauma, therefore, cannot be considered to be in the same category with focal etiologies, although focal effects have been observed.

OVERVIEW: NEUROLOGICAL EXAMINATION

The neurologist can examine the basic status of sensory, motor, and cognitive systems in a brain-injured patient in about thirty minutes. His or her goals are to determine whether there is impairment of the nervous system, the nature of impairment, and the location of impairment. In order to confirm a preliminary diagnosis of type and site of lesion, the physician may request laboratory tests such as an angiogram, brain scan, or CT scan (see Chapter 3). Once the diagnosis is determined, the neurologist develops an overall plan of medical and rehabilitative treatment which results in referrals to physical therapy, occupational therapy, and/or speech-language therapy. If surgery is a possible treatment, the neurologist will consult with a neurosurgeon.

The diagnosis begins when the patient enters the examination room and the physician initiates conversation. Level of consciousness reflects status of the reticular activating system (RAS), and alertness and orientation reflect status of internal cerebral structures and general level of cortical function. The initial interview yields a great deal of information pertaining to localizing signs such as memory loss, muted affect, language impairment, motor speech deficit, drooling, and paralysis or incoordination of the extremities.

In the formal clinical examination, sensory and motor systems are tested according to functional levels which are indicative of status of the peripheral and central nervous systems. The visual system receives considerable attention, partly with examination of sight in each eye and to each visual field. Wolf (1980) omits the traditional tuning fork screening of hearing because "we have competent audiology laboratories . . . to diagnose the site of hearing loss at all levels of the anatomy of hearing" (p. 369). Simple reflexes from head to toe are surveyed, with hypoactivity indicating peripheral damage and hyperactivity indicating central damage. Control of voluntary movement and balance provide an indication of cerebellar function. Motor and sensory impairment of one side reflects damage in one cerebral hemisphere, and deficits localized to particular body parts reflect damage to locations within the motor and sensory strips (pre- and postcentral gyri) of the cortex. Degree of impairment is determined by using the unimpaired side as a standard, and the neurologist systematically compares left and right sensation, left and right reflexes, and so on.

3 Language Function and the Brain

Structurally, the left and right cerebral hemispheres have a comparable appearance; functionally, they are similar with respect to sending impulses to muscles and receiving input from sensory receptors. However, with respect to programming the muscles to move for particular purposes and to interpretation of sensory input, the two hemispheres behave very differently. While the previous chapter dealt primarily with what the hemispheres share in common, this chapter addresses the uniqueness of each hemisphere, with an emphasis on control of the language function. The study of the brain correlates of language function is called *neurolinguistics,* which includes people with aphasia as a principal source of data. This is a discipline within *neuropsychology,* the study of brain-behavior relationships.

THE MIND-BODY PROBLEM

The relationship between the body and behavior has intrigued philosophers and physicians for centuries. It was obvious that the ears are for hearing, the eyes are for seeing, and the muscles of the arms and legs are for manipulating objects and moving about. Much less obvious has been the

relationship between mental functions and human anatomy. By the middle of the nineteenth century scientists were agreeing that the brain plays some role in intellectual and emotional activity, but satisfactory evidence had not been presented.

Differing views of the relationship between the brain and mental activity, according to Campbell (1970), arise from a dilemma created by the logical incompatibility of four initially plausible statements:

1. The human body is a material thing.
2. The human mind is a spiritual thing.
3. Mind and body interact.
4. Spirit and matter do not interact.

The human body can be seen, handled, and measured, while the human mind eludes all of these possibilities. Disorders of memory and language consequent to brain injury are evidence that the mind and body interact in some way. However, demonstrating a causal relationship between mind and body is hampered by the logical and scientific impossibility that spirit and matter interact in any way.

Several philosophical solutions to the mind-body dilemma have arisen largely from the logical compatibility of any three of these statements and rejection of a fourth statement. Dualism, for example, accepts (1) and (2) as true; and two versions of dualism depend on acceptance of either (3) or (4). These conceptualizations admit the reality of a nonmaterial mind as well as a material body. Interactionist dualism accepts a causal interaction between mind and matter. The other version of dualism maintains that mind and body operate in a parallel fashion. Parallelism accepts a correlation between brain and mind functions but does not accept a causal relationship. A third view, materialism, is very different from dualism by virtue of its acceptance of statements (1), (3), and (4) and its rejection of (2). By rejecting (2), materialism accounts for all mental activity in terms of physical and chemical phenomena. Finally, radical behaviorism demolishes the problem by rejecting the existence of anything mental, an acceptance of only (1) as true. Most of the scientific thinking represented in this chapter can be considered to be some form of dualism, with the parallelist version being a somewhat safer position.

LOCALIZATION OF FUNCTION

During the Renaissance, as seen in a drawing by Leonardo da Vinci (Blakemore, 1977), the nonmaterial mind was thought to inhabit the caverns of the lateral and third ventricles. In the eighteenth century the French medical community was the stronghold for a belief that the material brain has something to do with psychological processes, and the physician Cabanis had concluded by 1802 that "... the brain secretes thought as the liver bile ..." (Berlin, 1956, p. 269). Elsewhere in Europe, materialistic explanations of the soul were discouraged by a powerful clergy.

Broca in 1861 and Wernicke in 1874 discovered focal brain damage related to speech and auditory disorders (Broca,

1960; Wernicke, 1977). As a result of numerous autopsies, proof was found for a relationship between mental function and the brain. Many physicians became convinced that specific language functions are controlled by specific areas of the brain. However, debate arose between advocates of strict localization and advocates of an antilocalization position. *The two positions in the localization issue are (1) that specific psychological functions are controlled by (localized in) certain brain areas and (2) that psychological functions are controlled by the brain acting as a whole and, therefore, are distributed throughout the brain.* Reviews of this issue have been prominent in the aphasia literature (Schuell, et al., 1964; Eisenson, 1973). As Brookshire (1978b) pointed out, *the truth probably resides somewhere between these positions.*

One barrier to a resolution of the localization issue has been a limitation in our understanding of cognitive or mental processes in general, and of language processes in particular (see Chapter 4). The problem is partly one of defining the processes to be localized; the "what" question. In the eighteenth century, certain psychologists divided the mind into a variety of discrete components called faculties. The mental faculties included various aspects of reason, memory, emotion, and will. Specific faculties included hope, courage, prudence, love of home, love of life, and attraction to wine. Broca demonstrated the location of what he called the "faculty of articulate speech." A concept of brain "centers" was developed with respect to the modalities of language function. Several investigators diagrammed models of brain function based on associations among auditory, visual, spoken, and graphic language centers (Bastian, 1897; Bramwell, 1906; Broadbent, 1878; Lichtheim, 1885). In effect, all of auditory comprehension was located in one place, and all of writing was located in another place.

Contemporary subdivisions of the language function maintain some identification with respect to modalities. However, certain language processes are common to all modalities. The language function has been divided into *linguistic components* such as the phonological, semantic, and syntactic and into *psycholinguistic processes* such as perception, short-term memory, retrieval from long-term memory, organization of long-term memory, and concept comparison. The relationship between linguistic components and psychological processes still is being determined, so that we cannot be certain about what is to be related to the brain. Furthermore, appropriate concepts of brain structure and function should be applied to establishing mind-brain relationships. Caplan (1981) advised: "... the localization of functions in grossly defined areas of the brain—convolutions and parts thereof—is at best a convenient shorthand. Working at this level of neural description cannot, in the face of what we know about nervous function, allow us to frame the most important questions about language-brain relations in ways amenable to investigation" (p. 129). Cognitive processes and structures should be related to neural processes (physiology) as well as to neural structures (anatomical regions).

The anti-localizationist position has been a positive expression of a different orientation to mental and cerebral function. Instead of looking at the mind and brain as collections of separable parts, critics of strict localization have taken a "holistic" view of these functions. The incredible complexity of brain structure is emphasized, especially the interconnections among its different parts. One component should not be considered to function in isolation. Rather, its function depends on teamwork with other components. The connections among brain structures are considered in current approaches to localization, causing theorists to be more careful than the early proponents of cortical centers. The antilocalization arguments arose primarily as a

criticism of a particular method of mind-brain investigation, namely, the lesion or deficit method.

METHODS: BRAIN-IMPAIRED SUBJECTS

Inferences about the cerebral location of normal cognitive functions are made from observing the behavior of patients with damaged brains. The study of brain-impaired subjects must contend with a basic problem of interpretation. The researcher can never be confident that the relationship between a deficient function and locus of lesion represents the location of the normal realization of that function. Ideally, the researcher wants to observe the normal brain in order to explain normal function. As will be shown later, several methods for studying the normal brain have been developed.

The Lesion Method

The lesion method (also, deficit method) formed the basis for nineteenth-century theories of localization. It continues to be the primary source of data concerning the differentiation of functions within a cerebral hemisphere. The method involves two basic steps: (1) identification of a specific impaired function and (2) determining the site of lesion. Improvements in the lesion method have come from increased sophistication in the comprehensive observation of deficits and greater accuracy in identifying the site of lesion near the time of behavioral observation, rather than much later upon autopsy.

Double Dissociation. The concept of *dissociation* is used in the identification of an impaired function which is to be related to a site of lesion. A dissociation is observed when one function is impaired while another remains intact or when one function is clearly more impaired than others.

For example, if reading is impaired and auditory comprehension and other language functions remain relatively spared, then the investigator may be able to relate the reading function to a site of lesion. As concepts of cognitive and language functions have changed or become more precise, researchers have proposed a variety of dissociations, such as verbal from nonverbal short-term memory or syntactic from semantic language processes.

Glassman (1978) described a minimal criterion for inferring a mind-brain relationship from deficit-lesion data. This criterion is called *double dissociation,* in which two different observations of behavior and two differently located lesions are required: lesion X produces deficit A which is greater than deficit B, while lesion Y produces deficit B which is greater than deficit A. Perhaps the most common double dissociation in mind-brain research occurs when left-hemisphere damage (X) produces a deficit in verbal behavior (A) which is greater than any deficit in nonverbal behavior (B), while a right-hemisphere lesion (Y) produces the opposite effect. When this double dissociation occurs we can infer that a single dissociation of A-more-impaired-than-B occurs, not merely because function A is more susceptible to any brain damage, but because the area of lesion X possesses some characteristic which produces this dissociation. Also, we may conclude that function B has a special relationship with the area of lesion Y. The criterion of double dissociation is illustrated in Table 3–1 with function-location relationships which will be mentioned later in this chapter and in subsequent chapters.

Glassman (1978) noted that the ideal would be to achieve multiple dissociations in relating a deficit reliably to a site of lesion. He remarked: "It is interesting that the criterion of double dissociation is not generally demanded of a lesion study before publication" (p. 17). Glassman provided an instructive perspective on the scientific process of theory building in this arena of investigation: "Everyday perception involves the integration of multiple cues with past experience. In science, *single* cues take much effort to obtain. In this way, it can be seen that the double-dissociation criterion for lesion studies is really a special case of the search for converging information" (p. 3). Numerous reports based on fairly precise location of lesion sites have been published which have allowed this convergence to take place.

TABLE 3-1. The criterion of double dissociation in localization research (Glassman, 1978) is related to some common double dissociations which have been suggested in various investigations. A single dissociation occurs when a lesion site X yields a deficit A which is greater than a deficit B.

Lesion Site X	→	Deficit A	>	Deficit B
Lesion Site Y	→	Deficit B	>	Deficit A
Left hemisphere (LH)	→	Verbal tasks	>	Nonverbal tasks
Right hemisphere (RH)	→	Nonverbal tasks	>	Verbal tasks
Temporal LH	→	Language	>	Music
Temporal RH	→	Music	>	Language
Anterior LH	→	Speech fluency	>	Comprehension
Posterior LH	→	Comprehension	>	Speech fluency
Anterior LH	→	Syntax	>	Semantics
Posterior LH	→	Semantics	>	Syntax

Left and Right Hemisphere Comparison. A common research paradigm involves the comparison of two groups of subjects, each group defined according to the cerebral hemisphere that is damaged. A nonbrain-injured group often is included so that the presence of a deficit can be demonstrated in either damaged group. These studies are intended to investigate asymmetry of function between left and right hemispheres without precision as to the site of damage within a hemisphere. Sometimes the evidence for unilateral damage is based on clinical neurological examination by noting the presence of aphasia, hemiplegia, hemianopsia, and so on.

Lesions within a Cerebral Hemisphere. Identification of specific lesion sites has been accomplished by postmortem examination and observation during surgery (Hecaen and Angelergues, 1964) and by determination with X-ray of the site of missile penetration in many cases of traumatic injury during World War II (Luria, 1966; Russell and Espir, 1961). Russell and Espir reviewed medical records of 1,166 brain-injured patients; Luria examined over 800 cases; and Hecaen and Angelergues focused on 214 right-handed patients with left-hemisphere lesions. Traumatic injury may not be the best source of data on site of lesion because of the devastation to brain tissue that can be caused by a bullet or piece of shrapnel. Malignant tumors may infiltrate a vast region of tissue. Cerebral infarcts, on the other hand, may damage a small region of cortex with relative precision depending on the site of occlusion within the arterial system. Advances in neuroradiological diagnostic procedures have enabled researchers to identify the location of these lesions with relative inconvenience to the subject.

Angiography or *arteriography* has not often been used as a research tool, because it is an invasive procedure (injection of a foreign substance into the body) and may have "infrequent but potentially serious consequences" for the patient (Wolf, 1980, p. 23). It is an X-ray procedure for observing the blood vessels of the head and neck. Injection of an iodinated opaque fluid into the arterial system allows the cerebral arteries to be seen on an X-ray. Vessels cannot be seen on the angiogram beyond the point of an occlusion. Space occupying lesions are indicated by distortion of the pattern of arteries.

The *brain scan* has been used more frequently in reports of lesion-deficit relationships (Benson, 1967; Karis and Horenstein, 1976; Kertesz, 1979, 1981). Other names for this procedure include "isotope scanning," "radionuclide scanning," and "radioisotopic encephalography." Brain scans were popular as a diagnostic tool between 1965 and 1975 (Oldendorf, 1978). A radioisotope called technetium-99m is injected intravenously, and emission of gamma rays from this medium is detected with a scintillation camera or gamma camera. Damaged tissue is detected because of its greater permeability for the radioisotope. The brain scan, though invasive, is a relatively safe procedure with complete absence of morbidity (Wolf, 1980).

Computerized Tomography (CT Scan) was announced to the public in 1972 with the EMI Scanner from England and, in essence, "permits the clinician to perform a gross brain autopsy at any time during the course of an illness" (Oldendorf, 1978, p. 531). The CT scan is accurate, safe, and easy to administer; it can be done on an outpatient basis if necessary. It uses narrow beams of X-rays to obtain readings of tissue density in successive layers of the head. With the EMI model, 160 readings are taken per 180-degree transversal of the scanner as it rotates around the head. A total of 28,800 readings are fed into a computer which transforms the X-ray data into absorption coefficients. Results of the computer analysis are displayed as a digital printout representing 6,400 small blocks of tissue. The printout provides a picture of the shape, size, and position of a particular plane of brain structure. Normal EMI scans were analyzed by Gawler, Bull, DuBoulay, et al., (1975). Pathologic tissue is indicated by alterations in the normally expected densities. The procedure may be completed in thirty minutes.

The value of CT scan for localization lies in its power of resolution of the lesion and its detection of longstanding CVAs. Infarcts are shown as decreased tissue density and hemorrhages are shown as increased density. Identification of an infarct can be enhanced with intravenous injection of a contrast material (Wing, Norman, Pollack, et al., 1976). Mazzocchi and Vignolo (1978) described a procedure for mapping lesions observed with a CT scan onto a standard lateral diagram of the brain. They found satisfactory reliability among three clinicians who recorded lesion site in this way. Sources of variation and possible error were mentioned: (1) standard diagrams do not take into account the individual differences among human brains and (2) clinicians may have different criteria for outlining the area of damage especially with acute infarcts within three weeks postonset. Gado compared CT and brain scans of forty CVAs and found comparable results (Gado, Coleman, Merlis, et al., 1976). The CT scan was superior in distinguishing between an infarct and an intracerebral hemorrhage. The CT scan is not infallible; Messina (1977) found that it missed 11 percent of lesions in cases scanned two weeks before death.

The popularity of CT scanning is reflected in numerous studies of lesion-deficit relationships (Hayward, Naeser, and Zatz, 1977; Kertesz, 1979, 1981; Naeser and Hayward, 1978; Mazzocchi and Vignolo, 1979; Naeser, Hayward, Laughlin, et al., 1981). Its effect on clinical neurology has been dramatic because it is a cost-effective procedure which replaces many other diagnostic procedures including the neurological examination, at least for the purpose of locating and identifying the lesion (Oldendorf, 1978).

Limitations of the Lesion Method. Relating a deficit to normal function and then relating both to a site of lesion seem to be a relatively straightforward means of determining the functional organization of the normal brain. On the contrary, there are several reasons for exercising care in interpreting lesion-deficit data.

Historically, the holistic viewpoint of the antilocalizationists has largely been a critique of the lesion method rather than an argument against the possibility that cognitive functions can be related to regions of the brain. Because language and brain functions consist of interacting components, Henry Head (1920) argued that a disturbance of one component necessarily has some consequence for other components. Advocating an "organismic approach," Kurt Goldstein (1948, 1960) interpreted each behavior of an aphasic as an expression of the whole organism. A symptom was viewed as a combined result of the lesion and of the rest of the organism's adjustment to that lesion. Therefore, a patient's symptom pattern cannot be attributed solely to the damaged region. Rather, symptoms reflect what the whole system does without a particular region (Glassman, 1978).

Caplan (1981) suggested that some aphasic behavior may not best be analyzed as deficits but rather as brain lesions producing new functions. The aphasic deficit is not necessarily an impaired normal function but, instead, represents a process which does not exist in normal cognitive machinery. Caplan's example was phoneme substitutions in phonemic paraphasia, which can be seen as representing an added set of phonological processes rather than a deficit of normal processes.

Regarding the views of Head and Goldstein, Glassman (1978) noted that "it would be dangerous to take too seriously the holist criticism, which smacks of naive realism as much as do interpretations in terms of centers. The holist criticism is an overreaction to the overinterpretation of lesion data, which leads to talk of centers" (p. 8). Caplan's (1981) comments point to the need to consider possibilities besides a correspondence between deficit and normal function. It should be proved that a symptom represents an impairment of the normal before normal function can be inferred from the patient's language behavior.

The early localizationists, who relied on autopsy to localize lesions, left themselves open to methodological criticism other than what comes from hindsight and the advance of theory and technology. Head (1915) cited clinical observations that were often incomplete or emphasized symptoms which tended to support the language center concept. Relatively recent investigations have been characterized as "unbalanced" presentations which were clear in anatomical findings but incomplete in syndrome description (Green and Howes, 1977). Certain methodological considerations are unavoidable artifacts of dealing with brain dysfunction. For example, symptom patterns change over time as a result of the recovery process. Therefore, interpretation of the deficit may depend on when the deficit is observed (Mohr, 1976, 1980; Caplan, 1981).

tional roles associated with specific regions of the brain.

Sodium amytal injection is used to determine hemispheric laterality of speech in a patient prior to brain surgery (Wada and Rasmussen, 1960). The drug is injected into the left or right common or internal carotid artery resulting in a temporary "paralysis" of one hemisphere. Lateralization of speech is determined by having the patient count, say days of the week, and name objects after the injection. If the drug has immobilized the hemisphere responsible for speech, then the patient's counting is halted or seriously disrupted. Several cases for whom this preoperative procedure was employed were surveyed in order to determine the relationship between handedness and hemisphere asymmetry (Branch, Milner, and Rasmussen, 1964). Musical abilities of each hemisphere were investigated with this procedure by Bogen and Gordon (1971).

Penfield and Roberts (1959) developed a method of artificially stimulating cortical gray matter while it is exposed during surgery, called *cortical mapping*. Tiny electrodes are placed on different regions of the brain and effects of electrical stimulation are observed. The patient is conscious during the procedure, performing various verbal and nonverbal tasks. Stimulation may interfere with a behavior or activate a particular behavior. Sophisticated observations of word retrieval and short-term memory related to cortical and subcortical electrical stimulation have been provided by Ojemann, Fedio, and Van Buren (Fedio and Van Buren, 1975; Ojemann, 1975, 1978; Ojemann and Whitaker, 1978).

Procedures Accompanying Surgery

Surgical removal of a portion of the brain may be accompanied by procedures which permit study of functional asymmetry between hemispheres or of func-

Postsurgical Investigations

Surgical procedures have been used usually to remove an epileptic focus or to keep seizure activity confined to one hemisphere. Surgery is considered when seizures have been shown to be resistant to medication and often is performed in clinics with research programs where long-term follow-up can be pursued (Solomon and Plum, 1976). Surgical procedures permit functional comparison between hemispheres and sometimes between specific areas within each hemisphere.

Lobectomy is the complete or partial removal of a lobe. Milner (1967) compared functional abilities before and after surgery, and turned attention to the special capacities of the nonverbal (usually right) hemisphere. Verbal and nonverbal auditory tasks were presented to patients with left and right temporal lobe excisions. Each subject served as his own control because preoperative performance was measured to determine postoperative sparing or reduction of function. Left temporal lobectomy resulted in reduction of verbal recall and sparing of musical tone discrimination, while right temporal lobectomy resulted in reduction of music discrimination and sparing of verbal recall. Milner's findings are a clear example of double dissociation (see Table 3–1) between verbal and nonverbal auditory processes. Others have studied short-term memory (Samuels, Butters, and Fedio, 1972) and deductive reasoning (Read, 1981) following unilateral temporal lobe removals.

Hemidecortication, in which one hemisphere is removed, has been investigated extensively by Dennis (1980a, 1980b) and Zaidel (1976, 1977). Three of Dennis' subjects were left with one hemisphere prior to five months of age because of Sturge-Weber syndrome, which is congenital calcification and atrophy of cortex producing seizures. This procedure, also called a hemispherectomy, has provided a rare opportunity to study some of the unique properties of each hemisphere and the capacity of each hemisphere to develop language.

Another opportunity to study the unique properties of each hemisphere

appeared first in 1961, when a forty-eight-year-old war veteran underwent an operation which completely separated the two hemispheres from each other. The *split-brain* operation, also called commissurotomy, produces independently functioning hemispheres by cutting all commissural fibers connecting them, thereby confining uncontrollable epileptic seizures to one hemisphere. The first successful procedures on humans were performed by Vogel and Bogen in California, and a few cases have been investigated extensively over several years in order to determine the receptive and expressive capabilities of each hemisphere. Most early behavioral investigations were directed by Sperry and Gazzaniga, with Sperry winning a Nobel prize in 1981. Gazzaniga (1967) observed that "the operation produces no noticeable change in the patient's temperament, personality or general intelligence" (p. 118). Patients did report unusual experiences such as pulling trousers up with one hand and down with the other. During an argument with his wife, one patient grabbed and shook her with the left hand while restraining that side with his right hand (Gazzaniga, 1970). However, such occurrences were rare (see Springer and Deutsch, 1981).

Zaidel (1978a) delineated three chronological periods of research with split-brain subjects. The first, from 1961 to 1968, established that each hemisphere possesses a dominance for particular kinds of tasks, the left hemisphere (LH) generally for language and the right hemisphere (RH) generally for spatial-constructional tasks. The second period followed with elaboration of right hemisphere superiority on a variety of nonverbal spatial tasks involving tactile or tactile-visual stimuli. The third period, beginning in 1972, launched special techniques for simultaneous visual presentations to each hemisphere which have been applied to the study of normal subjects.

In the basic research technique, a

stimulus is presented to either the left or right hemisphere via the contralateral visual field or tactile modality. Output from either hemisphere is through the contralateral hand or is oral-verbal which is assumed to be generated from the left hemisphere. Linguistic and nonlinguistic stimuli were presented to each hemisphere, and linguistic or nonlinguistic responses were made with either hand. A picture of an object to the right visual field or an object held in the right hand (LH) could be named by the split-brain subject, but these stimuli to the left side (RH) could not be named. A printed word in the left visual field could be identified with left-hand selection of the object but not with the right hand. This indicated that the right hemisphere can comprehend single words but may not be able to generate speech.

An incomplete independence of hemispheres following commissurotomy was illustrated by one of Sperry's female patients, who was being presented geometric figures at random to the right and left visual fields. A nude pin-up was included in the otherwise mundane series of shapes and was flashed to the left field (RH). The patient blushed and giggled but could not report what she saw. Still giggling she said, "Oh, Dr. Sperry, you have some machine." Somehow, the verbal left hemisphere got the idea that the right had seen something special, but the left was still ignorant of what that special something was. There may be some "cross-cueing" from one side to the other by way of other channels of stimulation.

METHODS: NORMAL SUBJECTS

Although each cerebral hemisphere after hemidecortication or commissurotomy can be considered to be undamaged, each is still separated from its normal functional context, that is, its communication with the opposite hemisphere. Penfield and

Roberts (1959) could not be sure of the effect of artificial electrical stimulation itself on the responses observed during cortical mapping. As stated previously, inferences about normal brain function from the dysfunction of damaged brains is, at best, an indirect route to a model of normal function. However, the 1970s saw a proliferation of techniques for studying the functional characteristics of undamaged hemispheres capable of sharing information. Some of these techniques have confirmed left-right asymmetries of function which correspond to asymmetries inferred from brain-impaired subjects. Other techniques have measured cortical activity directly while subjects perform various tasks.

Input and Output Modality Bias

Several procedures take advantage of the structural contralaterality between the hemispheres and the input and output modalities. Investigators generally start with assumptions about the predominant function of each hemisphere, then examine whether this asymmetry has some effect on the processing of stimuli presented simultaneously to each hemisphere or has some effect on the production of certain motor behaviors.

The body of research with *dichotic listening* has become massive; healthy reviews were provided by Berlin and McNeil (1976) and Krashen (1976), and the journal *Brain and Language* devoted two issues to the procedure in 1974 and 1975. Dichotic listening involves indirect comparison between normal left and right temporal lobes. In this procedure, two different stimuli are presented simultaneously, one to each ear. The subject is asked to report what is heard. When brief verbal stimuli such as two digits were presented by Kimura (1961), she found that subjects reported hearing the digit to the right ear most of the time. This right ear advantage (REA) has been considered to indicate dominance of the left hemisphere for language processing (Kimura, 1967).

As noted in Chapter 2, the human visual system is structured so that the occipital lobe of each hemisphere receives input from the contralateral half visual field. A stimulus presented to one half field will be received first by the opposite hemisphere. Simultaneous *hemifield presentation* of different visual stimuli, if it is to reach contralateral hemispheres as in dichotic listening, must minimize ocular scanning which would prevent experimental separation of the hemispheres. Ocular scanning was controlled with split-brain subjects by having the patient fix his gaze on a point in the center of the visual field. Also, stimuli were shown no longer than one hundred milliseconds with aid of a tachistoscope to avoid shifts of gaze. McKeever and Huling (1971) required normal subjects to report a centrally fixed digit before responding to simultaneous hemifield stimuli. Schmuller and Goodman (1979) wanted to avoid memory decay during a digit report, and so they placed an arrowhead between the left and right-field stimuli. Subjects responded first to the field indicated by the arrow's direction. To insure input to one hemisphere, Zaidel (1975) developed a special visual apparatus called the "Z lens." This apparatus permits the viewing of stimuli for longer than one hundred milliseconds so that complex linguistic material can be presented.

Amidst refinements of procedure, a right visual field (RVF) advantage has been found for simultaneous presentation of verbal material (McKeever and Huling, 1971), and a LVF advantage has been shown for nonverbal visual stimuli (Hannay, 1979).

A *dichaptic task* was developed by Witelson (1974), who presented objects to each hand simultaneously within a box in order to isolate the tactile modality. Pointing responses were made to two choices.

She observed left-hand input superiority for nonverbal spatial forms and absence of laterality with letters.

With direction of gaze to the left or right, we begin to consider lateralized motor activity as a sign of hemispheric asymmetry of function. Penfield and Roberts (1959) alluded to eye shifting in response to electrical stimulation of either hemisphere. Investigators have come to believe that direction of *conjugate lateral eye movement* (CLEM) is indicative of selective activation of the hemisphere contralateral to the direction of gaze. Direction of eye orientation has been related to type of question or problem with right-handed subjects: a significant tendency for right direction during verbal or analytical problems such as "Divide 144 by 6" or "Define prejudice," and left direction during problems of spatial orientation such as "Which way does George Washington face on a quarter?" (Kinsbourne, 1972; Kocel, Galin, Ornstein, et al., 1972). An even distribution was observed with left-handed subjects. Gur (1975) found, however, that this phenomenon depends on the experimental situation. Task-dependent contralateral gaze shifting occurred when the experimenter sat behind the subject, as in Kinsbourne's research, but did not occur when the experimenter sat in front of the subject.

Asymmetry in motor activity has been studied with *verbal-manual time sharing tasks.* According to White and Kinsbourne (1980), when a person performs two unrelated tasks at the same time, he does better if the tasks are controlled by different hemispheres than if both tasks are controlled by the same hemisphere. Subjects, while silent, balanced a dowel rod on the right hand longer than on the left, but while talking they balanced the rod longer on the left hand (Kinsbourne and Cook, 1971). It was as if the region for speech in the left hemisphere interfered with the motor area for the hand within the same hemisphere. Speaking and even humming have been shown to interfere with right-handed finger movements but not with the left hand (Hicks, Bradshaw, Kinsbourne, et al., 1978).

Measurement of Cortical Activity

Looking for laterality effects relative to input and output channels is motivated by an assumption that asymmetry of the periphery reflects asymmetry of cerebral activity. The possibility of direct access to cerebral processes, however, is an exciting development in mind-brain research, because now the cognitive processes assumed to underlie different tasks can be related to electrophysiological processes while by-passing assumptions about what is going on beneath the skull.

Electroencephalography (EEG) has for decades provided a record of the electrical activity of the brain. At the time of Schuell's investigations of aphasia in the 1950s, it was about the only routine laboratory tool available to neurologists for localization of brain damage. EEG has been a relatively crude but safe diagnostic tool. It has been replaced to a great extent by angiography, brain scan, and CT scan for the localization of focal lesions. The site of a focal lesion in the cortex can be estimated by comparing recordings of brain wave patterns obtained from electrodes placed on the skull at locations corresponding to each lobe of each hemisphere. A pattern from one region which is diferent from more regular patterns of other regions is indicative of a focal lesion. EEG continues to be useful for diagnosis of seizure type, determination of death, follow-up after trauma, and diagnosis and prognosis of certain slow viral infections (Wolf, 1980).

The EEG has found new status as a research tool. The alpha rhythm, a regular wave pattern eight to thirteen cycles per second, is pronounced during decreased levels of processing, such as during sleep. It is attenuated during active processing, when the brain is engaged in a particular task. Just as CLEMs have been a behavioral sign of predominant hemisphere activity during a task, EEG *alpha suppression* has shown that the left hemisphere (LH) is active during verbal-analytical tasks while the right hemisphere (RH) dominates during nonverbal spatial and musical tasks (Galin and Ornstein, 1972; Galin and Ellis, 1975; McKee, Humphrey, and McAdam, 1973; Morgan, MacDonald, and Hilgard, 1974; Moore and Haynes, 1980b). The EEG technique has been extended to the study of stutterers (Moore and Haynes, 1980a; Pinsky and McAdam, 1980).

The *averaged evoked potential* (AEP) is a refinement of the EEG measurement in that it represents a more localizable electrophysiological response in conjunction with a specific behavior or assumed cognitive process. The AEP also is known as the averaged evoked response (AER), evoked potential (EP), or event-related potential (ERP). A 1980 issue of *Brain and Language* was devoted to a survey of this technique. The AEP is derived from a sorting of the complex continuous electrical activity of the brain. It is that part of the ongoing EEG that is time-locked to onset of a specific stimulus event. EEG recordings from the scalp are fed to a computer. If a stimulus has a consistent specific effect on cerebral activity, this effect will be summated by the computer while all irrelevant cortical activities will cancel each other. The summated activity appears on a recording as a visible peak or spike representing the averaged evoked potential.

The usual left-right asymmetry has been observed: a greater left-hemisphere AEP to verbal stimuli and a greater right-hemisphere AEP to nonverbal stimuli (Neville, 1980). Broca's area (LH) has shown a greater AEP during speech production than the corresponding RH region, while the converse has occurred for making nonverbal noises (McAdam and Whitaker, 1971). A greater AEP over Wernicke's area (LH) was observed as a cortical response to auditory verbal stimuli (Kutas and Hillyard, 1980). Posterior LH responses have been recorded in association with semantic decisions (Thatcher and April, 1976) and connotative judgments (Chapman, McCrary, Chapman, et al., 1980).

Measurement of *regional cerebral blood flow* (rCBF) as an indicator of differences in cortical activity within each hemisphere is based on the physiological process of tissue metabolism. Functional activity of a region produces an increased demand for oxygen and glucose from the blood supply, and so rate of blood flow increases at the region of increased activity in order to meet this need.

Methods for measuring rCBF have been invasive or noninvasive. In the invasive method, an isotope called xenon-133, is injected into the internal carotid artery (Lassen, Ingvar, and Skinhoj, 1978). In the noninvasive method xenon-133, a colorless and odorless gas which emits gamma rays, is mixed with air and other bases and then is inhaled using a face mask (Stump and Williams, 1980). Among five hundred patients, Lassen found eighty who were considered to have a normal brain. They suffered from severe headaches, generalized epileptic seizures, and other transient neurological symptoms which were not associated with permanent lesions. Blood flow patterns from this group were displayed in dramatic color in *Scientific American* (Lassen, et al., 1978). Like a brain scan, these patterns were obtained with 254 externally placed scintillation detectors. The noninvasive method, surveyed in a 1980 issue of *Brain and Language,* makes it easier to study neurologically normal individuals. A comparison of the *Brain and Language* articles reveals that thirty-two (sixteen per hemisphere), twenty-four, or sixteen detectors may be used.

In the article by Lassen, et al., (1978) functional activation of a cortical region was shown as bright red and yellow against a background of blue and green depicting minimal activity. As a subject was counting to twenty, a concentration of red and yellow appeared in Wernicke's, Broca's, and motor speech areas of the left hemisphere; the rest of this hemisphere looked blue. Halsey, Blauenstein, Wilson, et al., (1980) observed a bilaterally diffuse pattern of activation in twenty-three normal right-handed subjects while "they were speaking spontaneously about banal topics" (p. 57). Halsey expressed a holistic view of normal function based on rCBF data: "... it seems probable that both hemispheres of the brain participate actively in many, if not most, tasks which have been viewed in clinical neurology as focal ..." (p. 59).

The rCBF measure holds some promise as a differential diagnostic aid. "The differential diagnosis of organic dementia against pseudo-dementia seems to be the most important clinical use at present" (Risberg, 1980, p. 31). The procedure is in the youth of its development; inconsistencies in results of research with normals may be due to inconsistencies of detection methods and some inefficiency with inhalation as a means of introducing xenon-133 into the brain. Patients with dementia have shown a diffuse diminished CBF, and patients with Broca's aphasia have shown a failure of response in the left frontal lobe (Meyer, Sakai, Yamaguchi, et al., 1980). The injection method was used to locate lesions in twenty-six cases of aphasia (Maly, et al., 1977). The location of flow disturbances did not always correspond to the site which might be expected with classifications of motor, sensory, and anomic aphasias.

Limitations of Methods
with Normal Subjects

The most frequent and consistent conclusions from studies of normal adults pertain to the functional level of left-right asymmetry more than the level of regional function within a hemisphere. However, we can infer that dichotic listening and hemifield presentation reflect posterior temporal and occipital asymmetries. CLEMs and manual tasks may reflect a link between posterior asymmetries and lateralized control of motor functions.

In their comprehensive survey of left-right brain asymmetries, Springer and Deutsch (1981) discussed weaknesses of the indirect and direct indicators of cerebral activity. Dichotic listening has been unreliable, with repeated testing of the same subjects, and has underestimated the usually high incidence of left-hemisphere control of language in right-handers. Hemifield asymmetries have not correlated highly with dichotic asymmetries and have been susceptible to individual subject strategies. There has been little direct evidence that CLEMs are tied to activation of one hemisphere. Right-movers and left-movers did differ in rCBF in the expected directions (Gur and Reivich, 1980). Findings with CLEMs and manual time sharing have not been replicated occasionally. Direct measures of cortical activity are valuable because the investigator does not have to rely on inferences from behavioral responses. However, measures of EEG alpha can be difficult to relate to specific stimulus events; some findings with AEPs have not been replicated; and rCBF measures have been somewhat insensitive to rapid variations of cortical activity. Regarding EEG and AEP studies, Springer and Deutsch (1981) acknowledged inadequacies of design, conduct, or analysis: "The problems range from an unwise selection of the aspects of electrical activity that are measured, to failure to control for individual differences among subjects, to the use of tasks that do not in fact differentially involve the two hemispheres" (p. 93).

FUNCTIONAL ASYMMETRY
OF THE HEMISPHERES

These several methods of mind-brain research have contributed to a convergence of multiple observations onto a few well-established facts about location of function. In most people the two cerebral hemispheres function differently, each with its own specialties. History of the fascination with our two brains can be characterized broadly as movement toward an appreciation of the equivalent importance of each hemisphere to our cognition. Until around 1965, investigators had thought in terms of "dominance" of one hemisphere over the other, with the dominant hemisphere being the one that controls language. After 1965, chapter and book titles on brain function began to reflect a replacement of this idea of dominance with a perspective defined as "specialization" or "asymmetry." The other hemisphere has come to be thought of as special, too, but in a different way. Now, "dominance" applies to each hemisphere with respect to the tendency of each to control particular types of behavior and to possess its own mode of processing information. Either hemisphere may dominate the other, depending partly on the task performed by the individual.

Verbal and Nonverbal Hemispheres

In the surveys of cases with unilateral brain lesions since World War II, the frequency of resultant aphasia firmly established that language function is controlled by the left hemisphere in most people. Only a small percentage of people have right-hemispheric or bilateral representation of language function. These conclusions represent observations of primary capacity or control rather than of exclusive capacity or control, because the "nonverbal" hemisphere possesses some linguistic capabilities. For convenience, the left hemisphere (LH) is usually identified as the verbal half of the brain and the right hemisphere (RH) as the nonverbal half. Most of this section deals with the RH, while details about language in the LH are reviewed later.

Specialization for Stimuli. Each hemisphere is suited for dealing with particular kinds of stimuli. Among the earliest evidence of hemisphere differences was from the extensive standardized testing of brain-damaged patients conducted by Weisenburg and McBride (1935). While LH-damaged patients were more impaired on the verbal tests, RH-damaged patients were more impaired on tests involving recognition and reproduction of visuospatial configurations. When split-brain subjects permitted the direct comparison of independent hemispheres, the unique visuospatial capacity of the RH became apparent. These subjects could match colored blocks to a geometric design quickly with the left hand (RH), but they made many mistakes with the right hand (LH). Studies of EEG alpha show greater RH-involvement in reproducing a geometric pattern from memory than in writing a letter (Galin and Ornstein, 1972). The RH is most likely to dominate when visuospatial stimuli are not easily labeled.

Similarly, the RH has a proclivity for recognizing *un*familiar faces, which has been shown in comparisons of RH and LH-damaged patients (Cicone, Wapner, and Gardner, 1980) and in hemifield presentations to normal subjects (Strauss and Moscovitch, 1981). Recognition of familiar people probably involves the labeling capacity of the LH, which is why prosopagnosia (see Chapter 1) usually results from bilateral damage instead of focal RH damage.

Milner's (1967) studies following lobectomy and Kimura's (1964) dichotic listening technique established that the RH is superior for recognizing music. In measures of EEG alpha, the RH was shown to be more active in recognizing a repeated theme from an unfamiliar Bach concerto than during reading from the Congressional Record (McKee, et al., 1973). Searleman (1977) reviewed a few studies of adults without LHs in which subjects were able to sing with the remaining RH and yet were unable to speak propositionally.

RH damage produces deficits in the recognition and expression of emotion, while basic verbal abilities remain relatively intact (see Tucker, 1981). RH-damaged groups have difficulty recognizing happiness, anger, or sadness in verbal expressions (Schlanger, Schlanger, and Gerstman, 1976; Tucker, 1981); but aphasics have shown an equivalent impairment. However, DeKosky, Heilman, Bowers, et al. (1980) found RH-damaged subjects had more difficulty naming emotional scenes, such as children drawing tic-tac-toe on a living room wall, than did LH-damaged subjects. RH-damaged groups have trouble recognizing the emotion in faces (Cicone, et al., 1980; DeKosky, et al., 1980), and Cicone felt that impaired facial recognition may be partly responsible.

Studies with normals substantiate these indications from the deficit method. A left visual-field superiority was found for recognition of happy, sad, and surprised faces (Strauss and Moscovitch, 1971). Of four tasks defined as verbal or spatial and emotional or nonemotional, the spatial/emotional tasks produced the most frequent leftward eye movements (RH): "When you visualize your father's face, what emotion first strikes you?" (Schwartz, Davidson, and Maer, 1975). Tucker, Roth,

Arneson, et al. (1977) replicated this study and found that stress-inducing instructions further enhanced the leftward direction of gaze. In considering research on emotional arousal, Tucker, et al. (1977) noted: "It does seem clear that the two approaches to inducing emotional arousal were different. The emotional questions involved recalling and reporting personal material, while the stress manipulation involved a response to the immediate situation" (p. 699).

As will be discussed in later chapters, methods for treatment of aphasia have capitalized on spared capacities of the RH: visuospatial, musical, and emotional. The influence of these factors on recovery of language is not clear, and future investigations might examine, for example, the effect of emotional arousal on aphasic verbal behavior, whether emotions are recalled or are actually experienced.

Specialization for Cognitive Processes. The CLEM studies cited previously have involved the presentation of verbal instructions which results in left eye movement suggestive of RH dominance in the activity. On the surface, this appears contradictory if verbal-nonverbal functional asymmetry is contingent upon differences in stimuli per se. Actually, subjects were instructed to process mentally in certain ways: by visualizing or by conjuring up an emotion. Furthermore, LH superiority is indicated sometimes when nonverbal, visuospatial stimuli are presented. For example, pictures of objects might be presented to each visual field, and a right field (LH) advantage occurs when the subject is instructed to name the stimuli (Schmuller and Goodman, 1980). As Springer and Deutsch (1981) put it, "What seems to be more important than the nature of the stimulus is what the subject does with the stimulus" (p. 73).

Each hemisphere is actually specialized for the way it mentally represents (codes)

and processes the stimuli it receives. The LH is more active when subjects are thinking of words beginning with *t*, while the RH becomes more involved in imagining a sheep climbing a ladder (Morgan, et al., 1974). Seamon and Gazzaniga (1973) employed the hemifield technique to test subjects on word recall. Subjects were instructed to remember words either by a visual imagery strategy or by a subvocal verbal rehearsal strategy. Words which had been presented to the left field (RH) were recognized faster with the imagery strategy, and words presented to the right field (LH) were recognized faster with the rehearsal strategy. Specialization for coding strategy can make visuospatial stimuli easier for the RH to manage and linguistic stimuli easier for the LH. However, the determining factor as to the dominant activation of a hemisphere is not task stimuli but rather is the manner in which stimuli are to be processed.

Structure and Style

What is it about the two hemispheres that makes each one become specialized for particular functions? Though their general physical appearance suggests that the right and left halves mirror each other in structure, there is evidence to indicate that structural differences do exist. Geschwind and Levitsky (1968) examined one hundred brains. The planum temporale, which is the upper posterior surface of the temporal lobe, was larger on the left in 65 percent and larger on the right in only 11 percent. This region forms part of Wernicke's language comprehension area in the LH. The angular gyrus appears to be larger in the RH than in the LH (Rubens, 1977a). A structural basis for functional specialization has not been clearly established. Ratcliff, Dila, Taylor, et al. (1980) reviewed the structural evidence and noted that certain structural asymmetries are evident in areas without clear functional significance. Also, posterior asymmetries have been found in 73 percent of cases studied, which is below the expected prevalence of functional asymmetry.

Another approach to explaining the lateralization of functions involves an attempt to define differences in the innate mode or style of processing between the two hemispheres. These differences represent cognitive styles that are more general, or basic, than either verbal processing or spatial recognition. For example, the LH may be equipped to process information sequentially and analytically, while the RH processes simultaneously and intuitively. If this is so, then the temporal nature of language would find a home more naturally in the LH. This issue has been expressed more frequently as to whether hemisphere asymmetry is innate or develops over time. Dennis (1980b) pressed for a different orientation: "... there is an extensive data base for the time course of left-hemisphere ascendancy over the right but almost no information about the processing features that enable the left hemisphere to develop the rich and flexible structures of mature language" (p. 159).

One test of the idea that the LH is equipped to process sequentially has involved comparing left and right unilateral damage with respect to processing nonverbal input. In perception of sequences of tones, clicks, and lights, a damaged LH has shown greater difficulty than a damaged RH (Van Allen, Benton, and Gordon, 1966; Carmon and Nachshon, 1971; Lackner and Teuber, 1973). The classic study in this line of research was Efron's (1963) observation that aphasic subjects were impaired in recognizing the sequence of lights and pure tones. Swisher and Hirsch (1972) contradicted some of Efron's conclusions concerning anterior and posterior lesions, but aphasics still had some problems reporting order of nonverbal inputs. These lesion studies indicated that the LH may be more inclined than the

right to process sequentially, whether the stimuli be linguistic or nonlinguistic.

The two hemispheres have come to be distinguished quite often with respect to contrasting cognitive styles (Ornstein, 1972; Galin, 1976). These contrasts are summarized in Table 3-2. The verbal-analytical style of the LH is associated with a tendency to break information down into parts, while the spatial-holistic style of the RH is associated with a tendency to perceive relationships, to integrate many inputs simultaneously.

Galin (1976) warned of excessive tendencies to divide the mind into two parts, what he called "dichotomania": "The specialization of the two halves of the brain is being offered as the mechanism underlying everybody's favorite pair of polar opposites. . ." (p. 46). Functional asymmetry has been used to explain differences between the Freudian conscious and subconscious, between the masculine and the feminine, and between classroom performances of the middle class and the urban poor. Jaynes (1976) suggested that the two halves of the brain had split the consciousness of ancient humanity between "language of men" in the left hemisphere and "voices of gods" in the right hemisphere. Watzlawick (1978) explained psychotherapeutic change as a process of blocking analytical and rational language from the LH and of unlocking usually inhibited RH language patterns of emotion and fantasy. Edwards

TABLE 3-2. Contrasting cognitive styles have been attributed to the two cerebral hemispheres.

Left Hemisphere (LH)	Right Hemisphere (RH)
Temporal	Spatial
Sequential	Simultaneous
Successive	Parallel
Linear	
Analytic	Holistic
Rational	Intuitive
Logical	Emotional

(1979) taught drawing as a "shift from the ordinary verbal, analytic state to the spatial, nonverbal state" (p. 46). She called it shifting to the "R-mode," or "drawing from the right hemisphere."

A Working Relationship

We know that the two hemispheres are different, especially when their function and dysfunction can be examined separately. However, in normal function, the hemispheres are not disconnected; stimuli arrive at both ears and eyes; and many of our activities have verbal and spatial components. We do not know very much about how the hemispheres work in relationship to each other. Measures of cortical activity with EEG and rCBF have shown that both hemispheres activate to some degree upon verbal and nonverbal stimulation. Some tasks produce a greater activation of one side over the other. Some EEG studies have indicated that the activation of one hemisphere may be accompanied by an inhibition of the other hemisphere. The two hemispheres may interact with each other in various ways, depending on the person's preferred strategy and on the nature of a task.

Galin (1976) proposed several possibilities. One is that the left and right hemispheres operate in alternation; they take turns depending on the situation or depending on the cognitive style chosen by the individual. While one hemisphere is dominant, the other is inhibited. Moscovitch (1976a) proposed that the LH inhibits linguistic capacities which have been discovered in the RH. "A variant of this relationship might be that the dominant hemisphere makes use of one or more of the subsystems of the other hemisphere" (Galin, 1976, p. 43). The unused systems of the other hemisphere are inhibited. A third possibility is that the less active hemisphere is disconnected in some way from the one in dominant use at any time. A fourth possibility is different from the others in that the two hemispheres may sometimes function fully together. Integrated use of the two hemispheres has been associated with creativity. Also, certain complex activities may involve both hemispheres working in rapid alternation or simultaneously. As Galin explained, high-level mathematics may require spatial and sequential modes, and a dancer may analyze individual steps and integrate them into a fluid artistic expression.

LOCALIZATION OF LANGUAGE IN THE BRAIN

Language in the Left Hemisphere (LH)

The syndromes of aphasia are related to lesions in different areas of the LH. These different symptom patterns have led neurolinguists to attribute functional responsibilities to these areas. The relationship between patterns of aphasia and sites of lesion is one subcategory of mind-brain investigations employing the lesion or deficit method. Functions have been shown to be more differentiated as to location in the LH than within the RH.

Chapter 2 began with Luria's three functional levels of the central nervous system (see Figure 2–1). Two of these levels are similar to a traditional sensory-motor division within each hemisphere. Reception, analysis, integration, and storage of language are handled posterior to the central sulcus; planning and initiation of speech are managed anterior to the central sulcus. The circumscribed cortical zones which receive sensory stimuli and send impulses to the muscles are commonly referred to as *primary zones*. Other cortical regions, comprising most of the cortex, are called *association areas*. Interpretation and integration occur in these areas.

Geschwind (1970, 1979) proposed a traditional and still prevalent model of language organization within the anterior and posterior regions of the LH. Whitaker's illustration in Figure 3–1 is representative of models of functional centers and connections between them. The boxes indicate concentrations of functional responsibility in the cortex, and the connecting arrows represent subcortical association tracts and their primary functional directions. Geschwind's conception was drawn largely from lesion studies, Penfield and Roberts' cortical mapping, and post-surgical studies. Damasio (1981) and Kertesz (1979) provided comprehensive discussions of lesions responsible for the aphasia syndromes. The rCBF measures of Lassen, et al. (1978), indicated that

many of these centers activate simultaneously during a simple speech activity, reinforcing the idea that the subprocesses of language operate in an integrated manner.

The expression of language through speech is associated with *Broca's area* (see Figures 3–1 and 2–4), located in the posterior third frontal convolution immediately anterior to the primary motor cortex. Broca's aphasia, which includes agrammatic and awkward speech with relatively good comprehension, is usually associated with damage to this left frontal region. Mohr argued that Broca's aphasia is produced by a larger lesion, however, which includes Broca's area, the oper-

Figure 3–1. Functional regions of the left hemisphere responsible for language are connected by subcortical association tracts. *(Reprinted by permission from Selnes, O., and Whitaker, H. A., Neurological substrates of language and speech production. In S. Rosenberg (Ed.),* Sentence Production: Developments in Research and Theory. *Hillsdale, N.J.: Lawrence Erlbaum Associates, 1977)*

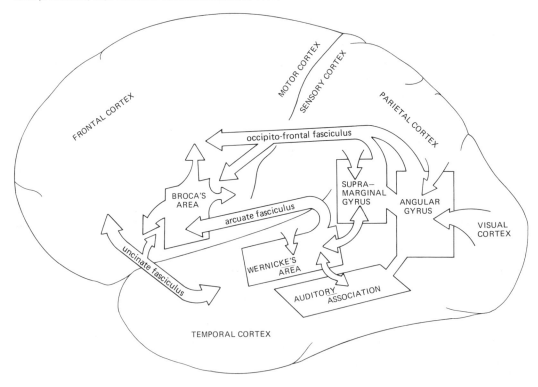

culum, insula, and adjacent cerebrum, all supplied by the upper division of the middle cerebral artery (Mohr, 1976, 1980; Mohr, Pessin, Finkelstein, et al., 1978). His review of recent autopsy findings, CT scans, and the literature since 1820 indicated that only an initial mutism followed by rapid recovery to an apraxia of speech results from damage to Broca's area alone. Mohr referred to these syndromes as "big Broca" and "baby Broca" aphasias. An implication is that Broca's area is responsible for motor speech programming and that a broader region is responsible for the syntactic level of linguistic expression. Kertesz's (1979) brain scan and CT scan studies tend to support Mohr's conclusions: "There is a spectrum of syndromes produced by Broca's area infarct. More than just initial mutism and verbal apraxia, the larger lesions produce the full-blown symptom complex of Broca's aphasia . . ." (p. 187).

Another motor center is sometimes represented in diagrams such as Figure 3–1. *Exner's center,* superior to Broca's area in the left frontal lobe, has been associated with written language.

Auditory comprehension of language has been associated with *Wernicke's area,* located in the posterior superior temporal gyrus. The serious comprehension deficit and neologistic speech of Wernicke's aphasia suggests that the link between the semantic component and auditory images of speech is related to this posterior region. However, Wernicke's area appears to be primarily responsible for speech perception, and semantic/syntactic comprehension requires additional cortex. Kertesz (1981) found neologistic jargon to be associated with damage to the temporoparietal junction, including the supramarginal gyrus and the posterior parietal operculum. Perecman and Brown (1981) suggested that a lesion in the superior and middle temporal gyrus produces neologistic forms of Wernicke's

aphasia. Semantic and syntactic processing for sentence comprehension probably involves the auditory association area and supramarginal gyrus shown in Figure 3–1.

According to Geschwind, Wernicke's area plays a role in verbal expression by generating the form (perhaps, an auditory-based image) of the utterance. The *arcuate fasciculus* is a bundle of subcortical association fibers connecting Wernicke's and Broca's areas. Geschwind (1979) stated that "the underlying structure of an utterance arises in Wernicke's area" (p. 187). He continued, "It is then transferred through the arcuate fasciculus to Broca's area, where it evokes a detailed and coordinated program for vocalization."

The dissociation of repetition from other language functions in conduction aphasia has been attributed to a lesion through the arcuate fasciculus since Wernicke's paper in 1874. However, this relationship has not been well supported with CT scan research (Kertesz, 1979; Mazzocchi and Vignolo, 1979). Upon reviewing the literature, Green and Howes (1977) concluded that damage to the left temporoparietal region, above and below the posterior Sylvian fissure, produces conduction aphasia. Damasio (1981) has observed that lesions in the primary auditory cortex, Wernicke's area, and sometimes the insula and its subcortical white matter produce this syndrome. Perecman and Brown (1981) observed: "No cases of exclusively subcortical lesions have been reported, controverting the classical arcuate fasciculus model of this disorder" (p. 219).

Finally, according to Geschwind's model, the *angular gyrus* is associated with reading and writing, because damage to this region bordering the occipital lobe results in the syndrome of alexia with agraphia. Comprehension of the written word is impaired because of a disconnection between the left occipital lobe and

Wernicke's area. Also, damage to this general posterior region has been associated with the syndrome of anomic aphasia. However, anomic aphasia has eluded clear localization (Goodglass and Kaplan, 1972); it was called a "nonlocalizing syndrome" by Benson (1979a). The process of word retrieval has been correlated with most of the perisylvian language area, especially in studies involving electrical stimulation of the cortex (Ojemann and Whitaker, 1978).

Benson (1979a) classified the aphasias as perisylvian syndromes (Broca's, Wernicke's, and conduction) and borderzone syndromes, which include transcortical motor and sensory aphasias. Lesions producing transcortical motor aphasia occur anterior and superior to Broca's area, while transcortical sensory aphasia results from lesions posterior to Wernicke's area around the anterior boundary of the occipital lobe (Damasio, 1981).

A similar concept of language localization was provided by Luria. His concept maintains a differentiation of language functions but contains a lesser degree of separation into centers and direct connections between centers. He focused on the posterior region of the brain, which he organized into a hierarchical arrangement of zones surrounding the three primary receptive zones. Luria (1970a) proposed three levels of function: "a primary zone that sorts and records the sensory information, a secondary zone that organizes the information further and codes it and a tertiary zone where the data from different sources overlap and are combined to lay the groundwork for the organization of behavior" (p. 67). Primary zones correspond to the three primary sensory areas where multiple sensory stimuli are separated into the reception of somesthetic, visual, and auditory information. The secondary zones, adjacent to the primary zones, are responsible for recognition of stimuli within each modality. Wernicke's area would be a secondary zone. The ter-

tiary zone consists of additional association areas of cortex. At this level, the individual is able to deal with the semantic-syntactic relationships of language. Tertiary zones would include the middle temporal gyrus and the temporoparietal junction.

Language in the Right Hemisphere (RH)

Considerable speculation has been addressed to right hemisphere (RH) participation in recovery from aphasia (see Chapter 4). Before discoveries of its unique propensities, the RH was thought of as "just a rather stupid spare for the left" (Galin, 1976, p. 28). Capacity of the adult RH to learn language was once suggested to be minimal (Lenneberg, 1967). However, split-brain, hemidecortication, hemifield, and evoked potential research has indicated that the adult RH possesses some language skills. These findings have enhanced interest in its role in recovery and have fueled a relatively new interest in its contribution to residual language function in aphasia.

The discovery of RH language skills was greeted for a while with considerable enthusiasm. The RH of split-brain subjects in the 1960s could comprehend simple nouns in the left visual field and, with the left hand, could pick out an object that was described verbally. One patient was able to spell simple words by arranging plastic letters with the left hand. Moscovitch (1976a) concluded that "a wide range of linguistic skills" (p. 47) had been revealed. Zaidel (1976) wrote that "the disconnected right hemisphere comprehends language surprisingly well" (p. 191); it was surprising, because the RH had been labeled so confidently as being "nonverbal." However, early language testing of the right hemisphere was extremely limited, especially if we consider the extent to which language function can be explored psycholinguistically. Early hemifield stimulation of hundred-milli-second duration permitted only a simple level of linguistic input. Also, there has been a tendency for investigators to extend generalizations to language as a whole from restricted language testing. Moscovitch (1976a) drew conclusions about the functional organization of language in normals partly from hemifield presentations of a few letters.

One method with a surprisingly untapped potential is the deficit method. The vast array of linguistic investigations of aphasia due to LH damage seldom have included a RH-damaged group, except in studies of speech perception and short-term memory. More recent studies of RH damage, reviewed later in Chapter 6, indicate that the RH may participate in language processing when the spatial-holistic cognitive mode is involved in the language task. After all, eyes shift right much less often while answering questions such as "Which way does Lincoln face on a penny?" or "How many edges are there on a cube?" (Galin and Ornstein, 1974).

A ceiling to the language skill of the RH was quickly realized. Gazzaniga reported that split-brain subjects did not respond as well to verbs given as simple printed commands, such as "smile" or "frown," as they did to nouns. The RH had trouble recognizing basic grammatical relationships, including tense and plural markers (Gazzaniga and Hillyard, 1971). In addition to limits in comprehension, split-brain subjects were rarely able to verbalize accurately about information presented to the RH. The linguistic limitations of the RH were not ignored by Moscovitch and others; but other opportunities to probe the RH and improvements in the hemifield technique permitted a more thorough examination of this hemisphere's language capabilities.

Zaidel (1976, 1978b) gave several tests of word comprehension to two split-brain subjects and one left-hemispherectomy subject, permitting observation of three

right hemispheres. Two right-hemispherectomies provided four left hemispheres for comparison. Surgeries had been performed at ten years of age or older for the RHs tested, and so their language development had been completed. Contrary to Gazzaniga and Hillyard's (1971) results with rapid tachistoscopic presentation, Zaidel's RHs comprehended verbs as well as nouns. Also, normal hemispheres were equivalent with both word categories in a hemifield study (Koff and Riederer, 1981). In spite of these specific comprehension abilities, the RH generally comprehended less than the LH on varied word comprehension subtests from standard aphasia examinations (Zaidel, 1976). The RH understood 67 to 88 percent of the test items.

The RH can comprehend sentences but at a fairly low level. Gordon (1980) showed that the RH of split-brain subjects can follow simple commands to the left ear upon dichotic presentation. The commands, such as "Turn the knob" and "Scratch the smooth disk," required simple responses with the left hand (RH). Zaidel (1977, 1979) gave the Token Test to his subjects. The Token Test measures auditory comprehension with a series of instructions for identifying and manipulating tokens of varying color, size, and shape (see Chapter 8). The tokens were presented to each visual field, and the RH performed at the level of a four-year-old child. On other standard language comprehension tests for children and adults, the RH had particular difficulty with lengthy sentences of more than three critical elements ("lady blowing the horn"). Short-term memory was the principal downfall of the RH with the Token Test as well.

Investigators have begun to focus on specific syntactic/semantic features of RH sentence comprehension. In hemifield presentation to normals, the RH was equivalent to the LH in identifying the subject and object in pictures of one fish biting another (Segalowitz and Hansson, 1979). Though subjects did not have to comprehend subject(S)-verb(V)-object(O) sentences, the study indicated that the perceptual basis for this structure is available to the RH. Heeschen and Jurgens (1977) presented sets of three words dichotically to split-brain subjects. Some sets were syntactically structured (S-V-O), and others were unstructured; some were semantically probable, and others were improbable. Heeschen and Jurgens concluded that the LH dominates the RH with respect to syntax but that both hemispheres are sensitive to semantic plausibility. LH superiority for syntactic processing was evident to Dennis (1980a; Dennis and Kohn, 1975) in studies of hemispherectomy done at least at 9:1 years of age. The LH and RH were equivalent in comprehending simple active and active-negative sentences. The LH was superior in comprehending passive and passive-negative sentences. The passives were reversible sentences such as "The girl is pushed by the boy"; and so, although the RH comprehended passives, the RH seemed to be less suited than the LH for processing variations from S-V-O order. Dennis (1980a) concluded that the two hemispheres decode passive sentences in different ways. The RH has "an inability to integrate interpretative rules with surface structure syntax, despite a capacity to find each component separately" (p. 315).

The most unequivocal language trait of the RH lies in its superiority of comprehension over verbal expression. Nonverbal is an appropriate description for this hemisphere, when we think of it as referring to expression only. The RH in split-brain subjects has been unable to talk about what is presented to it. After left hemidecortication in adults, the RH can sing or engage in nonpropositional speaking but is severely limited in its use of propositional language (Searleman, 1977; Selnes, 1976).

The level of language representation in the RH was expressed by two analogies: linguistic age and comparison with aphasic patients (Zaidel, 1976, 1977, 1978b). When compared with age norms, the RH was much "older" when comprehending words (eight to sixteen years) than when comprehending sentences (four to five years). Comparisons with aphasia are of interest clinically, because RH capacity may contribute to sparing of some language and to some reorganization of function in recovery. In tests of word comprehension, the RH displayed some variability in comparisons with aphasics. On one vocabulary test, the RH average score was lower than average aphasic performance obtained by Goodglass, Gleason, and Hyde (1970). On one aphasia test, the RH level was comparable to anomic and Broca's aphasia, in which the comprehension deficit is mild to moderate. On another aphasia test, RH performance at the word level was superior to the average for aphasia.

In sentence comprehension, the RH was comparable to aphasics below the 50th percentile of performance (Zaidel, 1977, 1978b). Patients with LH damage showed a different pattern of comprehension from the linguistically limited RH. One test permitted analysis of errors with respect to familiarity of vocabulary, sentence length, and syntax. The RHs were much worse than aphasics in dealing with variables of vocabulary familiarity and length. While both groups performed poorly relative to the syntax variable, the RHs did slightly better than LH-damaged subjects. These results, so far, are not optimistic with regard to the role of RH language in, at least, compensating for reduction of function in the LH. This conclusion is supported further by the stability of RH Token Test scores found by Zaidel (1979). Moscovitch (1976a, 1976b) maintained that the connection between hemispheres in aphasia enables the LH to inhibit RH language which is released from inhibition in cases of split-brain and hemidecortication. Selnes (1976) argued against this view. The RH still may be of assistance to cases of severely impaired language from LH damage.

Subcortical Structures No! and Language *Left*

The thalamus consists of several components, each with connections to specific areas of the cortex, anterior and posterior. Its central relationship to these regions beneath the cortex has led investigators to believe that it must serve a role in speech and language function. A special issue of *Brain and Language* in 1975 and a review by Ojemann (1976) provide evidence to support this belief. The evidence came from deficits after thalamic tumor and hemorrhage, stereotaxic stimulation and surgically placed lesions to alleviate motor disorders, and electrical stimulation of different locations in the thalamus. Hemorrhage presents uncertainty of localization because of mass effects on adjacent projection fibers.

Lesions produce speech difficulties, and electrical stimulation disrupts object naming from the ventrolateral nucleus and, primarily, the pulvinar of the thalamus. The pulvinar is located in the posterior portion of the thalamus. Language and other cognitive deficits following hemorrhage are often temporary. Mohr, Watters, and Duncan (1975) found periods of intact language and periods of extended paraphasia "rapidly fading into an unresponsiveness resembling sleep" (p. 16). Surgically placed lesions resulted in impaired arousal and motor organization of speech, while language changes were temporary. Relationships between the thalamus and verbal behavior have largely been lateralized to the left thalamus. Luria (1977) concluded that symptoms of thalamic lesions are very different from aphasia. The processes associated with the thalamus seem to be more basic than specific language processes. Luria tied the thalamus to attention or vigilance as it is applied to the speech processes. Ojemann (1976) interpreted responses upon electrical stimulation as indicative of a thalamic role in short-term memory and attention.

Subcortical Structures No! and Communication

In Chapter 1, language function was characterized as one servant of communication. Emotion, for example, flavors our messages and is conveyed nonverbally as well as verbally. Lamendella (1977) widened considerations of neurological structure that would account for relationships between language and communication. He argued that traditional fixation of attention on language disorders and localization of language functions "provides too narrow a theoretical foundation because grammatically organized, phonologically structured verbal encodings of messages constitute only one of many levels and types of human communication." He added that there has been "an unhealthy reliance on the term *language* as a catchall for widely divergent aspects of communication" (p. 157). A network of cortical and subcortical structures, called the *limbic system* (see Chapter 2), may play an important role in the communicative process.

Lamendella (1977) advised that the limbic system "has often been thought of only in relation to its regulation of emotion and motivation, but in fact its range of functional responsibilities is quite large and includes major segments of our social and communicative behavior" (p. 159). He explained that communication is carried out through integration between cortical and limbic systems. Lamendella delineated three levels of communication which are supported in part by the limbic system: (1) the *appetitive* subsystem, the most basic communicative activity resulting in automatic sign behavior that reflects internal sensations and drives; (2) the *affective* level, the regulation of social interaction through emotion and motivational states; and (3) the *volitional* subsystem, the intentional component of propositional communicative behavior.

INDIVIDUAL DIFFERENCES

The lateralization of verbal-analytical and spatial-holistic functions described in previous sections cannot be attributed to everyone. Some people possess control of language in the right hemisphere. Others appear to possess more diffuse or bilateral representation of all major cognitive functions. Furthermore, there may be differences in the general population as to the preferred use of each hemisphere, no matter where verbal and nonverbal functions are represented. Because these differences may introduce variation in severity of aphasia and course of recovery, the signs indicating hemispheric lateralization and preferred use become important to the clinician. Multilingualism is one factor which is ignored in this discussion, but Albert and Obler (1978) provided a comprehensive survey (also, see Paradis, 1977).

Handedness Scan!

Interest in the correlation between preferred hand and lateralization of language has a long history. Branch, Milner, and Rasmussen's (1964) data typifies findings from many studies of unilateral brain damage and normal modality biases. With sodium amytal injection, most right-handers possessed language control in the contralateral hemisphere (90 percent LH, 10 percent RH), while left-handers were mixed in the distribution of language function (48 percent LH, 38 percent RH, 14 percent bilateral). Ambidextrous individuals were a heterogenous group, as

were left-handers. Estimates of ipsilateral language specialization in left-handers have been higher, with 72 percent of left-handers having aphasia after surgery in the left hemisphere in Penfield and Roberts' (1959) study. A related variable which appears to indicate degree of lateralization is familial history of left-handedness (sinistrality). Familial sinistrality correlates with more bilateral representation in right-handers and with stronger unilateral representation in left-handers (Hardyck, 1977); it may be related to ear and hand preference in dichotic and dichaptic tasks (Nilsson, Glencross, and Geffen, 1980).

Left-handers are of considerable interest theoretically because of their heterogeneity, and clinically because of the relationship between functional organization and focal disorders. Aphasia may be less severe, accompanied by "RH" symptoms, and have a better prognosis in left-handers (Hecaen and Sauguet, 1971; Humphrey and Zangwill, 1952; Subirana, 1958). The clinician may infrequently see a case of *crossed aphasia,* in which the lesion is in the hemisphere ipsilateral to the preferred hand. Crossed aphasia is more likely to occur in left-handers; however, seven cases of crossed aphasia in right-handers were described by Carr, Jacobson, and Boller (1981) and Yarnell (1981). Satz (1980) analyzed twelve studies reporting the frequency of aphasia following unilateral brain damage in left-handed adults. While right-handers were characterized with a unilateral model of language specialization, left-handers seemed to be "bilateral and variable unilateral." Language of left-handers is distributed as follows: 40 percent in the left hemisphere, 20 percent in the right hemisphere, and 40 percent bilateral (Satz, 1980). Therefore, at least 80 percent of left-handers possess some representation of language in the ipsilateral hemisphere.

The clinical problem posed by left-handers is how to identify the differences among them. Witelson (1980) suggested three factors: familial sinistrality, strength of handedness in the individual, and hand posture in writing. Familial history of left-handedness increases the likelihood of contralateral hemispheric control of language in left-handers; for example, a left visual-field (RH) advantage for picture naming was shown for left-handers with familial sinistrality (Schmuller and Goodman, 1980). Strength of handedness should also be positively correlated with degree of contralateral control of language. Right-handers possess a standard hand posture when writing, the "under" posture (Witelson, 1980). About 40 percent of left-handed undergraduates surveyed by Searleman, Tweedy, and Springer (1979) possess an inverted or "hooked" posture in which the hand is curled above the line of writing. The inverted posture has been associated with less pronounced lateralization. Levy and Reid (1976) made the strong prediction that inversion by left-handers would indicate ipsilateral language control (LH). However, most evidence indicates that 60 percent of left-handers possess contralateral language control, while Searleman, et al. (1979) found that only 40 percent of young adult left-handers use the inverted writing posture. Searleman's findings are consistent with Satz's model of asymmetry for left-handers.

Age No!

Most evidence now suggests that the left hemisphere's propensity for verbal-analytical processing is present at birth (Kinsbourne, and Hiscock, 1977) and that organization of function is developed further at least through childhood (Kinsbourne, 1975). Structural differences between the hemispheres are present in infancy (Rubens, 1977a). Verbal stimuli result in reduced right-limb, but not left-limb, tremors in premature infants (Segalowitz and Chapman, 1980). Child-

ren five months of age have left hemisphere AEPs to speech stimuli (Molfese, 1977). REAs for speech in dichotic listening have been found in children as young as three years of age (Kinsbourne and Hiscock, 1977). The degree of LH lateralization in verbal-manual time sharing tasks is invariant between ages three and twelve (White and Kinsbourne, 1980). The evidence runs against Lenneberg's (1967) proposal that the hemispheres are equipotential for language at birth, with the LH developing dominance over the RH during the period of language development.

Hemispherectomy before two years of age has shown that the RH is equipped to develop language at this early age; this capacity decreases as the child becomes older. However, the innate asymmetry of the hemispheres is evident when left hemispherectomy is performed before five months of age, because complete language development does not appear to occur in the RH even with such early surgery. Dennis (1980b; Dennis and Whitaker, 1976) studied three children with left and right hemisphere removals in infancy. By at least nine years of age, the left and right hemispheres were similar in phonemic and semantic abilities, but the RH was incomplete in several syntactic abilities. "The matrix of interrelationships among words appears less well integrated in the right hemisphere than in the left . . ." (Dennis, 1980b, p. 181).

The development of cerebral organization into the circumscribed zones of function shown in Figure 3–1 may be a lifelong process (Brown, 1976; 1977; Brown and Jaffe, 1975). Concentration of speech programming in Broca's area may not be complete until middle adulthood. Concentration of auditory language processing in Wernicke's area may not be complete until later adulthood. Focal lesions in childhood, including Wernicke's area, tend to produce mutism or agrammatism, with maintenance of good auditory comprehension. Wernicke's aphasia appears to be a syndrome of older adults. Four studies have shown that patients with this syndrome are older than other aphasics (Harasymiw, Halper, and Sutherland, 1981; Holland, 1980a; Kertesz and Sheppard, 1981; Obler, Albert, Goodglass, et al., 1978). Generally, Wernicke's aphasics were about twelve years older than Broca's aphasics.

Sex

Research on differences in functional asymmetry between males and females usually indicates that males are more lateralized than females for verbal and spatial abilities (Levy and Gur, 1980; Witelson, 1980). Attention has been focused on spatial skills assumed to reflect RH function (Harris, 1978). Stronger lateralization in males has been seen more consistently for spatial skills than for verbal skills (McGlone, 1977). However, in a hemifield study, males showed a stronger left-hemisphere preference for digit recall (Kail and Siegel, 1978). Right-handed males had a stronger tendency to shift eyes right (LH) during verbal tasks (Gur and Gur, 1980). The opposite trend was found by Moore and Haynes (1980b), who measured EEG alpha suppression during verbal and nonverbal tasks. Females showed a stronger lateralization in both tasks. Females have faster and stronger auditory brain stem responses to auditory nonverbal stimuli (Seitz, Weber, Jacobson, et al., 1980).

If men have a stronger lateralization of language function, then we might expect more sparing of function and, perhaps, better recovery in women who suffer the same focal lesion as men. We have little information on this possibility because most clinical research on aphasia has ignored the sex factor. Research in Veterans Administration Medical Centers ensures a sampling bias toward males. McGlone (1977) found a higher incidence of aphasia in males than females, but each group had

equal severity of aphasia. Verbal intelligence and verbal memory were more impaired in males. McGlone concluded that bilateral language representation is more common in females.

Preferred Cognitive Style

Most of us possess two modes of cognitive activity which are separated by the cerebral commissure. These modes were described earlier as (1) analytical, rational, logical, and verbal and (2) holistic, intuitive, emotional, and spatial (Table 3-2). These characterizations of left and right hemisphere function may correspond to preferred cognitive style and to personality traits of two different people. Some people may prefer to use the analytical-rational mode in solving most problems, while others may prefer the holistic-intuitive mode. The former may be more self-inhibitory of emotion, while the latter may be more spontaneous and impulsive (Galin, 1974). Dichotic listening, conjugate lateral eye movement (CLEMs), and EEG alpha suppression have been observed in order to determine whether individuals have a preference for one hemisphere.

Individual differences in experience and training with a task may determine the extent to which a cognitive mode and, therefore, a cerebral hemisphere might be utilized. Studies of ear preference for melody recognition have shown that student musicians score better with their right ear (LH) and student nonmusicians score better with their left ear (RH). Student musicians may tend to listen to music in an analytical mode. However, faculty musicians did not have an ear preference, indicating that their greater experience allowed them to develop a more integrated approach to melody recognition (Wagner and Hannon, 1981). Ornstein and Galin (1976) speculated that the middle class and urban poor employ different cognitive modes based on different cultural experiences. The former's verbal-analytic style is more compatible with the traditional educational system than the latter's spatial-holistic style.

Day (1964) and Bakan (1969) suggested that some individuals consistently shift gaze in one direction regardless of task, indicating a preferred cognitive style. Among undergraduate students, "right-movers" (LH) were more likely to major in science and engineering, while "left-movers" (RH) were more likely to major in literature and the humanities. Right-movers have been characterized as verbal, intellectual, and analytical; left-movers have been described as spontaneous, emotional, and intuitive. Hysteric personality types engaged in more left eye movement than did obsessive-compulsive types (Smokler and Shevrin, 1979). Right-movers preferred to sit on the left side of a classroom and left-movers preferred to sit on the right (Gur and Gur, 1977).

Kinsbourne (1972) presented data indicating that eye shift and, therefore, cognitive mode are a task-dependent instead of an individual characteristic. Gur (1975) showed that task-dependent shifts occur with the experimenter seated behind the subject, while individual tendencies are prominent when the experimenter is in front of the subject. The latter circumstance was thought to induce anxiety, which might cause the subject to resort to preferred style rather than to a task-induced style. On the other hand, stress may influence gaze only in a leftward direction because of the RH capacity for emotion (Tucker, et al., 1977). Hiscock (1977) replicated Gur's findings with face-to-face positioning of the experimenter, but found that task-related eye movement occurred only for certain types of analytical and spatial questions. Lawyers and ceramicists differ in direction of gaze, but the difference appears more in a vertical dimension than in a horizontal dimension (Galin and Ornstein, 1974). Some CLEM studies show mainly a problem-type effect on eye

directionality; others show consistent individual cognitive styles; and others show both effects (Gur and Gur, 1980). In critical analyses of CLEM research (Ehrlichman and Weinberger, 1978; Otteson, 1980), the task-relatedness and individuality of eye movement have been found to be equivocal.

Galin and Ornstein have studied individual differences of cognitive style indicated by EEG alpha suppression (Galin and Ornstein, 1972; Ornstein and Galin, 1976). Lawyers were compared with sculptors and ceramicists on verbal and spatial tasks. Several comparisons were not significant, but lawyers differed from artists in the extent to which they used the LH on both tasks. Dumas and Morgan (1975) compared engineers and artists and found task-related differences between hemispheres but not individual differences. A person's use of one hemisphere may depend on a number of factors, including preferred style and nature of the task. Dumas and Morgan (1975) concluded that "when a person has a dominant cognitive style, he does not necessarily use one hemisphere, but rather has differential aptitudes in lateralized functions and perhaps seeks out environments in which the more developed mode is utilized more" (p. 227).

CLINICAL ASSESSMENT AND IMPLICATIONS

The neurologist quickly examines several cognitive functions which provide clues to location of the lesion. Asking the patient questions and observing verbal behavior may provide evidence of LH damage. Questions about time and place may expose RH damage. While examining sensory functions, the physician looks for indications of modality-specific disorders of recognition from damage to association areas surrounding primary areas. These and other disorders are summarized in

Table 3–3. Thorough testing by a speech-language pathologist is helpful in locating lesions within the LH. A neuropsychologist examines cognitive functions and emotional qualities associated with both hemispheres. When a patient has multiple or diffuse lesions, the neuropsychologist can be very helpful to the speech-language pathologist by identifying disorders which may interfere with a language treatment program. Emotional problems, in particular, should be identified as existing prior to brain damage, due to brain damage, a psychological reaction to brain damage, or as a combination of these.

Certain principles of language treatment capitalize on the functional organization of the brain. Aphasia results from destruction of a part of the brain, and preserved brain structure supports certain spared functions. Because of the intricate connections among the different regions of the cortex, the spared regions still may operate at a reduced efficiency, especially

those areas which are closest to the destroyed area. Treatment may be geared toward improving efficiency of functions for which cortical tissue remains to support them. Also, treatment may be directed toward the maximally functioning areas, capitalizing upon whatever contribution they might make toward improvement of depressed functions and enhancement of communication. Treatment directed toward improving the performance of the deficient processes of aphasia was said by Holland (1977b) to be based on a "medical model." She described it as an effort to fix up what is wrong with the patient; improving auditory comprehension, word retrieval, or the richness of grammatical detail. However, another orientation toward treatment is possible, namely, maximizing the use of spared functions which can be used to convey messages. In summary, treatment is based on three factors of impairment relative to cortical structure and function: (1)

TABLE 3-3.   Specific disorders are associated with their most typical site of lesion.

	Left Hemisphere (LH)	Right Hemisphere (RH)
Frontal	Apraxia of speech Broca's aphasia Transcortical motor aphasia	
Parietal	Astereognosis Constructional apraxia	Astereognosis Constructional apraxia
	Ideomotor apraxia Acalculia Finger agnosia Right-left disorientation	Spatial disorientation Dressing apraxia Muted emotions Unilateral neglect
Parieto-temporal	Conduction aphasia Anomic aphasia	
Temporal	Pure word deafness Wernicke's aphasia	Amusia
Temporo-occipital	Transcortical sensory aphasia	Agnosia for unfamiliar faces
Occipital	Alexia without agraphia Color agnosia	
	Bilateral Lesions Auditory agnosia Prosopagnosia Visual object agnosia	

certain deficits arise from the reduced efficiency of intact areas, especially those close to the permanent damage; (2) other areas of the brain, such as the opposite cerebral hemisphere, remain essentially intact; and (3) the different areas of the brain are interconnected in complex ways, directly or indirectly.

Individual differences in asymmetry of cortical function may complicate plans for treatment based on functional organization. Researchers are certainly becoming more aware of the need to consider handedness, familial handedness, age, sex, and experience with a task when studying lateralized responses in dichotic listening, hemifield presentation, and eye movement. Clinicians are generally aware of using handedness as a sign of possible diffuse functional organization. The relationship of age, especially throughout adulthood, and sex to functional organization is not as well established. Preferred cognitive style may indicate a patient's readiness to use the RH in the reorganization and compensatory processes of improving communicative ability. Investigation of cognitive style is characterized more by its potential than by its establishment of fact. Nevertheless, its potential raises some new questions. For example, does an analytical lawyer respond to language treatment in the same manner as an impulsive artist?

4 Theoretical Foundations

A complete theory of treatment should include a set of assumptions about the nature of language function, aphasia, and recovery. It provides rationales for treatment procedures, enabling the clinician to identify "what" is being treated and "why" a particular procedure is selected. A set of assumptions, whether the clinician is aware of them or not, always forms the basis for the selection of stimulus content and the manner in which stimuli are presented. The clinician's rationales generate the clinician's behavior, determine judgments and evaluations, provide the substance of goals, guide the perception of individual patients as examples of particular generalizations, and enable the clinician to provide individualized treatments which are consistent with the essence of aphasia and language function; they are the foundation for creative treatment.

Theory-building involves an intimate interaction between theory and experimentation, and so the separation of Chapters 4 and 5 into theory and research is an artificial one. Some research will be cited in Chapter 4 in order to explain the status of theories; theoretical positions will be reiterated in the next chapter in order to explain results.

NORMAL LANGUAGE FUNCTION

Understanding the normal leads to understanding the deficit. The reverse is also true; linguists, psycholinguists, and neurolinguists have examined aphasia meticulously in order to find clues to an understanding of the normal mind and the normal brain. The ideal situation would find us defining aphasic impairment partly in terms of a complete model of normal language structure and processes. We would use the same vocabulary to talk about aphasia and normal language. That is, if normal speakers mentally recode passive sentences into an actor-action-object format to facilitate comprehension, then it is possible to have an impairment of "recoding." Conversely, if aphasics have an auditory impairment called "slow rise time," then rise time should be a component in a model of normal language comprehension. Aphasic word retrieval might be elucidated with a model of the cognitive machinery in normal word retrieval.

However, as was pointed out in Chapter 3 with Caplan's (1981) analysis of the lesion method, aphasia may not be explained entirely as an impairment of the normal. Aphasia may include modified or new processes which are unique to the disorder. Furthermore, a theory of normal language function should correspond to concepts of neurological function. The absence of neurophysiology in formulations of the language function may be one reason why a few clinicians have not chosen prevailing psycholinguistic theories as a basis for their clinical methods. For example, Porch (1981b) has used the vocabulary of cybernetics in discussing the breakdown and reestablishment of "brain circuits." Also, aphasia was defined as a breakdown within the "speech cycle" from a servo-system model (Mysak, 1976); treatment "is geared toward the activation of the organism's intrinsic self-adjusting processes" (Mysak and Guarino, 1981, p. 215).

Because there is no comprehensive model of normal language comprehension and expression, a review of the subject requires addressing varied approaches to developing such a model. Reviews are available elsewhere (Clark and Clark, 1977; Foss and Hakes, 1978; Paivio and Begg, 1981). The remainder of this section is devoted to an orientation to normal language that might be useful for thinking about aphasia and its treatment.

Clinical Rationale

There is a strong clinical rationale for maintaining a theory of normal language. The clinical aphasiologist's manipulations are directed to the language behaviors of their patients. Accurate and efficient use of language is the direction toward which the clinician leads the patient. Therefore, assumptions about the nature of language function necessarily pervade the clinician's planning and implementation of treatment. The following statement provides a general orientation toward considerations given to treatment of aphasia:

Communication with language is carried out through two basic human activities: speaking and listening. These are of particular importance to psychologists, for they are mental activities that hold clues to the very nature of the human mind. In speaking, people put ideas into words, talking about perceptions, feelings, and intentions they want other people to grasp. In listening, they turn words into ideas, trying to reconstruct the perceptions, feelings, and intentions they were meant to grasp. . . . Speaking and listening, however, are more than that. They are the tools people use in more global activities. People talk in order to convey facts, ask for favors, and make promises, and others listen in order to receive this information. These actions in turn are the pieces out of which casual conversations, negotiations, and other social exchanges are formed. . . . (Clark and Clark, 1977, pp. 3–4)

Language behavior is a product of certain cognitive structures and processes, and is used for a variety of purposes and in a variety of contexts. A complete treatment program exercises the mental activities of language use with respect to the varied intentions of speaking and to the kinds of circumstances in which language is used.

Approaches to Normal Language

There are three general approaches to the study of language: linguistic, behavioral, and cognitive (Paivio and Begg, 1981). "Linguistic approaches," according to Paivio and Begg, "focus on language itself as the object of study, viewing it as an abstract system that underlies linguistic behavior" (p. 3). Linguists describe rules of the system which people share in order to communicate. They have provided aphasiology with methods for describing aphasic behavior. However, linguistic theories are generally constructed without consideration of how the rules are used by the mind or brain for comprehension or expression. Psycholinguists have had a difficult time trying to mold psychological theories out of purely linguistic ones (see Davis, 1978b).

Linguistics was influential in shaping treatment plans in the 1960s and 1970s, primarily as a means of sharpening detection of subtle differences among structures in order to improve planning of task hierarchies. Treatment programs sprouted which leave the impression that certain linguistic structures are to be stimulated in all aphasic patients. However, in the last decade individual differences in language use have received more attention:

> Linguists take a tolerant and anti-chauvinistic attitude toward languages and dialects that differ from their own. In the same way, when anthropologists go to study another culture, they do not do so with the intent of converting members of that culture to their own cultural values. Their intent is rather to describe and explain the culture as they find it. There is no room in their work for a view that one culture is inherently superior to another. So, too, with linguists and psycholinguists. They are trying to explain what they find, not to change it. There is no place for the myth of a "pure" language or for linguistic chauvinism. (Foss and Hakes, 1978, p. 7)

The natural use of language involves individual differences of dialect, social status and setting, personal style, and sophistication with language (see Fillmore, Kempler, and Wang, 1979). We cannot train a Southerner to eliminate "might could" as a modal form or to say "press the button" instead of "mash the button." Stimulating language in aphasia treatment implies that the clinician elicits vocabulary and syntax which the patient already knows and has used naturally.

The behavioral approach takes many forms, but behaviorists are basically concerned with observable linguistic events. Language behavior is explained in terms of associations between stimuli and responses and of consequences of responses.

Learning theory, a major component of the behavioral approach, has contributed to the development of treatment styles (see Chapter 10).

Cognitive approaches accept the reality of mind; and their concepts include ideas, imagery, mental organization, and process. In effect, this orientation is directed toward inferring what goes on inside "the black box" between stimulus and response. The goal is to specify the mental structures and processes which may turn out to correspond with neuroanatomy and physiology and which are just as hidden inside our heads. Models of mental structures and computations used to comprehend and produce language are constructed. The mental computations are sometimes referred to as processes. The remainder of this section follows a cognitive approach.

A Cognitive Approach

Definition of terms is in order. Terms such as model, function, and process are tossed about a great deal in this book, and we sometimes feel uncomfortable with what they mean.

Function: "Language function" or "language functions" have been used frequently. This term is difficult to distinguish from "process," but there is a small difference. A function is a particular class of behaviors. It refers to the outcome of a process; and, therefore, a function is realized because a process has occurred. Language function is a general class of behaviors. More specific functions include comprehension and naming. Naming is one functional outcome of the processes of lexical search and retrieval.

Process: A process is the means by which a behavioral outcome is achieved; the mental activity that results in comprehension and expression. The function of a car, for example, is to transport a person from point A to point B. Combustion is a process which results in that movement. Fortunately, we can open the hood of a car anytime to examine this process. The problem with this concept as applied to human behavior is that, even if we could open up anyone's skull to look inside, we still could not observe mental processes.

Model: A model is a representation of another entity, and becomes valuable when that entity is difficult to discern by simple observation. Depicting mental structure and processing necessarily entails the development of models. A model may be a set of interrelated statements depicting a structure and its processes, or it may be an analogy for the entity. Computers have been proposed as analogies or even replicas of human cognition, while other models have consisted of assumptions, propositions, boxes, and arrows.

The cognitive view of language function considers mental structure and activity to be no less real than the brain. Models of its organization and processes are being developed and tested through careful experimentation and inference. Clinical aphasiologists sometimes discuss cognition, memory, and language as if they were three independent entities. However these concepts overlap considerably.

All cognitive processes, including those which involve language, are carried out within a memory structure (Figure 4–1). Sensory information is received initially in each modality and arrives independently at each primary receiving area of the cerebral cortex. At this level of memory, called *sensory memory* or preattentive storage, a large amount of information is received from the environment and held for a fraction of a second (Norman, 1976). This information is coded with respect to modality; *iconic* memory consists of visual images and *echoic* memory consists of auditory images. We cannot act upon all input at once, however, and so an attention mechanism selects a small portion of sensory information to be held several seconds longer for further processing.

This further processing, which, for example, results in language comprehension, takes place within the constraints of *short-term memory* (STM). STM has a small capacity; and, unless its information is rehearsed or specially coded in some way, information in STM is held for only twenty to thirty seconds. The activity of cognitive processing takes place "within" STM; this component of memory does not appear to correspond to a particular location in the brain but rather corresponds to activation of the brain for particular purposes. Many investigators refer to it as

Figure 4-1. Three levels of memory have implications for language function. Processing for comprehension and production takes place within the capacity and time constraints of short-term memory, also called "working memory." The knowledge-base for communication is housed in long-term memory. *(Reprinted by permission from Smith, A. D., and Fullerton, A. M., Age differences in episodic and semantic memory: Implications for language and cognition. In D. S. Beasley and G. A. Davis (Eds.),* Aging: Communication Processes and Disorders. *New York: Grune & Stratton, 1981)*

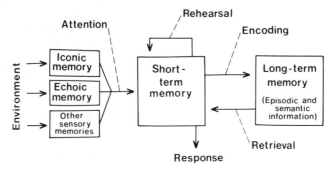

"working memory." The importance of this point pertains to the tendency of clinical aphasiologists to consider STM or "immediate memory span" as a variable of interest which is separate from language comprehension and production. It is as if STM can be exercised in addition to comprehension. However, the processes of comprehension comprise part of the load placed on STM. STM defines the time and capacity constraints upon comprehension and production.

Our knowledge of the world, our memories of particular experiences, and our knowledge of language are stored in *long-term memory* (LTM). *Semantic* memory consists of abstract concepts which represent our knowledge of the world, and *episodic* memory consists of specific events which have been recorded. Words appear to be stored separately in *lexical* memory. LTM possesses an enormous capacity, and its information is retained for years and decades. The feature of LTM which is of importance to cognitive processing is its organization which makes speedy access to its content possible. Several theories of the organization of semantic and lexical memory have arisen, based on measuring response time in tasks requiring the comparison of two concepts (Collins and Loftus, 1975; Glass and Holyoak, 1975; Smith, Shoben, and Rips, 1974). Models of LTM organization are sometimes called semantic and lexical networks. Figure 4–2 illustrates the elaborateness of such models derived from a few simple rules for representing concepts and relationships between them. This small portion of a semantic network represents information contained in the following sentences: *Luigi's is a tavern, Louise drinks wine, Bob drinks wine, Mary spilled spaghetti on Sam,* . . . (Lindsay and Norman, 1977, pp. 396–397). This sample contains elements of semantic and episodic memory.

It may not be accidental that the network model looks like a pattern of neurons interconnected by axons and dendrites. This is *not* to suggest that concept nodes correspond to nerve cell bodies and that relationships correspond to nerve fiber tracts. Instead, the complexity of organization and the movement about the material and mental networks may be similar. In searching for a concept or a word, mental "impulses" may scurry about among network patterns in tiny fractions of a second. Collins and Loftus (1975) outlined some assumptions about search and retrieval in semantic and lexical memory which have a neurophysiological tone. Their model was called the "spreading-activation theory."

Aphasia is generally viewed as an impairment of access to the lexical network. The content and structure of episodic and semantic memory are basically intact. However, as shown in the next chapter, some questions have been raised as to whether semantic memory might be changed in aphasia, affecting the word retrieval process.

Processes underlying language comprehension and production remain a mystery, especially because these processes occur with the rapidity of a neural impulse, thus escaping conscious awareness. Certain treatment procedures have been aimed at making the aphasic patient more aware of strategies for analyzing utterances (Luria, 1970).

To explain comprehension, the problem for investigation is what goes on between speech perception and realization of meaning. Linguistic and psychological approaches, according to Paivio and Begg (1981), "are faced with the problem of translating theoretical concepts into empirical ones that can be observed and measured . . . the theoretical concepts must be operationally defined before they can be tested" (p. 73). As one example, models of mental operations underlying response time patterns in sentence-verification tasks have been developed (Carpenter and Just, 1975).

Certain mental processes within work-

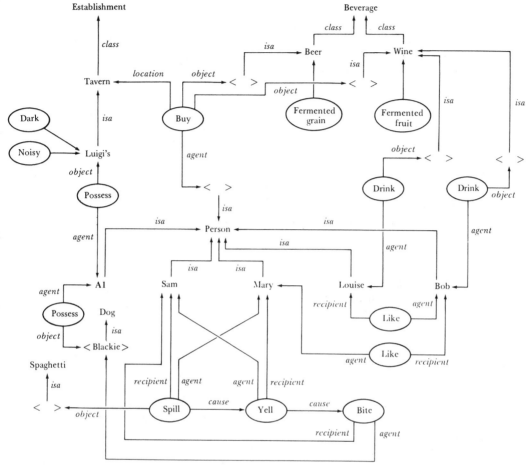

Figure 4-2. This depiction of a network of concepts in semantic memory is indicative of the complexity of semantic organization. Connections between concepts are defined by a few types of relationships. A person may search through a network like this to retrieve a word. *(Reprinted by permission from Lindsay, P. H. and Norman, D. A., Human Information Processing, 2nd ed. New York: Academic Press, 1977)*

ing memory seem to be mandatory, and these processes are inferred from measurements of response time in milliseconds. *Coding* forms a mental representation of attended stimuli and of input from long-term memory. There may be dual coding, with sensory-based images and linguistic codes. There may be a common code in which all input to working memory is represented in an abstract form which theorists describe as propositions, a

linguistic format used for convenience of explanation. Another process is *comparison* of inputs to STM; a linguistic stimulus is compared with information from a picture in a treatment task or from semantic memory in everyday conversation. A third process is *scanning* a mental representation so that constituents of mental representations can be compared sequentially, perhaps, one at a time.

Our ability to select a treatment procedure which exercises a normal language process is limited to our knowledge of these processes. Paivio and Begg (1981) provided a succinct status report of our knowledge of auditory comprehension:

> Our review of the research evidence suggests that associative, linguistic and cognitive processes are used in comprehension. The evolution of scientific thought in the area has shown an increasing emphasis on the importance of semantic and contextual factors, including nonverbal ones such as imagery and the concrete situational context. Moreover, it is increasingly recognized that comprehension operates at different levels, from a relatively superficial grasp of the meaning of a message to a deep detailed understanding . . . Thus, comprehension is a complex business . . . Finally, it must be acknowledged that our scientific understanding of the nature of comprehension is itself still relatively superficial and primitive . . . A detailed theoretical interpretation of how such factors operate to result in the "click of comprehension" is yet to be written. (p. 169)

Language comprehension is certainly more complex than the strictly linguistic conceptions of the 1960s; yet diagnostic and treatment methods continue to rate difficulty in terms of linguistic complexity without consideration of contextual variables. There are situations in which passive sentences are easier to process than active sentences (Olson and Filby, 1972).

APHASIA

If a treatment program is to be derived from an explicitly stated theory of aphasia, the program should logically follow from that theory and should not necessarily follow from other theories. This point can be demonstrated by certain theoretical positions on the nature of aphasia. With aphasia viewed as a language disorder instead of as a speech disorder, the choice of

stimuli for word retrieval practice would be based on considerations of semantics such as familiarity. A former secretary may say "telephone" as easily as "pen." If aphasia were a speech disorder, the clinician would be concerned more with syllable length and articulatory difficulty in selecting the words to be practiced. Student clinicians, who are familiar with articulation therapy, are sometimes surprised when an aphasic patient writes "daughter" instead of "girl" to label a picture of a young female.

Loss or Interference

Hughlings Jackson (1879) was the first to recognize that aphasics may not have lost words from lexical memory but probably have a reduced ability to retrieve them at the propositional level of word usage. Schuell, Jenkins, and Jimenez-Pabon (1964) concluded that "the language storage system is at least relatively intact" (p. 336). Schuell, et al. preferred to think of aphasia as an interference with the processing of verbal messages rather than as a loss of previously stored language. Although it is difficult to find a clinical aphasiologist who has believed in the loss theory, several writers have pursued the loss-versus-interference distinction as a major issue (Eisenson, 1973; Martin, 1978; LaPointe, 1978a). This issue has been of concern because of the possibility that a treatment strategy can be derived from the loss view, which is different from a strategy derived from an interference view.

There is one example of an approach to treatment based on the loss view. Mills (1904) described his treatment of a patient with apparent Broca's aphasia:

> A language primer and a grammar were next employed, the patient being instructed as much as a child would be in the nature and use of parts of speech, in the methods of

conjugating verbs and of giving the cases of nouns . . . The patient, in other words, was retaught, insofar as possible, the grammar which he had learned in childhood and which had slipped away from him as the result of the cerebral lesion. (p. 1941)

Sarno (1975) observed that early treatment of aphasics after World War II was based partly on methods from the field of education. Without a well-developed theory of aphasia, it is possible that early efforts to teach spelling and arithmetic were derived from an assumption of loss, as if the aphasic were a child learning new things.

In characterizing an orientation to treatment based on an interference with language processing, Eisenson (1973) stated that the role of the clinician is that of "a stimulator or an *agent provocateur.*" Schuell, et al. (1964) wrote that "the clinician's role is not that of a teacher. . . . Rather, he tries to communicate with the patient and to stimulate disrupted processes to function maximally" (p. 338). Eisenson (1973) explained that the clinician helps the patient " . . . retrieve what he knows more readily than if he were left to his own devices" (p. 134). Principles of aphasia treatment are based primarily on the assumption of interference. Nevertheless, some specialized approaches to treatment do involve new learning for the patient. Some patients are taught new strategies for communicating that had not been used before, including unique gestural symbols and nonverbal symbol systems.

Clinicians have drawn somewhat different kinds of implications as to the treatment that is implied by a loss or interference view. Martin (1978) suggested that "stimulus-response therapy" or programmed approaches follow from a loss view. Seron, Deloche, Bastard, et al. (1979) placed the contrast in operational terms and then compared two approaches with two small groups of patients. They stated that one approach involves training a great number of lexical items geared toward the patient's relearning of each lexical item missing in his or her vocabulary; the other approach was described as intensive, concentrating on a small set of lexical items and stressing "access strategies to lexicon" (p. 150). The latter approach, based on an interference view, was found to be more effective. Brookshire (1978b) advised: " . . . we do not advocate teaching the patient vocabulary words. Instead, we feel that treatment should be directed toward the process which appears to underly deficient naming. We do not advocate teaching the patient certain grammatical constructions. Instead, we feel that treatment should be directed toward those basic language processes which are necessary to understand and use those grammatical constructions" (p. 147). With respect to treatment of auditory retention, Brookshire added: "The clinician should in most cases avoid extended drill on a small list of stimulus materials" (p. 149).

One could argue that the loss view implies training on a large number of words to replace all that is assumed to be missing, or that it implies drill on a small set of words until the patient can comprehend or produce those particular words. The size of the lexicon used in treatment may not be pertinent to this issue. Also, both orientations involve stimulus-response interaction and some degree of programming. The distinguishing feature appears to be how the deficit is defined and then translated into treatment goals. Treatment based on interference is directed toward an impaired process and not toward particular words or grammar. For example, Brookshire (1978b) recommended exercises toward expanding the patient's STM capacity and that the lexicon employed should change from day to day.

A Unidimensional
or Multidimensional Disorder

Two somewhat different approaches to the characterization of aphasia have produced some lively debate in clinical aphasiology (Canter, 1972; Duffy, Ulrich, and Bisantz, 1977; Smith, 1972, 1977) to the point where these approaches have been portrayed as being contradictory. Instead, these approaches can be complementary.

The two approaches can be termed the unidimensional and multidimensional characterizations of aphasia. The multidimensional approach identifies components of the language process, where at least one component may be disrupted to create a particular symptom pattern. One consequence of this view is that qualitatively different types of aphasia are considered to be possible depending on which component is impaired. Different versions of the multidimensional view arise from different ways of defining the components of the language process. The unidimensional approach, on the other hand, does not entail a differentiation of components of the language process. The various manifestations of aphasia are thought to come from differences in degree of interference with a unitary language process. Qualitatively different types of aphasia are not recognized or are not considered to be possible. These two theoretical orientations could lead to different orientations toward treatment. That is, the multidimensional view implies that qualitatively different methods might be required for different types of aphasia, while the unidimensional view implies that the same procedures would be applicable to any case of aphasia.

Unidimensional Theory. Schuell's concept of aphasia has typified the unidimensional view (Green, 1969b). She concluded that one dimension of language impairment contributes to the deficits found in each modality and that different types of aphasia do not exist (Schuell and Jenkins, 1959). "All aphasic patients show some impairment of vocabulary and of verbal retention span, with a proportionate amount of difficulty in formulating and responding to messages at some level of complexity" (Schuell, et. al., 1964, p. 114). She classified patients into five basic categories, but only one category represented a pure aphasia and the remaining categories reflected aphasia complicated by modality-specific perceptual or motor impairments. Schuell believed that aphasia involves a general reduction of language and that differences among cases represent differences in degree of impairment. Darley (1982) maintained this point of view by relegating types of aphasia to clinically useless adjectives which arise from "special interests" and incomplete or biased observations.

To test the validity of these conclusions, Schuell and Jenkins (1959) used the Guttman scaling technique to analyze results of Schuell's test given to one hundred aphasic patients. The purpose of any scaling procedure is to construct a continuum or dimension on which persons or objects are located. If a rank order of different subtest performances can be found, it is assumed that the tests examine one general behavior at different degrees of complexity. Schuell and Jenkins (1959) found that performances on eighteen subtests could be rank ordered and concluded that this reflected a unidimensional language deficit underlying the variations among their one hundred patients. Jenkins and Schuell (1964) replicated this technique with a larger sample of aphasic patients and found similar results.

Jones and Wepman (1961) suggested that the use of only eighteen subtests and the Guttman scaling technique were predisposed toward finding a single dimension of language underlying subtest performances. They reasoned that a factor analysis of test results would instead reveal separate clusters of language skills contributing to the multidimensionality of language deficits in aphasia. These investigators administered thirty-seven subtests of a different aphasia test to 168 persons with aphasia. Jones and Wepman found six clusters of correlated performances and concluded that six components of language function contribute to performance on the thirty-seven tasks of their test battery. One factor or component was independent of modalities and was interpreted as reflecting general language comprehension ability. Four factors were related to input-output transmission functions.

Schuell and Jenkins (1961a) responded with a letter to the editor in the *Journal of Speech and Hearing Disorders*. They suggested that Jones and Wepman's factors actually supported the Schuell and Jenkins position. The language comprehension factor could be closely allied with the general language function proposed by Schuell. The four transmission factors could reflect the sensory and motor problems cited by Schuell as frequently accompanying aphasia. In addition, Schuell conducted a factor analysis of her own, using her test administered to 155 patients (Schuell, Jenkins, and Carroll, 1962). She found five clusters, one of which represented a general language factor and three of which reflected modality-specific visual and motor impairments. The fifth factor appeared to be related to disturbances of general cognitive functioning which Schuell, et. al. (1962) associated with the most severe forms of aphasia. Schuell and Jenkins argued, therefore, that scaling and factor analyses of formal test results could be interpreted readily as reflecting a unidimensional impairment underlying all cases of aphasia.

Factor analysis of test results may not only be followed by different interpretations, but also may yield different results depending on the statistical procedure used. Clark, Crockett, and Klonoff (1979b) examined scores from the *Porch In-*

dex of Communicative Ability (see Chapter 7). One analysis produced a general language factor consistent with the unidimensional theory. Another analysis produced three separate factors: a fluency-nonfluency dimension, a receptive dimension, and a graphic dimension. *yes*

Multidimensional Theory. The multidimensional orientation specifies distinct components of the language process. Each component may be controlled by different locations within the language area of the cerebral cortex. Depending on the location and size of a brain lesion, the pattern of symptoms of a particular aphasic patient may be due to disruption of at least one component of the language process. Because the language function is considered to be composed of multiple parts or dimensions, different types of aphasia are possible depending on which dimension is affected. The multidimensional orientation has taken two different forms *depending on how the components of language function have been defined.* One version, earliest in the history of aphasia study, has been in direct conflict with Schuell's unidimensional orientation. The other, more recent in development, can be considered to be compatible with the data used to support the unidimensional view.

The earliest version of the multidimensional approach involved dividing language into parts defined in terms of input and output modalities. Four components were described as "centers," each with a corresponding location in the brain, which contain auditory, visual, spoken, and graphic images of words. It was popular to diagram these centers with connections between them, as was discussed regarding localization in Chapter 3. The discoveries by Broca and Wernicke led to what Smith (1971) described as the "classical dichotomy" between motor and sensory aphasias. To the extreme, motor aphasia was considered to be an impairment of the speech component, and sensory aphasia was considered to be an impairment of the auditory component. This tradition has lingered in that the presence of comprehension deficits in all aphasias continues to be used as an argument against the validity of syndromes. Darley (1982) viewed syndromes this way: "It should be noted that profiles of different 'types' of aphasia are never based on the *absence* of impairment in particular modalities but rather on *relative differences* in degrees of impairment between different modalities" (p. 42). However, observing aphasia in terms of degree of impairment within modalities makes it difficult to discern differences among patients which may truly exist but on a different basis.

Head (1920, 1926) insisted that the language function is composed of multiple processes functioning in a highly integrated manner. He proposed that these processes are central in relation to the separate modalities and are involved in both receptive and expressive use of language. Furthermore, a disturbance of one of these language components would necessarily have some consequence for the functioning of other components. Though Head did not clearly identify the nature of components of normal language function, he did propose that there are four types of aphasia that reflect impairments of individual components. He chose linguistic terminology rather than modality-based terms in order to be suggestive of the predominantly impaired language component in each type. Head described nominal, semantic, verbal, and syntactic aphasias, each of which involved deficits in each modality.

Head's reworking of the multidimensional concept was the beginning of the identification of language components in linguistic terms for the purpose of defining the bases for different types of aphasia. One subsequent example was Jakobson's (1955, 1971) specification of similarity and contiguity disorders reflecting disruption of paradigmatic and syntagmatic language

processes, respectively. Lesser (1978) suggested that the concept of language function as a central process can be maintained with a division of labor among components of language attributed to organizational levels of *syntax, semantics,* and *phonology.* Each of these components is somewhat independent of modalities and, therefore, applies to the use of language through each modality. In this way, if different aphasic deficit patterns can be attributed to one or another of these linguistically defined components, then the concept of aphasia as a multidimensional phenomenon can be aligned, at least, with Wepman's notion of aphasia as a central disorder. This approach to multidimensionality encourages the realization that language function is a complex process of interdependent parts.

The most frequently used contemporary classification of aphasias is the Boston system presented in Chapter 1. Some confusion may arise with these classifications because some of the classical terminology is retained, such as "Broca's aphasia" and "Wernicke's aphasia." However, these terms have taken on new meanings based on linguistic descriptions of spontaneous speech patterns (paraphasias, syntax) rather than on modality-oriented test interpretation. Comparisons between Broca's aphasia and other syndromes have led to proposals that the syntactic and semantic components of language are aligned with different processes which can be isolated in aphasia (Caramazza and Berndt, 1978; Zurif, 1980). That is, syntactic processes may be impaired in one case, while semantic processes may be impaired in another (see Chapter 5). The main point here is that this division represents a revision of thinking and not necessarily the true explanation of differences among aphasias.

It is not mandatory that impairment of syntax (agrammatism) or semantics (anomia) be observed strictly in pure form in order for this theory to be valid. As Darley suggested regarding modalities, "isolation" of a component is based on *relative differences* between impairments of syntax and semantics. Head's emphasis on the interaction among components, whatever they may be, should be kept in mind when considering multidimensional theories of any kind.

In conclusion, the unidimensional concept of language deficit in aphasia captures the centralized nature of the disorder and its impact on all language modalities. Like the concept of symbolic dysfunction, it identifies aphasia as being different from modality-specific disorders. The multidimensional approach simply adds more detail to the concept of central dysfunction. It specifies that aphasias can assume qualitatively different forms because the language function is composed of multiple components interacting to comprehend and produce utterances. When these components were defined in terms of modalities, the corresponding types of aphasia did not reflect the multimodality impact of the disorder as revealed by complete clinical evaluations. However, when the linguistic aspects of spontaneous speech were described more carefully, different types of aphasia became more apparent even though all modalities showed deficits. The components of language that could be independently disrupted were redefined in linguistic terms which were compatible with the notion of central dysfunction. In effect, the unidimensional view specifies what is common among all instances of aphasia, while the multidimensional view points out the individual differences among aphasic patients.

Language Competence and Performance

Theoretical frameworks used to depict normal language function have been applied to describe and to explain aphasia. Conversely, some investigators of language function have turned to the study of aphasia for clues to the identity of normal language structures and processes (Forster, 1978; Green, 1970; Schnitzer, 1978; Whitaker, 1970). For example, the separation of syntax and semantics in aphasia has led to the conclusion that these components of language are functionally independent in normal language-processing (Caramazza and Berndt, 1978; Lesser, 1978; Zurif, 1980). The most frequently applied theoretical construct from the study of normal language has been the dichotomy between linguistic competence and performance. This dichotomy drags numerous issues with it into the investigation of aphasia and is an extension of the multidimensional orientation. It is also the normal construct underlying the ideas of loss and interference.

Competence and performance refer to two aspects of the cognitive basis for language function. Competence, as defined by Chomsky (1965), is the speaker-listener's knowledge of his own language, namely, its rules of structure and its lexical content. Certain linguists believed that their descriptions of the syntactic, semantic, and phonological components of language correspond to the idealized mental representation of the knowledge of language stored in long-term memory. Performance, on the other hand, refers to the processes of comprehending and expressing utterances. In normal performance, comprehension sometimes may fail and utterances may contain deviations of grammar, because mechanisms of attention and memory, for example, limit use of the idealized knowledge described by linguists.

The question has arisen as to whether aphasia is an impairment of competence, performance, or both (Schuell, 1969). The loss view can be related to the disappearance of knowledge from the patient's linguistic competence, and interference can be related to disrupted performance. However, there has been a variety of opinions as to whether competence or performance is impaired, and some of this variation has been based on different definitions of competence. For example, the nature of competence has been linked to the notion of language function as a central process. Moreover, there has been some doubt as to whether the competence-performance distinction is appropriate at all in characterizing the cognitive bases for language function. In the rest of this section, we shall wade through this potentially confusing state of affairs.

Lenneberg (1967) and Weigl and Bierwisch (1970) argued that aphasia is a disruption of some aspect or aspects of performance and that competence remains intact. Therefore, symptoms of aphasia are to be explained relative to active processes such as attention, perception, coding, scanning, or retrieval. Lenneberg suggested that "neither discrete words nor discrete grammatical rules are neatly eliminated from the store of skills" (Lenneberg, 1967, p. 207). Rather, the processes of performance are interfered with; or, more specifically, a defective timing device regulating inhibition and retrieval interrupts the process of turning language plans into utterances. Linguistic competence must be present if language can be understood at least some of the time and if words, not retrieved at one time, can be retrieved at another time. Also, under conditions of "deblocking" when a weak modality is preceded by a stronger one (see Chapter 10), linguistic content once unavailable can be retrieved. Weigl and Bierwisch concluded that because deblocking of linguistic content exposes an intact linguistic competence, aphasia demonstrates the neuropsychological validity of the competence-performance distinction.

If competence is neuropsychologically real, then it should be affected to some extent by brain damage. Taylor and Anderson (1968) had decided that there is a competence-performance continuum and aphasic impairment may occur anywhere along it. Schuell (1969) concluded that

aspects of competence are less impaired than components of performance, "as evidenced by the aphasic's spontaneous application of the rules of his language as his available vocabulary increases, and his utterances increase in length and fluency" (p. 119).

Looking for a deficit of linguistic competence is bound to be a frustrating enterprise if such a deficit is thought to be a disappearance of all knowledge of language structure. Aphasia could involve a loss of some part of competence such as knowledge of either syntactic, semantic, or phonological rules. A competence deficit could entail a loss of only part of syntactic knowledge. Furthermore, damage to competence could involve a disorganization of one component rather than a loss of that component. As Schnitzer (1978) pointed out, if a knowledge of language structure is represented in the human mind, then "it must be represented in some way in the functioning of the human brain" (p. 352) and, therefore, be susceptible to brain injury. He suggested that linguistic competence can be an empirically verifiable "neurophysiological construct."

A deficit with respect to linguistic competence can be inferred, according to Schnitzer (1978), if all possible performances requiring a certain aspect of linguistic knowledge are analyzed. These performances include artificial linguistic activities in addition to ordinary comprehension and expression. Such linguistic activities include sorting words into well-formed sentences, transforming sentences, and correcting linguistic errors. All of these activities require a knowledge of the structure of language. A performance deficit would affect one or a few of these activities but not all of them. "A deficiency which affected all of the linguistic abilities," wrote Schnitzer (1978), "would have to be either a remarkable coincidence or (more likely) a deficiency in the linguistic competence underlying all modalities" (p. 347). In one study, subjects primarily with syntactic (Broca's) aphasia were asked first to recognize sentences as grammatically correct or incorrect and then to correct the errors (Bliss, Guilford, and Tikofsky, 1976). The subjects' abilities with these tasks indicated to the investigators that aphasia is an impairment of performance.

There are two paths of escape from the dilemmas associated with the competence-performance distinction. One, described by Lesser (1978), is the differentiation of competence into "competences." Another is to abandon the notion of a competence-performance dichotomy and replace it with a model of cognitive structures and processes involved in language function.

Though aphasic patients demonstrate knowledge of language and rule-based production errors, this does not preclude the possibility that linguistic competence might be disturbed in some way. Lesser (1978) outlined an expanded and more differentiated view of competence that is consistent with this possibility. First, speaker-hearers possess an additional competence which includes knowledge of the rules for social discourse, namely, what is socially acceptable and appropriate in the use of language. This competence appears to be retained with aphasia (Holland, 1977). Second, linguistic competence is differentiated among levels, including phonology, syntax, and lexical organization. Receptive and expressive processes make different uses of these levels. For example, syntax may be more crucial for planning of expression than for extracting meaning in comprehension. Some persons with aphasia may have lost some aspect of syntactic knowledge having more obvious impact on expression than on comprehension (Zurif and Caramazza, 1976).

A further point made by Lesser (1978) also takes into consideration the role of linguistic competence as a part of human cognitive structure. Within a language community there is a range of language knowledge and skill among individuals as a function of social class, education, age, and other differences. This realization about competence contrasts with the idealized descriptions of competence put forth by linguists. Lesser (1978) stated: "The aphasic adult's linguistic competence is being compared not with that of an ideal speaker but, theoretically, with his linguistic competence before he became aphasic" (p. 49).

The notion of competences risks an encroachment into the territory of performance. Lesser (1978) made a distinction between competence for speech and competence for comprehension: "comprehension is probabilistic whereas speech must be at least partially pre-planned" (p. 50). That is, using guessing strategies, general semantic information, and extralinguistic cues, a person can comprehend, in effect, more than he can produce, without attending to the syntactic details used in producing a sentence. Yet these differences could be due to the processing characteristics of comprehension and expression rather than to competences for each. In fact, it would be cumbersome to store in permanent memory a knowledge of language for comprehension and another one for speech. The costs to clear understanding of language function by broadening the domain of competence are that active processes become attributed to linguistic structures and performance processes are relegated to "limitations of memory, distractibility, inattentiveness, and the variability of behavior . . ." (Lesser, 1978, p. 52). Certain linguistic orientations to language function make the processes of performance appear to be accessory functions that keep a person from using a set of linguistic rules perfectly, instead of being processes that are inherent to the psychological activation of comprehension and expression.

The term "competence" is general enough to invite a variety of interpretations and applications, and its meaning has been stretched beyond the static structures of knowledge. The term is being replaced in the aphasia literature with terms more directly oriented toward specifying the static cognitive structures of linguistic and conceptual knowledge. Instead of linguistic competence, Zurif and Caramazza (1976) referred to variations of the phrase "tacit knowledge of English." Goodglass and Baker (1976) referred to "semantic field organization," while Caramazza and Berndt (1978) referred to "structure of the lexicon." These references to semantic and lexical organization reflect the distinction between storage of concepts and storage of words in long-term memory described earlier in this chapter. Though replacing the competence-performance distinction with a distinction between cognitive structures and processes appears to be simply a change in terminology, at least the mixing of structure and process that has been associated with "competence" might be minimized. Furthermore, we might get away from associating comprehension with competence and production with performance. A syntactic problem in a patient's comprehension and production does not necessarily imply a loss of knowledge (competence), but, rather, it may reflect a problem in the mental processing (performance) related to this linguistic component.

The Regression Hypothesis

On occasion, a hypothesis has been entertained that aphasia represents a regression of language to a stage of language development, a kind of language development in reverse. This hypothesis has produced studies in which linguistic features of adult aphasia and child language are compared. Jakobson (1968) has proposed that "the dissolution of the linguistic sound system in aphasics provides an exact mirror-image of the phonological

development in child language" (p. 60). Dennis and Wiegel-Crump (1979) explained the issues and reviewed the evidence concerning this theory. They wrote: "The issue is not whether there exists an absolute correspondence between adult dissolution and ontogenetic growth of language ... but whether there is enough in common to make the regression hypothesis a tenable account of language function" (p. 211). Dennis and Wiegel-Crump explained that there is a strong version of the regression theory in which a mirror image of language development is proposed, and a weaker version which claims only parallels between the two processes. Their review led to the conclusion that adult aphasia and child language are different and that regression of an ontogenetic process is an untenable explanation of aphasia.

A variant of regression theory relates levels of aphasia to levels of species or phylogenetic development, a kind of evolution in reverse. Hughlings Jackson held this view in the late nineteenth century. Brown (1976, 1977; Brown and Jaffe, 1975) proposed simply that there are parallels between aphasia, evolution of language, and a lifelong process of localization of function in the brain. The stage at which a brain lesion intercepts the specialization process determines the resultant type of aphasia. Brown suggested that this theory explains why a lesion in a particular location may not produce a deficit at one age, while it may produce that deficit at an older age.

EXPLANATIONS OF RECOVERY

Whether or not an aphasic person receives treatment of the language deficit, at least a small amount of recovery is inevitable in most cases. Called *spontaneous recovery*, it may occur only in the hours or weeks immediately following onset or for a few months. It may be reflected merely in a heightening level of awareness of surroundings, or in a return to some level by specific functions such as language comprehension or word retrieval. Explanations of this recovery consist of proposed adjustments or changes in the brain and of proposed modifications of cognitive functions underlying language.

Explanations of recovery are distinguished between the physiological processes associated with etiology, which occur during the acute phase of recovery, and the theories of function returning independently from these short-term physiological sequelae of the specific etiology. The latter explanations account for changes occurring after the acute phase. The time frame of the acute phase has been defined variously as the five days subsequent to onset (Kohlmeyer, 1976) or as the first month to six weeks after onset (Duffy, 1972; Kertesz, 1979).

Improvements subsequent to the waning acute phase may be attributed either to sparing of function or to recovery of function. Sparing refers to a failure to detect any loss of function probably related to undamaged regions of the brain, while recovery is the return to a certain level of efficiency of initially impaired functions. In stressing the importance of differentiating between means and ends when defining function, Laurence and Stein (1978) indicated that recovery could involve the actual restitution of a function or the substitution of new means (strategies) for achieving the same goal of a function. Sparing of function would be observed early in the recovery process, while recovery would be observed to evolve from the acute phase to several months afterward.

The Acute Stage

Ischemic strokes are accompanied by edema or swelling which diminishes during the first week postonset. This swelling causes increased intracranial pressure and compression of brain structures affecting the hemisphere contralateral to the infarction. Reduction of swelling is considered to be responsible for some of the recovery occurring soon after onset.

The phenomenon of temporary suspension of functions dependent on intact ipsilateral and contralateral hemispheric structures remote from the infarct is called *diaschisis,* first defined by von Monakow, a Swiss neurologist, in 1914. The "term has been rather loosely applied to a wide range of phenomena" (Laurence and Stein, 1978, p. 385), including early spontaneous recovery. This generalized reduction of function has been attributed to tissue swelling and to a bilateral reduction of cerebral blood flow following infarction within one hemisphere. Meyer et al. (1970) found that this reduction of blood flow in the healthy hemisphere disappears within two or three weeks after onset. According to Laurence and Stein, diaschisis is an explanation of loss of function rather than of recovery of function. In effect, it explains how, upon onset of ischemia, a shroud is cast temporarily over the regions of damaged and undamaged brain which are responsible for the later-appearing patterns of specific deficient and retained cognitive functions.

Another phenomenon which may be related to early recovery from thromboembolic occlusions was described by Kohlmeyer (1976). He administered carotid angiography twice within two to four weeks after onset to fifty-seven cases with occlusion of the middle and posterior cerebral arteries. He demonstrated that thromboembolic occlusion may be only temporary in some cases. *Spontaneous recanalization,* through which some blood flow resumes, sometimes occurs "rarely after a few hours, more frequently after a few days" (p. 83). Recanalization occurred in thirty-nine of the fifty-seven cases (68 percent), but it was not observed in cases with occlusion of the internal carotid artery. The incidence of early spontaneous recovery of language function was much higher when recanalization occurred than when it did not occur.

Although recanalization did not occur in the internal carotid artery, complete recovery within one month was observed in 33 percent of the patients with occlusion of this artery in the neck. Kohlmeyer attributed this recovery to *collateral circulation* through the Circle of Willis at the base of the brain. Barr (1974) stated that normally little blood is exchanged between the major arteries through the communicating arteries of the Circle of Willis. However, compensatory blood flow can occur through the communicating arteries when one of the arteries from below is occluded. These alternative routes are frequently insufficient to prevent infarction, especially in elderly persons in whom the connecting arteries are narrowed by vascular disease (Barr, 1974).

Reduction of tissue swelling, return to normal circulation in the undamaged cerebral hemisphere, recanalization, and collateral circulation are suggestive of an unstable medical condition soon after onset which produces an uncertain picture of the behavioral impairments produced by infarction of a certain area of the brain. When studying the effects of an infarct including recovery, investigators often wait until at least one month postonset, when a clear delineation of the language disorder is assumed to be most possible at the earliest time.

Sparing of Function

Once the shroud of diaschisis has been lifted, the effects of focal brain damage leave a pattern of impaired and spared sensory, motor, and cognitive functions. For example, a patient may present a deficit in word retrieval and a retention of normal limb strength and movement, normal hearing perception, and relatively mal hearing perception, and relatively normal auditory comprehension of language. This pattern does not necessarily mean that these receptive and motor functions have recovered; but it may mean that, because of the way functions are organized in the brain, damage to one area does not appreciably affect the functional integrity of undamaged areas. Concepts of spared function are tied directly to concepts of localization of function in the intact brain. Therefore, information on brain function (in Chapters 2 and 3) provides a foundation for predicting what functions would be impaired and spared given a lesion to a particular area. With reference to the previous example, concepts of recovery account for improvements in word retrieval, while concepts of sparing account for retention of motor strength and auditory processing.

Laurence and Stein (1978) described two explanations of sparing, both of which represent theories of how functions are localized in the brain. These theories represent static conditions instead of a process of change in brain structure or function subsequent to damage. Both theories account for how a function can be retained in spite of damage to an area which is responsible for that function.

The first explanation is *redundancy of organization,* from which it is possible "that a part of a neural system may adequately mediate the function normally subserved by the system as a whole" (Laurence and Stein, 1978, p. 373). That is, part of region A may perform a function just as well as all of region A, so that damage to part of brain region A may have little or no effect on function. Laurence and Stein stated that the concept of redundancy is similar to Lashley's concept of equipotentiality in which, within a given region, a function is accomplished by all tissue in that region. Also similar is an analogy of memory storage in the brain proposed by Pribram (1971), who compared it to a photographic process called holography. Holography has been described vividly by several authors in books about the brain (Blakemore, 1977; Furst, 1979; Restak, 1979). "The hologram . . . corresponds to a jigsaw puzzle of which any piece, after removal from the completed puzzle, can be used to reconstruct the whole puzzle" (Restak, 1979, p. 225). Penfield and Roberts' (1959) finding that a tiny electrode touching a spot on the cortex can stimulate a complex of memories is suggestive of a form of memory storage in the brain like that of the hologram. However, the sparing of function in the human brain has not been proved to be based on such a phenomenon. Laurence and Stein added that investigations of the redundancy theory are weakened because of the possibility that behavioral measurements may not be sensitive enough to detect a mild deficit resulting from damage to region A.

The second explanation is *multiple control* of function, in which a specific function is considered to be controlled by more than one location in the brain. The destruction of one center leaves the other intact, and the intact center maintains the function at a premorbid level. For example, if the left and right hemispheres are capable of comprehending single words, then in spite of damage to the left hemisphere the intact right hemisphere may be responsible for sparing comprehension at this level. Osgood and Miron (1963) invoked a similar concept to account for spontaneous recovery. They claimed that if there is "replication of function" between sites A and B in the brain, then damage to site A would result in spontaneous recovery as long as B is intact. However, following the reasoning of Laurence and Stein, replication of function or multiple control should be an explanation of sparing and not of recovery. They concluded that this proposition is weak theoretically because it is "untestable and therefore unfalsifiable" (Laurence and Stein, 1978, p. 376). That is, one could simply propose additional control centers to explain any maintenance or "recovery" of function.

Recovery from Deficit

While explanations of sparing pertain to the state of functional organization in the brain prior to onset of aphasia, explanations of recovery specify changes in structure or process which occur after onset. While sparing entails the maintenance of a function at normal or near-normal levels once the acute physiological processes of etiology have cleared, recovery involves the improvement of a function which is observed to be deficient at the end of this early phase. This improvement may take several weeks or months to be completed. Some theories of recovery specify changes in the organization of cognitive functions associated with regions of the brain. They characterize, for example, modifications in interaction between left and right hemispheres. Other explanations are purely mechanistic, including proposals of changes in brain anatomy and physiology which occur subsequent to damage (see Laurence and Stein, 1978; Kertesz, 1979). The mechanistic proposals do not necessarily relate changes in the brain to functional changes, though there may indeed be a correlation. Not enough is understood about the relationships between neural physiology and cognitive function in order to specify these correlations with confidence.

A common explanation of recovery is **functional substitution,** which is closely related to the notion of multiple control. Instead of two functional subsystems mediating the same function, one subsystem which normally does not mediate a given function takes over the function of the damaged subsystem. This theory has been related to regions of the brain, as in the proposition that the right hemisphere (RH) may take over functions which are normally accomplished by the left hemisphere (LH). According to Laurence and Stein (1978), the replacement subsystem need not perform the function in the same manner as the usual subsystem; it need only accomplish the same goals. For example, auditory comprehension of language may improve because of a gradually developed, spatially organized cognitive strategy mediated by the RH as a replacement for a crippled sequentially dominated process of the LH. Research on language in the RH (see Chapter 3) suggests that the RH comprehends sentences differently from the LH. Similar levels of comprehension between the RH and aphasia is, according to Zaidel (1976), "consistent with the radical conjecture that the right hemisphere may in fact support auditory language comprehension functions in some aphasics" (p. 206). In this vein, Gazzaniga (1974) argued that recovery "is the result of preexisting behavioral mechanisms not necessarily previously routinely involved in a particular act now covering for the mental activity under question" (p. 205).

The substitution process may operate in two ways: (1) a subsystem, perhaps one in the RH, undergoes some adjustment in order to accomplish different goals, or (2) a new subsystem emerges in the brain in response to injury (Laurence and Stein, 1978). One possible consequence of functional substitution is that the substituting subsystem might become crowded trying to serve its own ends as well as new ends, thus reducing the efficiency of its usual function.

Osgood and Miron (1963) suggested a similar process based on an assumption of functional organization in the brain called "vicarious functioning" between sites A and B. In the normal functioning of the intact brain, site B would not participate in the function of site A. However, when site A is damaged, site B may have the capacity to take over the impaired function.

These authors used this theory as a basis for retraining a function. That is, they predicted that damage to site A would not be followed by spontaneous recovery and that retraining of function could occur as long as site B is intact. Nevertheless, it is possible that a site B can reorganize itself to perform a function without treatment directed at the impaired function.

Quadfasel, in Osgood and Miron's (1963) report, described what might be a crucial test of any theory involving functional substitution, especially of the RH for the LH. The test would involve retraining an aphasic patient with a LH lesion and then inducing aphasia by nembutal injection into the right carotid artery. One might also happen upon a serendipitous test of this theory if, after retraining, a second stroke were suffered in the RH, producing deficits in the retrained language functions. Kinsbourne (1971) examined two aphasic patients who happened to receive sodium amytal injections to the RH. All residual speech was arrested following the injection. This did not occur, however, with other aphasic patients; the RH may take over for some but not others.

The possibility of a shift or transfer of language function to the RH has been investigated with the dichotic listening technique (see Chapter 3). Darley (1972) recommended using this procedure to study recovery because the lateralized ear effects are suggestive of specialized functioning by each hemisphere. When verbal stimuli are presented simultaneously to both ears of normal subjects, the stimuli to the right ear are perceived better than stimuli to the left ear. This right-ear advantage (REA) for verbal material is considered to be indicative of verbal function by the LH. Some aphasic subjects have demonstrated the normal REA, while others have demonstrated a left-ear advantage or LEA for verbal stimuli (Sparks, Goodglass, and Nickel, 1970).

Three investigations were conducted to determine whether a LEA in aphasic patients represents a shift in receptive language function over time to the RH. Johnson, Sommers, and Weidner (1977) questioned whether the magnitude of a LEA in twenty posteriorly damaged aphasic subjects (fluent aphasia) would be related to initial severity of aphasia, time since onset at which the dichotic test was given, or the amount of improvement in receptive performance on an aphasia test given initially within one month postonset. First, they concluded that the LEA demonstrated by their aphasic subjects was indicative of a shift to the RH for auditory-verbal recognition. Second, magnitude of the LEA was greater for the severely impaired subjects, suggesting a greater reliance on the RH. Third, the magnitude of LEA was the same for subjects tested before and after six months postonset. Finally, magnitude of LEA was correlated with amount of recovery only for the ten subjects tested within six months after onset. Johnson, et al. concluded that the suspected shift to the RH is related to spontaneous recovery within six months after onset. Pettit and Noll (1979) retested a mixed group of twenty-five aphasic subjects with verbal dichotic listening tasks with an average two-month interval between tests. They did not indicate the time postonset of testing. These subjects improved in language performance during this interval, exhibited a LEA on first test and retest, and had significantly better left ear scores on retest. Since premorbid ear preferences were not taken with these subjects, it is difficult to be certain that a true shift in ear preference actually occurred (Searleman, 1977). If a shift did occur, it pertained only to word recognition ability.

The third study was conducted by Castro-Caldas and Botelho (1980) who compared fluent and nonfluent aphasia with three dichotic tasks, one of which was a word comprehension paradigm involving pointing to a picture. Forty of 117 subjects were retested during the first year after onset, and only a few of these were given all three tests twice. Like Johnson, et al., Castro-Caldas and Botelho compared subjects tested either before or after six months postonset. However, contrary to Johnson's results, fluent aphasics showed a tendency toward an increased REA. The same pattern was observed in those subjects who were retested. These contradictory findings may have been due to differences in design of these studies and to differences in the composition of fluent aphasic groups. Because fluent aphasia represents a variety of syndromes and can be defined by researchers with reference to either site of lesion (posterior) or symptoms (fluency), the opportunity for conflicting results is inevitable until researchers either agree on the use of this term or describe their subjects more completely.

A second functional approach to the explanation of recovery is associated with the terms **plasticity** and **reorganization** (Laurence and Stein, 1978). Instead of a simple takeover or substitution by one functional subsystem for another, these terms refer to a global reorganization of neural systems in response to brain damage. Plasticity refers to "a kind of morphological flexibility" which has been accounted for by anatomical changes after damage such as axonal regeneration or sprouting. Perhaps, because of the functional potential attributed to structural adjustments in the brain, plasticity has referred to the capacity of undamaged structures to assume new functions. The term has been used to refer to recovery phenomena of early childhood. Children younger than age four have demonstrated a remarkable degree of recovery and learning of language even after complete removal of the left hemisphere (Lenneberg, 1967). Such recovery is not found in older children and adults with similar lesions. Explanations of this age-related difference in degree of recovery have included the concept of greater plasticity of brain structures in early childhood.

Reorganization of language function implies a rearrangement of existing component processes, perhaps creating a new system for achieving the same goals such as sentence comprehension or retrieval of a word. The component processes may include the mental representation of perceived sentences, the manner of organizing lexical items in memory, or the manner of searching the memory store for a word. It may include functional substitution with components previously not accustomed to participating now getting into the act. New and unimaginable components may be created. The result may be a novel cognitive basis for language processing, and the very novelty of it makes it difficult to describe its essential characteristics. Laurence and Stein (1978) remarked that theories of reorganization have been attractive because of their vagueness. Specific functional subsystems responsible for recovery often have not been specified, and this ambiguity has made it difficult to generate specific experimental hypotheses. Luria proposed a reorganizational theory which was linked to his concept of functional organization in the brain.

The clearest example of a theoretical basis for treatment strategy is Luria's (1970b) theory of spontaneous recovery. His concepts for describing natural adjustments of brain function in response to injury of one region are the same concepts used to explain the effect of treatment on brain function. His clinical procedures are a logical derivative from these assumptions. His view of spontaneous recovery consisted of two features: functional disinhibition and functional reorganization.

Like the holistic description of functional brain organization described in Chapter 3, Luria (1970b) ascribed to the interdependence among different functional systems in the brain and suggested that focal destruction of brain tissue results in "a dynamic inhibition or blockade of functional systems as a whole" (p. 375). He identified three factors of inhibition of function: (1) reduced or disrupted transmission of neural impulses in the area of destroyed tissue, (2) impairment of one link of a functional system resulting in a disruption of the whole system, at least temporarily, and (3) reaction of the whole system to the injury by avoiding use of the affected system. Treatment of inhibited functions, wrote Luria, "was directed toward restoring functions in *their original form*" (p. 381). He added, however, that this type of recovery is "the exception rather than the rule. . . ."

Given that the destruction of brain tissue is irreversible, Luria (1970b) emphasized that "recovery of the disturbed functional systems can be achieved only by *major reorganization* of cortical processes" (p. 381). The resultant restored function is derived from a cortical organization which is different from that of the original function. He described recovery from impairments of simple and complex functions:

> Damage to the primary projection areas of the cerebral cortex . . . leads *to loss of elementary forms of movement or sensation*. The elementary functions . . . are not recovered. The only means of compensating for deficits of this type is by transferring the functions to other structures or to other functional systems. Learning to use the other hand when one hand is paralyzed or learning to read Braille when the visual cortex has been destroyed are examples of such "substitutive compensation." (p. 381)

The second form of recovery relates more to complex disturbances such as aphasia:

> The injury does not result in loss of an elementary function but in the *disruption of complex functional systems*. The disintegration of such systems is irreversible, but they may be reorganized; the defective link may be

replaced by a new link so that the overall function is reestablished on a new basis. (p. 382)

Luria claimed that in man almost any cortical region can acquire new functional significance.

Two basic types of functional reorganization may be exploited by specific treatment procedures. One is **intersystemic reorganization,** in which one functional system, not ordinarily involved in an impaired function, is introduced to assist in the realization of the impaired function. Rosenbek (1978), for example, has had the apraxic patient use finger tapping as a means of facilitating the pacing of speech production. The other type of reorganization is **intrasystemic reorganization,** in which the impaired functional system is transferred to a new level of organization. This type involves remaining within the impaired system rather than borrowing from an ostensibly unrelated system. Usually it involves shifting a disturbed function down to a lower level, such as saying "seven" within the context of counting to ten instead of as an answer to a question. The principle of intrasystemic reorganization is similar to a basic concept behind progression from easy to difficult tasks in treatment:

> If an aphasic cannot bring forth an intended response by himself, it is sometimes possible to lead him to do so by eliciting a response first in a more automatic way and then in more and more voluntary ways by gradually withdrawing the facilitations incorporated in the stimuli. This passage from more automatic to more voluntary constitutes the core of rehabilitation (Basso, Capitani, and Vignolo, 1979, p. 192).

SUMMARY AND CONCLUSIONS

This chapter introduced a few theoretical orientations for subsequent topics. Hypotheses about normal language function have provided direction for several investigations of aphasic processing. For example, Chapter 5 will address rehearsal and scanning in short-term memory and the organization of semantic memory. Also, thinking about normal processes contributes to the task analysis which goes into interpreting deficient performances and planning tasks to exercise particular processes. Other theoretical orientations have appeared in speech-language pathology, such as cybernetics and servo-systems. However, one test of a theory's value is the extent to which it has been applied in the scientific arena for gathering data on normal and aphasic language. Concepts of normal language were selected for presentation here largely on this basis.

It is very difficult to examine specific processes such as scanning and comparison in the aphasic population, because the aphasic subject usually presents impairments which prohibit a clean examination of a process with the experimental paradigms created for normal subjects. Most theoretical issues in aphasiology are painted with broad, sweeping strokes such as questions of loss versus interference, syntax versus semantics, or competence versus performance.

One of the strongest differences of opinion is directed toward the validity of syndromes. Different conclusions come from two ways of observing pattern of deficit. When viewed relative to degrees of impairment among modalities (see Figure 6–2a), patterns among aphasic patients are similar. Defined in this way, syndromes are hard to find. When the patient is observed relative to characteristics of spontaneous speech and verbal repetition, qualitative differences among patients become more apparent. Syndromes are possible, especially given certain restricted sites of lesion.

Theories of sparing and recovery of function depend on theories of functional organization of the brain surveyed in

Chapter 3. Recovery by functional substitution and/or reorganization may be the foundation for observations of recovery surveyed in Chapter 9. Furthermore, treatment procedures may be justified as facilitators of substitution and reorganization processes. As will be seen in Chapters 10 and 11, treatment capitalizes on the sparing of some language functions and on the fact that brain damage ignores the right hemisphere in many cases of aphasia.

5 The Search for Primary Deficits

In this chapter, we shall turn our attention to what might be called *basic research* in aphasiology. This research is designed primarily to enrich our understanding of aphasia, with the dividend of learning more about the processes required for normal language function. Many investigators leave it to clinicians to figure out the clinical application of their methods and results. *Applied research* is directed toward development of practical procedures for effective differential diagnosis, assessment, and treatment. The methods of basic research sometimes can be clinically unwieldy; but, in addition to the knowledge gained from them, these methods might be refined in order to become practical at some later time. Basic research of any kind is important for rehabilitation because it is directed toward uncovering the primary deficits of aphasia. Also, as Darley (1982) demonstrated, basic research can be used as a data base for justifying the manipulation of certain stimulus variables in treatment.

PRIMARY DEFICITS

The clinician directs treatment toward primary deficits which underlie observed patterns of symptoms. Special investi-

gative procedures sometimes are needed in order to determine what the clinician should be looking for in diagnosis so that, in turn, the clinician will know what to treat. Luria (1958) made a distinction between primary and secondary symptoms, a concept which is based on a multidimensional view of aphasia. Focal lesions can be thought of as producing a primary breakdown of a single component of the cognitive system which supports language function, and the primary breakdown leads to a variety of secondary disturbances which appear during any thorough assessment. Luria defined these components with respect to each modality, namely, auditory, visual, kinesthetic, and motor systems of analysis and synthesis. An impairment within any one of these components "is a direct primary result of every focal lesion of the cortex" (Luria, 1958, p. 15). Damage to Wernicke's area, for example, might produce a breakdown of auditory language processing which is considered to be the primary deficit. Direct observations of auditory comprehension deficiency reveal the primary symptoms of a Wernicke's aphasia. Other symptoms of this disorder are the secondary effects of the primary breakdown; secondary symptoms in Wernicke's aphasia include repetition failures, lack of awareness of jargon, reading deficits and, possibly, the jargon itself. Secondary symptoms appear because a single component of the cognitive basis for language function, however defined, interacts with all other components in the use of language. A primary disturbance, therefore, simply upsets the sometimes delicate balance among these intimately related subsystems.

Whether a researcher holds a unidimensional or multidimensional view of aphasia, he or she is interested in finding common threads underlying all cases of aphasia. If all aphasic patients possess a primary deficit in short-term verbal retention, as Schuell suggested, then treatment would be directed toward stretching the capacity of short-term memory in all cases. Schuell also concluded that all aphasias include a word retrieval deficit. This appears to be true, and perhaps a better question would be whether all patients have the same kind of word-retrieval deficit.

Much of the research cited in this chapter is aimed at finding the primary deficits underlying particular symptom patterns. Is Wernicke's aphasia based on an impairment of phoneme discrimination, as Luria (1966) suggested? Is Broca's aphasia derived from a central disruption of syntactic processing which affects comprehension as well as expression? Is conduction aphasia basically an impairment of verbal short-term memory, or is it instead an impairment of a phonological production process? Do the different manifestations of anomia, such as paraphasias and circumlocution, come from deficits at different stages of a multifaceted word-retrieval process? Answers to these questions are vital for rehabilitation because they may mean that the clinician should focus on treating speech perception in some cases, syntax in others, and short-term memory capacity in others. In clinical assessment, the clinician compares secondary symptoms of each patient in order to infer one or more common threads underlying these symptoms.

RESEARCH STRATEGIES

Different types of questions can be answered depending on the subjects selected for an investigation. In order to produce conclusions which apply to a substantial population beyond the sample in the study, subjects are usually studied as a representative group and an average performance is obtained. With any group, a research question is answered by making at least one comparison. If a group of people with aphasia were studied, the researcher might want to know about the influence of syntactic structure on accuracy of comprehension and, therefore, may compare two different structures with the same task.

An aphasic group is compared with a normal group in order to identify the deficits of aphasia. If aphasics perform significantly worse (minimal overlap with normal range of performance) than the control group, then a deficit has been identified. The only difference between the two groups when they are selected is that the normals are without identifiable brain damage. Normal subjects are often patients in the same hospital, but are being treated for different problems. Normal controls are mandatory when the experimenter cannot be sure of what the normal standard of performance is on a task to be given to aphasics. In this case, the only way to conclude that the aphasics are deficient is to compare them with actual normal performance rather than comparing them against an arbitrary standard of success on the task.

Some questions pertain to whether a deficit is simply a result of brain damage per se no matter where it occurs, or is instead a unique result of damage to the perisylvian region of the left hemisphere. Answers to such questions refine our differential diagnostic capabilities. The comparison is between two brain-damaged groups, one which is probably aphasic and the other not aphasic. Frequently, left-hemisphere-damaged aphasics are compared with right-hemisphere-damaged nonaphasics. A normal group may be added so that levels of performance can be interpreted as to whether they represent deficits. As discussed in Chapter 3, accurate identification of different brain-injured groups has improved with development of brain scans and CT scans. Without such laboratory confirmation of lesion sites, left and right-hemisphere groups might be defined based on clinical signs such as side of hemiplegia. These signs do not ensure that the groups truly represent unilateral brain damage.

Subgroups of aphasia are compared for the purpose of answering more specific questions about aphasia. Many questions pertain to whether quantitative and qualitative differences exist among different patients. If such differences exist, the defining characteristics of a group can be used to predict the existence of certain primary deficits. Subjects may be divided based on levels of receptive and expressive functions, such as a high-comprehending group and a low-comprehending group; or subjects may be divided into four groups based on the interaction of two variables, such as level of comprehension and category of fluency. Increasingly common, however, is comparison among syndromes.

Syndrome comparisons may begin with the assumption that aphasics are already different in certain respects, and the investigator inquires into what makes them different. That is, the investigator is looking for a primary deficit unique to one syndrome. However, the researcher also may take the perspective that in certain respects the syndromes may not be different, and he or she sets out to examine this hypothesis. There are a few risks in this type of research. First, with the broad division

of subjects into nonfluent and fluent, the fluent group could represent a wide variety of aphasias, from relatively mild anomic aphasia to severe forms of Wernicke's aphasia. An average score from such a fluent group would rest between these syndromes and not be representative of any subjects in the fluent group. Second, unambiguous representatives of each syndrome may be difficult to find in many settings, making such comparisons impractical. As stated in Chapter 1, only half the cases may be categorized easily as specific syndromes, and conduction aphasia and anomic aphasia are relatively rare. As a result, group comparisons often contain a rather small sample size per group. A frequent sample size per group is five. Therefore, statistical comparisons should be interpreted with caution.

The value of studying well-defined subgroups of aphasia, no matter how small the group, is that the results can be related to specific patients more clearly than if the results come from a group described vaguely as simply aphasic. Objective criteria for maximizing homogeneity of group include pattern of performance on a standardized test battery and laboratory confirmation of type and site of lesion. Because definitions and observational methods have been refined over the years, it is risky to compare studies of one syndrome or one symptom that were done even a decade apart. After aphasic jargon, for example, became more precisely separated from schizophrenic language by the cutting edge of a linguist (Lecours and Vanier-Clement, 1976), definitions of jargon aphasia twenty years ago may be different from the jargon aphasia of today.

Case studies involve a thorough examination of one subject, and are valuable because observations of one case can readily be related to similar cases. Some research consists of multiple case studies, such as Buckingham and Kertesz's (1976) linguistic analysis of three cases with jargon and Yarnell's (1981) study of three cases of crossed aphasia in right-handers. Case studies differ from the increasingly familiar single case experimental design (Hersen and Barlow, 1976). Case studies are more descriptive, and there is little attempt to control for the influence of specific variables on well-defined responses as occurs with single case experimental designs.

Valuable information has come from the description of single cases. Case studies are especially informative when addressed to unusual or rare patients, such as Goldstein's (1964) report of an endentulous aphasic laryngectomee. Case studies are directed toward a thorough analysis of specific symptoms such as anomia (Wepman, Bock, Jones, et al., 1956), jargon (Brown, 1981a), agrammatism (Goodglass, Gleason, Bernholz, et al., 1972), and paralexia (Saffran, Schwartz, and Marin, 1976). Such studies may generate hypotheses to be tested later on a group of similar subjects, as was done after the case study of agrammatism (Gleason, Goodglass, Green, et al., 1975). Thorough investigation of language function in one syndrome, such as conduction aphasia (Caramazza, Basili, Koller, et al., 1981), may have implications toward finding the primary deficit. Case studies have also been influential in relating symptoms to lesion sites, especially with unusual cases of modality-specific disorders such as auditory agnosia or alexia without agraphia.

WORD RETRIEVAL

Retrieval of words from relatively permanent storage in long-term memory occurs in a variety of circumstances and for varied purposes. In conversation a word is retrieved amidst other words, and a speaker is free to choose his words within constraints imposed by topic, verbal context, and perceived knowledge of the listener. Words are retrieved to make statements, ask questions, and answer questions. Object naming is a special circumstance, in that it is demanded frequently of aphasic patients during clinical assessment and treatment of the more general word-retrieval process. Called "confrontation naming," object naming involves an elimination of many contextual influences, and demands a restricted range of possibilities for response. Its correspondence to natural word retrieval is limited indeed, but its clinical value lies in the ease with which word-retrieval deficits are exposed and analyzed.

Confrontation Naming

The confrontation-naming task is administered to see how well a patient is able to retrieve a word relative to the idea it represents. The idea is usually presented as a picture of an object, and the patient is asked to say its name. This has been described as a modality association between visual input and spoken output. The reading of words aloud (verbal visual input) is sometimes described as "word naming," but reading aloud is not considered here to be a word-retrieval task because the word is given to the speaker.

The Visual Referent. Recognition of the pictured object is the first step in a naming task, one which generally is not impaired by aphasia. Models of confrontation naming indicate that object recognition activates a region of semantic memory (conceptual knowledge) related to the word to be retrieved (Forster, 1978; Mills, Knox, Juola, et al., 1979). As will be discussed later, certain aphasics may have a problem with the structure of semantic memory, and the intimate relationship between the picture and the conceptual knowledge it evokes would suggest that the picture might play some part in the patient's naming.

Line drawings of objects have been compared with real objects as stimuli for evoking names (Benton, Smith, and

Lang, 1972; Corlew and Nation, 1975). In Benton's study, real objects were easier to name than small line drawings, but the authors questioned the clinical significance of the statistical difference. Corlew and Nation found no difference between objects and pictures of the same objects. They concluded: " . . . the physical characteristics of visual stimuli will not provide either theoretical or clinical insights into aphasic naming behavior'' (p. 1990).

Bisiach (1976) disagreed with Corlew and Nation by suggesting that there is a point where perceptual analysis will influence word retrieval. Bisiach (1966) had compared naming of realistic colored objects, line drawings of objects, and drawings obscured by superimposed lines. Aphasic subjects had no perceptual problem with these drawings, but their naming was reduced with the obscured drawings. If the redundancy of visual input is reduced, its evocation of words may be affected. Similarly, perceptually ambiguous pictures may reduce certainty of word selection, and enhancing redundancy may facilitate naming. Whitehouse, Caramazza, and Zurif (1978) considered this idea in a study which consisted of a picture recognition task. Perceptual ambiguity was created by varying dimensions of a cup, bowl, and glass, so that one picture, for example, could be either a cup or a bowl. Such ambiguity could be resolved with a contextual cue such as coffee pouring into a "cup." Broca's aphasics had normal sensitivity to "fuzzy" boundaries and context, while anomic aphasics were seen as having difficulty with this perceptual information.

Whitehouse, et al.'s study dealt with the *uncertainty* of a referent, which refers to the number of possible names that could be associated with it. When a clinician wants to evaluate naming accuracy, high uncertainty pictures are minimized so that judgments of accuracy can be unequivocal. Mills, et al. (1979) studied this factor by measuring aphasic's naming latency and accuracy. A picture of a cup was a low-uncertainty item, while a picture of a country home in winter was a high-uncertainty item which could be called "cottage," "house," "country," and several other names. Mills' subjects made more errors with high-uncertainty pictures. Mills concluded that uncertainty had its impact on the patients' lexical retrieval rather than on recognition of the picture.

Familiarity of the referent is usually considered by the clinician in selecting the semantic content of treatment. Rochford and Williams (1965) conducted a unique experiment in which common and uncommon referents for the same word were compared. For example, "teeth" could be the name for pictures of a mouth (common) or a comb (rare). "Eye" could be retrieved to a picture of seeing (common) or a needle (rare). Common concepts resulted in better naming than less common concepts.

Pictures in a naming task were studied by Gardner (1973) with respect to *operativity* of the item to be named. An object is perceptually operative if it is discrete and can be manipulated readily. An object is figurative if it is continuous with its surrounding context and not easily manipulable. Examples of operative objects would be a vase, hydrant, and rock; examples of figurative objects would be a ceiling, curb, and cloud. These categories were equated for word frequency, and aphasics named operative items more successfully. Better naming of operative items was attributed to multimodal experience with these objects.

Word Frequency and Grammatical Class. The frequency of occurrence of words has been estimated primarily from common reading material. Rochford and Williams (1965) and Gardner (1973) found that high-frequency (common) words were retrieved more readily than low-frequency (uncommon) words. High-frequency body part names (ear, nose) were easier to retrieve than low-frequency body part names (wrist, eyebrow, knuckles). Compound words were studied also with common-common words (lighthouse), common-rare words (sundial), and rare-common words (padlock). The influential factor was frequency of the first half. When it was common, naming was easier (Rochford and Williams, 1965).

Confrontation naming relative to grammatical word class has been examined mostly by comparisons between nouns (objects) and verbs (actions). Accuracy of naming objects and actions was correlated significantly, and verbs had the same frequency effect as nouns (Rochford and Williams, 1965). Broca's and Wernicke's aphasics had equal difficulty between nouns and verbs, while anomic aphasics did much better with verbs than with nouns (Goodglass, Klein, Carey, et al., 1966).

Naming Errors.   Schuell and Jenkins (1961b) observed a variety of incorrect picture-naming responses, called paraphasias in Chapter 1. The errors of sixty aphasic subjects were classified as related to the correct response in meaning (association), similar in sound (approximation), or irrelevant and "I don't know" responses. Current terminology would classify these errors as semantic paraphasias, phonemic paraphasias and apraxic substitutions, and a mixture of unrelated paraphasias and neologisms. Schuell and Jenkins' data lead to an important point: *pattern of group data for aphasia in general does not necessarily reflect patterns of individual patients.* Of all errors, the sixty subjects had 29 percent associations, 19 percent approximations, and 52 percent irrelevant or omitted responses. However, patients with minimal errors showed the opposite pattern from patients with many errors. Twelve patients making one error had 75 percent associations, while ten patients making sixteen to eighteen errors had 72 percent irrelevant and omitted

responses. As severity increased, errors shifted from semantic relatedness to unrelatedness.

Anterior, nonfluent aphasias often are characterized as giving appropriate responses in confrontation naming. The single word is usually within their production capacity, and the task simply does not tap into their syntactic deficit. Their word-retrieval difficulties are more apparent when they try to produce sentences. Gardner (1973) described naming "errors" of anterior aphasics as "synonymous and metonymic responses which were reasonably appropriate for the designated item yet not the required answer" (p. 218). These responses were probably functionally appropriate for communicative purposes. Broca's aphasics have been more accurate in naming pictures than posterior types, including Wernicke's and anomic aphasias (Goodglass and Stuss, 1979).

Errors of posterior fluent aphasia were catalogued by Buckingham (1979b). His categories overlap with the paraphasias defined in Chapter 1 and characterize errors in spontaneous speech as well. Anomic aphasia is characterized by sometimes long pauses before naming, "the definition" or circumlocution, and the "indefinite anaphora" such as "thing," "stuff," or "guy." These symptoms were considered by Buckingham to reflect a word-finding block. Wernicke's aphasia contains more "field errors," namely, semantic paraphasias, unrelated lexical errors, and neologisms.

Beyn and Vlasenko (1974) provided an analytical structure for the study of "action paraphasias," that is, errors in confrontation verb retrieval. They asked thirty-three aphasic patients in the Soviet Union to name the action in pictures such as of a blacksmith forging, a gardener planting a tree, and a peasant mowing. Most errors were classified as *static* or *dynamic.* Static errors were substitutions derived from a static element of the picture such as the actor or instrument in an action. "Forges" was replaced by "tongs," "hammer," or "blacksmith," all nouns instead of verbs. Dynamic substitutions were incorrect verbs such as "piercing" instead of "sewing" or "writes" instead of "draws." Dynamic errors were of two types depending on the aspect of the action apprehended by the subject. Either one part of the whole action was singled out, as in "piercing" for "sewing," or an equivalent or more general action was named, as in "writes" for "draws." Beyn and Vlasenko (1974) attributed these errors to "poor apprehension of the semantic structure of the verb" (p. 32).

Explanations. The confrontation-naming paradigm has been used to make generalizations about the source of word-finding difficulty in all circumstances, and a few investigators have tried to explain the impairment of picture naming itself. Theories which account for picture-naming deficits may generalize to all word retrieval. This section is focused only on studies which were addressed to the picture-naming process specifically by including this task as at least part of the experimental procedure. When different syndromes of aphasia are compared, the investigator is interested in whether there are different bases for naming deficits which contribute to differences among syndromes. Goodglass, Kaplan, Weintraub, et al. (1976) advised that "a raw score of picture-naming ability provides little clue as to type of aphasia or site of lesion" (p. 145), because all aphasics have a subnormal score on a thorough test of this function. Therefore, qualitative aspects of the process are examined, such as type of error.

Primary deficits for picture naming are proposed with respect to assumptions about stages in the process, such as visual recognition, access to semantic memory, and then access to lexical memory. Search through semantic and/or lexical networks is sometimes distinguished from retrieval of the word once it is found. Semantic paraphasias, for example, indicate that words can be retrieved but that the appropriate word cannot be found during the search phase. Circumlocutions indicate that search through semantic memory was accurate and that the slot which defines the correct word was found but that retrieval of the word is blocked. Phonemic paraphasias are suggestive of a problem at a later stage, where the correct word was retrieved but phonological formulation is impaired. Neologisms, according to Buckingham (1979b), may be replacements for inadequate searching in order to mask inevitable retrieval failure. Mills, et al. (1979) concluded that their ten aphasic subjects maintained adequate visual recognition and semantic (conceptual) network structure and that the basis for their naming delays and errors rested in impaired access to the lexicon.

Is the aphasic able to retrieve some properties of the target word when naming failure occurs? Without brain injury, we are able to think of the first sound or length of a word that is on the "tip-of-the-tongue." Barton (1971) inquired as to whether aphasics can achieve a similar TOT state. Sixteen subjects were instructed to point, upon picture-naming failure, to the word's first letter, to a number indicating number of syllables, and to the word "big" or "small" to indicate size of the word. Subjects guessed these properties accurately over 60 percent of the time in spite of being unable to say the word. Goodglass, et al. (1976) differentiated among syndromes and had subjects guess number of syllables by pointing to dashes instead of numerals. Overall, these aphasics were not nearly as successful guessing word properties as Barton's subjects, partly because vocabulary difficulty was greater in Goodglass' study. There were a few differences among the four syndromes. Conduction aphasics were the best at guessing first letters (34 percent) and syllable length (34 percent), while anomic aphasics exhibited almost total blocking of word retrieval (10 percent and 5.5 percent). Wernicke's subjects also possessed little information about the target word (13 percent).

An intriguing study by Goodglass and Baker (1976) represents the beginning of investigation as to whether word-retrieval deficits are based on damage to semantic and/or lexical organization in long-term memory. Aphasics' knowledge of conceptual relationships was tested with a unique word-recognition task. Subjects were first asked to name sixteen pictures. Then with each of these pictures a series of fourteen words was presented, and subjects indicated whether each of these words was related or not related to the picture. Seven words in the recognition task consisted of the object name (for example, *orange*) and six words bearing different relationships to the object concept including the name of another member of the same category (*apple*), a superordinate class (*fruit*), an attribute (*juicy*), a functional associate (*eat*), and so on. The other seven words were not related to the picture. All subjects recognized the name of the object, but the pattern of difficulty for recognizing associates in low-comprehending subjects differed from nonbrain-injured controls. High-comprehending aphasics showed a semantic structure that was similar to the controls. Furthermore, success in naming was related to success in associate recognition. Goodglass and Baker concluded that low-comprehending aphasics possess constricted semantic organization which contributes to their naming failures.

Verbal Stimulation
of Word Retrieval

Now we will begin to consider aphasic word retrieval in conditions other than confrontation naming. Verbal stimulation of single word retrieval is of interest clinically because it may facilitate confrontation naming and provides a broader range of conditions for exercising word retrieval. *Sentence completion,* for example, has been used in treatment as a cue to the correct name after a failure in picture naming. Barton, Maruszewski, and Urrea (1969) found that completions resulted in more accurate word retrieval than pictures in confrontation naming. They presented open-ended sentences such as "In order to tell the time, we usually wear a _____." Normative data from 280 aphasics for the *Porch Index of Communicative Ability* (Porch, 1971a) presents a different picture, however. Subtest IX presents short carrier phrases to stimulate retrieval of the same ten names in a confrontation naming subtest (IV). At all percentile levels of the aphasic sample, except for those at the 35 to 45 percentile levels, object naming and sentence completion resulted in the same level of word retrieval.

Word retrieval to *definitional statements* is more difficult than picture naming. Barton, et al. (1969) asked questions like "What is something for telling time, small enough to be carried in a pocket or worn on the wrist?" Goodglass and Stuss (1979) presented oral descriptions: "This animal lives in the desert. It carries people or bundles. It goes for a long time without water. It is a _____." These descriptions elicited fewer words primarily in Wernicke's and Broca's aphasia, while anomics were equally proficient in picture naming and naming the descriptions. However, Broca's aphasics were superior to the other groups in total number of words retrieved.

Rollin (1964) compared subtle variations of verbal requests for word retrieval. He presented questions ("What do people wear on their heads?"), imperatives ("Name what people wear on their heads"; "Tell me what people wear on their heads"), and carrier phrases ("On their heads people wear _____"). There were no differences in word retrieval among these types of stimulation for the aphasic group. However, Rollin's statistics revealed wide individual subject variation. This familiar phenomenon in aphasia research leads the clinician to check out such stimulus variations with each patient because group data often does not apply to the individual patient.

Another form of verbal stimulation is *free word association.* The subject is asked to say the first word that comes to mind in response to another word. Word association norms have provided an empirical basis for estimating distances between concepts in models of semantic memory structure (Glass and Holyoak, 1975). Frequent responses to a concept are considered to be "closer" to the concept than infrequent responses. Wyke (1962) found that four aphasics gave infrequent or idiosyncratic (not among normal associations) responses in an association task. A larger sample was studied by Sefer and Henrikson (1966), who presented words of different grammatical classes to fifty aphasics. Though aphasics expectedly retrieved fewer words than normal controls, the type of response was similar to normal in terms of whether a paradigmatic or syntagmatic response was given. A paradigmatic response is in the same grammatical class as the stimulus (apple-pear); a syntagmatic response is not in the same grammatical class and bears a syntactic relationship to the stimulus (apple-eat). Aphasic associations consisted of the same proportion of paradigmatic (called homogenous by Sefer) responses as those of normal adults, who generally produce more paradigmatic than syntagmatic responses.

Jakobson (1955) had proposed that aphasics are divided between predominantly contiguity (syntagmatic) and predominantly similarity (paradigmatic) disorders. This distinction corresponds to the more recent idea that aphasia can be manifested as an impairment of either syntax or semantics. In free word association, syntactic deficit would result in predominantly paradigmatic association responses because of impaired sequential constraints, while semantic deficit would result in predominantly syntagmatic responses because of impaired semantic structure. Sefer and Henrikson (1966) looked for such a division between agrammatic and anomic aphasics in their study, but did not find two different types of association behavior.

Divergent Word Retrieval

So far, word retrieval has been discussed as a single response to a particular stimulus. However, word retrieval can occur as a series of discrete lexical responses to a particular stimulus. Chapey, Rigrodsky, and Morrison (1976) characterized confrontation naming and verbal stimulation of single words as convergent semantic behavior requiring the patient to converge on one idea. Divergent semantic behavior, neglected in aphasia research, involves a quantity and variety of responses, generation of logical alternatives, and maintenance of relevance of varied output from the same source.

Chapey compared aphasics and normals with several divergent tasks. One of her five tasks involved responding with a series of words. The other four tasks allowed for production of a series of phrases or sentences. Object naming required subjects to list objects belonging to a class, such as all objects that roll. Calling this task "category naming," Grossman (1978, 1981) has analyzed aphasics' performance in thinking of a number of types of sports, tools, fruit, and so on. In the other tasks, subjects listed problems inherent to a common situation, uses for a common object, ways to improve usefulness or value of an object, and possible consequences of a hypothetical situation. On all five measures aphasics produced fewer relevant answers and a smaller variety of answers than normal controls. Chapey, et al. (1976) concluded: "The definition of the aphasic impairment should be broadened to include a divergent as well as a convergent component" (p. 673).

Word Retrieval in Discourse

The attention given to confrontation naming and verbal stimulation of words is understandable if we are to analyze word-retrieval deficit with any precision. Determining factors which might be responsible for this problem requires research in which variables are controlled. Such control is difficult to achieve when eliciting a series of utterances, and natural conversation provides almost no control at all. The severe-to-moderate forms of Broca's aphasia provide little spontaneous speech to study, which is a problem, particularly for syntactic analysis. Because paraphasias are most frequent in fluent aphasias, fluent speech has received increasing attention from linguists who are interested in word selection.

General Characteristics. Confrontation naming elicits words that are what Goodglass, Hyde, and Blumstein (1969) called "picturable." Words such as *bird* are picturable, and words such as *animal* are not picturable. Spontaneous speech samples were taken from patients with Broca's, Wernicke's, and anomic aphasia; and all groups used more nonpicturable nouns than picturable nouns. Goodglass' subjects tended to use words which are common in everyday conversation such as *time, year, week, wife,* and *people.* Picture naming may include objects that are commonly seen and used, but many of these items may not be the most typical lexicon of a conversation. At least, they do not correspond to most of the nouns spoken more naturally by aphasics.

A picture story test was employed in a comparison of spontaneous word usage between five Broca's and five Wernicke's aphasics (Gleason, et al., 1980). The test consisted of six different stories, represented by picture sequences. Broca's

aphasics produced 40 percent of the number of words per story produced by normals and Wernicke's aphasics. Analysis was focused on "target lexemes," main nouns and verbs. The reduced communicative content of Wernicke's speech was indicated in about 8 percent of their word total being target lexemes compared with 21 percent in Broca's aphasia and 28 percent from the normals. Wernicke's subjects also used many more verbs than nouns, while Broca's subjects used more nouns than verbs; this pattern was consistent among individual subjects. The lack of information in Wernicke's expression was shown further with the examination of *deixis,* which is verbal pointing with words such as *this, that, here,* and *there.* Of the total number of words, 4 percent were these indefinite words in Wernicke's aphasia, while proportion of indefinites in Broca's aphasia was 1 percent and, in normals, was 0.33 percent. Semantic jargon of the poor comprehending Wernicke's patient overlaps with anomic aphasia in this respect, consistent with Buckingham's (1979b) observation of indefinite anaphora in anomic speech.

Verbal behaviors upon retrieval failure in conversation were classified by Marshall (1976). He was interested in what eighteen aphasics did when they initiated an effort to retrieve a word. *Semantic associations* ("This is my rocking chair" for wheelchair) were used most often, followed by *description* or circumlocution ("You know that soft stuff that gets hard" for jello). *Delay* was used infrequently and tended to be used by higher-level subjects. Delay is a characteristic of anomic aphasia on confrontation naming.

Semantic Paraphasia. Semantic paraphasias are common in semantic jargon. The relationship between the error and the target word has been of interest to neurolinguists because of the clues it might provide to the structure of semantic or lexical memory. In examining a case diagnosed as Wernicke's aphasia, Buckingham and Rekart (1979) described five relationships between error and target: (1) synonymy, (2) membership in same category, (3) spatial contiguity, (4) instance of a category instead of the category, and (5) description instead of the object. They concluded that most errors were qualitatively similar to the "slips" of normal speakers. Aphasics differ from normals as to quantity of error, lack of self-correction, and the additional burden of associated problems such as motor and sensory deficits.

Buckingham and Rekart did not rely just on their one case to form their conclusions. They considered Rinnert and Whitaker's (1973) detailed inventory of error-target relationships from several cases. Rinnert and Whitaker compared these relationships to normal word association behavior. For 131 of 217 confusion pairs (60 percent), they found association norms for either the error or the target; and they concluded that "semantic confusions are more *like* than *unlike* normal word associations" (p. 66). In several instances when both words were found in association norms, at least one word, error or target, was a strong associate of the other. Therefore, semantic paraphasias appear to come from a relatively intact semantic organization.

Neologisms.   Neologisms found in picture naming usually enter the flow of spontaneous speech in Wernicke's aphasia. The issue of "Where do neologisms come from?" was reviewed by Buckingham (1981b, 1981c). The unrecognizability of neologisms lends itself to speculation. However, Buckingham provided a framework for finding an answer by suggesting some logical possibilities and some circumstances in which each possibility could be found.

First, neologisms might arise from defective phonological realization, the process which produces phonemic paraphasias. This was called the "conduction theory" by Kertesz and Benson (1980). For this to be the primary deficit, the patient "should NOT be simultaneously producing verbal paraphasia at other points in his speech output, or we could never, in principle, rule them out as possible inputs to the phonemic transformations" (Buckingham, 1981c, p. 50). Also, the patient should be producing some phonemic paraphasias in which there is an obvious relationship to the target. This theory would predict a progression of paraphasias from phonemic to neologistic within a patient. The conduction theory, however, was ruled out by Buckingham and Kertesz (1976) as a likely possibility, because their three subjects exhibited no "middle ground" between severe phonological permutations and a few obvious phonemic paraphasias.

A second possible origin of the neologism is a phonemic transformation of a word already selected incorrectly, a phonemic paraphasia of a hidden verbal paraphasia. Buckingham called this a "two-stage" error. In support of this explanation, verbal and phonemic paraphasias must be observed in conversation. Also, the patient should have a severe word-retrieval deficit. Buckingham implied that it would be a greater severity of deficit than would be associated with the first possibility.

A third possible source of neologism is perseveration of segments from a previously produced neologism. Buckingham (1981c) concluded that this dynamic process is a strong contributor to the masking of word-retrieval failures. Neologisms often consist of variations of a particular word form or of a particular few syllables. This has been called alliteration (words with the same initial sound) and assonance (rhyming). Also, neologistic jargon may include stereotypic use of a particular affix, such as in "I no thusly and loosely."

In a somewhat different discussion, Buckingham (1981b) entertained four possibilities. The fourth was that neologisms arise under conditions of a total word-finding block, rather than arising as a distortion of the intended word (also Butterworth, 1979). Neologisms may be " . . . strings of well-formed phonemes or syllables that fill in the gaps and compensate for words not retrievable from the lexicon" (p. 198).

A QUESTION
OF SEMANTIC DISORGANIZATION

On one hand, word-retrieval deficits have been associated with constricted semantic structure (Goodglass and Baker, 1976); and, on the other hand, a relatively normal associative structure may underlie semantic paraphasias (Rinnert and Whitaker, 1973; Buckingham and Rekart, 1979). The possibility of an impaired semantic structure places a primary deficit in the lap of one component of linguistic competence, namely, the static network of semantic relationships stored in long-term memory. A similarity between semantic errors in verbal expression and semantic errors in comprehension would indicate that a primary deficit is central to these modalities. Gainotti (1976) administered a word-comprehension test in which incorrect picture choices consisted of a phonemically related item, a semantically related item, and three unrelated items. Number of semantic paraphasias was correlated strongly with number of incorrect semantic choices on the comprehension test.

Investigators have begun to explore the possibility of an impairment in semantic memory or in the semantic organization of lexical memory as this central deficit. Buckingham (1981b) suggested that this research is indicating that " . . . brain damage will often loosen up the organization of the mental dictionary and thereby disrupt the system of verbal concepts" (p. 199). Issues have become more spe-

cific, especially as to whether fluent (posterior) aphasias differ from nonfluent (anterior) aphasia with respect to semantic organization. This was indicated at a perceptual level, when Broca's aphasics were sensitive to perceptual/conceptual boundaries while anomic aphasics were not (Whitehouse, et al., 1978). In some of these studies, type of aphasia has been unclear; the category of fluent or posterior aphasia is always ambiguous, and some subjects classified as having jargon or Wernicke's aphasia exhibited verbal expression skills which were too good for this classification.

The most direct look at conceptual organization in semantic memory comes from picture-sorting tasks in which language stimuli are absent. In two case studies (Green, 1981; Shanon, 1978), pictures were sorted in odd or vague ways by two fluent aphasics. One patient with "Wernicke's" aphasia, who could name 79 percent of 86 pictures of animals, sorted these pictures into piles of most similar items. The pictures were sorted into three broad categories, while normals divided them into twenty categories. The patient's semantic boundaries were not sharply defined. Chapey and Lubinski (1979) found that about half of their thirty aphasics would not sort pictures during a study period prior to verbal recall of the pictures.

We begin to see a double dissociation in tasks of conceptual organization which is similar to the double dissociation between semantics and syntax mentioned in Chapter 3. Seven Broca's and seven Wernicke's aphasics were compared in tasks involving *class* and *thematic* organization (Semenza, Denes, Lucchese, et al., 1980). In each task, a test picture was presented along with two choices, and subjects were asked to point to the picture most similar to the test picture. In the class-relation task, choices were in the same category as the test picture (fisherman: sailor, diver); in the thematic task, choices were related contiguously in space or time to the test picture (fisherman: fish, river). Error responses had been defined based on choices of ninety-four college students. The Broca's aphasics were equivalent to normals on the class-relation task but were impaired on the thematic task, while Wernicke's aphasics showed the opposite pattern. Mean number of errors illustrate this double dissociation: Broca's, thematic (7.57) more impaired than class (3.00); Wernicke's, class (8.28) more impaired than thematic (5.00). In a task requiring recognition of category membership with line drawings, Grober also found a difference between nonfluent and fluent patients (Grober, Perecman, Keller, et al., 1980). Semantic organization of the former was relatively intact, while semantic organization of the latter was impaired. However, Broca's and Wernicke's aphasics were impaired in a picture-matching task involving certain semantic relationships between different pictures (Cohen, Kelter, and Woll, 1980).

The dissociation, with semantic impairment concentrated in posterior aphasias, had been suggested initially from printed word-sorting tasks conducted by Zurif (Zurif, Caramazza, and Myerson, 1972; Zurif, Caramazza, Myerson, et al., 1974). In the latter study, anterior subjects were somewhat different from normal controls in that these aphasics sorted animal names according to *characteristic features* (experience-based, idiosyncratic) such as ferocity instead of *defining features* (species classification). Posterior subjects, on the other hand, showed little sense for semantic organization. In a later study with printed words, Broca's and Wernicke's aphasics had difficulty using class and thematic organizational strategies to facilitate recognition and recall (Zurif, Caramazza, Foldi, et al., 1979). Zurif restricted discussion to Broca's aphasia, and concluded that imposition of memory demands places a burden on otherwise well-formed conceptual organization.

Grossman (1978; 1981) provided a

glimpse of how a restricted or ill-defined semantic organization might be observed in word retrieval. He presented a divergent task in which nonfluent and fluent aphasics retrieved as many examples of a category (such as birds) as possible in sixty seconds. He looked for tendencies to provide prototypical examples of a category (robin) and atypical examples (chicken). Nonfluent subjects tended to provide prototypical examples "from the central portions of the referential field." Fluent aphasics started with examples of high typicality and progressed to examples of low typicality. "Their naming ranges over a broader portion of the centrality spectrum within a referential field, and they often cross the borders around a referential field" (p. 327). Grossman suggested that nonfluent aphasics are aware of conceptual boundaries, while fluent aphasics are less aware of these boundaries.

These varied research strategies with inconsistently defined subjects still exhibit a pattern, a convergence of multiple observations on a fairly consistent conclusion. Fluent and nonfluent aphasics have exhibited difficulty with semantic organization. The difficulty appears to be restricted to certain features in nonfluent, anterior aphasia (Broca's) and appears to be more devastating in fluent, posterior aphasia, especially Wernicke's aphasia. Generalizations from several studies are difficult to make because the composition of posterior or fluent groups is unclear. Furthermore, a conflicting conclusion was reached in a study involving semantic "primes" presented prior to a target word in a word-recognition study (Milberg and Blumstein, 1981). Wernicke's aphasics were aided in recognition by the priming words, leading the investigators to conclude that these patients possess "... a deficit in accessing and operating on semantic properties of the lexicon and not an impairment in the underlying organization of the semantic system used" (p. 381).

AGRAMMATISM

There has been some speculation about the basis for an absence of functors in the speech of anterior, nonfluent patients. Agrammatism is characterized by omissions of articles, verb auxiliaries, and morphemic attachments such as suffixes indicating verb tense and noun pluralization. It is observed in repetition and reading aloud as well as in spontaneous speech. This symptom of Broca's aphasia receives attention from treatment programs intended to retrain the use of syntax in richer detail.

Linguistic Description

Agrammatism has been studied for over twenty years by Goodglass and his colleagues. Goodglass and Mayer (1958) compared five nonfluent and five fluent aphasics. The nonfluent group made significantly more errors of word order ("When *he will* see his brother?") and used more coordinating constructions in place of subordinating constructions ("Eat your meat *an'* cut it" instead of "Eat your meat *when* you cut it"). These subjects tended to use more omissions and to simplify utterances. In a transformational grammatical analysis of three levels of agrammatism, Myerson and Goodglass (1972) observed (1) noun phrases (NP) produced more often than verb phrases (VP), consistent with a later finding by Gleason, et al. (1980), (2) negation indicated by "no" tagged onto the beginning or end of a phrase in the severe case, instead of between a NP and VP as in the milder cases, and (3) use of a possessive or demonstrative adjective before a noun only in milder impairment.

Case grammar was employed by Tonkovich (1979) in an analysis of sentence formulation by ten Broca's aphasics. In case grammar, the verb is central in a description of semantic categories, called case relations, which possess certain syntactic (word-order) constraints. Case relations, such as *agent* of an action or *object* of an action, are defined in relation to the verb. A consistent finding with agrammatism was described in terms of case relations; that is, agentive and objective cases (nouns) were produced more than other cases, such as those appearing in surface structure as prepositional phrases (instrumental and locative). There tended to be a rank order of case relations used as the grammatical subject; the agentive case appeared most often, and the objective appeared least often.

Order of Difficulty and Economy of Effort

If some grammatical elements or structures are used more frequently than others, treatment programs for Broca's aphasics could be based on the relative ease of producing these structures.

Two studies were focused on order of difficulty in producing morphemic word endings. Goodglass and Berko (1960) constructed a sentence completion task to elicit word endings. Plural (*-ez*) and comparative (*-er*) suffixes were the easiest to produce, and the possessive (*-ez*) was the most difficult. Middle ground was held by suffixes indicating past tense. DeVilliers (1974) ranked the use of eight morphemes in their obligatory contexts from samples of spontaneous speech of eight nonfluent aphasics. From easiest to most difficult, the morphemes ranked as follows: progressive (*-ing*), plural (*-s*), contractable copula (*I'm,* they*'re*), uncontractable copula (*were*), articles (*a, the*), past regular (*-d*), past irregular, and third person singular (*-s*). In spite of the differences in conditions of speech production, both studies suggested that plurals are more frequent than other suffixes and tense markers are of moderate difficulty. Order of difficulty did not correspond to order of acquisition by children and was not based on transformational or semantic complexity or on differential stress.

In a study of sentence repetition, functors were most likely omitted when unstressed and in the first position of a sentence (Goodglass, Fodor, and Schulhoff, 1967). With the additional observation that Broca's aphasics tend to initiate utterances with a stressed or salient word, Goodglass suggested that the increased effort required for speech production results in the elimination of less salient words such as functors. Goodglass (1976) concluded: "... a basic feature of Broca's aphasia is the increased difficulty of mobilizing the speech output system, which requires a stressed element to put it into action ... Another way of putting it is to say that the response threshold for the speech output system is raised and requires an emphatic or salient element in the message to overcome the elevated threshold and begin the flow of speech" (p. 252). This proposal can be linked to the idea of *economy of effort,* in which semantically impotent or redundant elements are omitted for efficient communication.

In order to determine the order of difficulty of a wide range of grammatical constructions in Broca's aphasia, the constructions must be elicited because they will not appear spontaneously in sufficient numbers to facilitate comparison. Goodglass and Gleason developed the Story Completion Test (SCT) for this purpose (Goodglass, Gleason, Bernholz, et al., 1972; Gleason, Goodglass, Green, et al., 1975); and the SCT has been utilized as an index of severity of agrammatism by Schwartz, Saffran, and Marin (1980), who called it the Syntax Retrieval Test. Tonkovich (1979) used a similar technique in which agrammatic subjects were asked to produce one sentence about information in a short story. The SCT, however, is "a series of 14 brief story-like introductions, spoken by a single examiner, de-

signed to elicit from the patient a specific response" (Gleason, et al., 1975, p. 455). The introductions elicit fourteen different grammatical constructions. For example, to elicit a yes-no question (*Did you call me?*) the examiner says: "John is in his room. He thinks he hears his mother call. So he goes downstairs to see if she called him, and he asks ..." (p. 453). To elicit a passive structure (*was killed by the train*), the examiner says: "A man was walking on the railroad tracks. A train came along. The man didn't hear it. What happened to him? The man ..." (p. 453).

Rank order of the fourteen constructions for eight subjects is presented in Table 5-1 along with the elements required for a correct score. This order for the group corresponded to the order by individual subjects. "It can therefore be concluded that the highest ranking items are the ones most likely to be available for severely agrammatic patients and the lowest ranking ones available only to the least impaired patients" (Gleason, et al., 1975, p. 457). This ranking tended to be related to sentence length, but there were some exceptions, as seen in Table 5-1.

TABLE 5-1. Rank order from easiest to most difficult of fourteen constructions elicited from Broca's aphasics with the Story Completion Test (Gleason, Goodglass, Green, et al., 1975).

Imperative Intransitive	*Sit down.*
Imperative Transitive	*Drink milk.*
Number + Noun	*Twelve cup.*
Adjective + Noun	*Funny story.*
WH Question	*Where put shoes?*
Declarative Transitive	*Dog chase cat.*
Declarative Intransitive	*Baby cry.*
Comparative	*She taller.*
Passive	*Was killed.*
Yes-No Question	*Did you call?*
Direct + Indirect Object	*Give friend dollar.*
Embedded sentence	*... them be quiet.*
Adjective + Adjective + Noun	*Small red car.*
Future Tense	*He will work.*

Consistent with deVilliers' (1974) interpretation of her rankings of morphemic suffixes, Gleason, et al. were unable to discern a single theoretically-based rationale for the relative difficulty of syntactic constructions. Transformational complexity has consistently been a weak predictor of processing difficulty in aphasia. Farmer and O'Connell (1980) concluded that "investigators have not uncovered a 'syntax of aphasia,' a hierarchy of structures typically absent or present, a system of phonological rules or semantic concepts that can be characterized as 'aphasic'" (p. 42).

Economy of effort continues to appear as a partial account for the simplification and omission occurring in agrammatism. In his case grammar analysis, Tonkovich (1979) observed some subtle aspects of agrammatic expression which were interpreted in terms of communicative efficiency. For example, the instrumental case relation was omitted, largely with respect to its semantic context. The instrumental case was more likely to be deleted from intended sentences such as "John is cutting bread with a *knife*" than from intended sentences such as "The lady hit the singer with her *shoes*." In the former sentence, "knife" is redundant because it can be inferred from "cutting bread"; while "shoes" is not likely to be predicted from its context. Broca's patients may try to convey the most information they can within constraints imposed by a crippled verbal-formation mechanism. Bradley, Garrett, and Zurif (1980) suggested that the plausibility of this explanation relies on the clinical impression of relatively spared auditory comprehension. However, even if a comprehension deficit is present, there is no reason to exclude some economy of effort as part of the patient's strategy to compensate for effortful speech, especially when apraxia of speech is so often present with agrammatism.

Word Order in Sentence Production

Reversals of word order—errors of commission instead of omission—have not been given much attention as a feature of motor agrammatism. Often Broca's aphasics do not say enough for such errors to occur. Goodglass and Mayer (1958) had indicated that nonfluent patients sometimes reverse word order in interrogative statements. Saffran, Schwartz, and Marin (1980) uncovered problems with word order in simple declarative statements. Five Broca's aphasics were asked to produce sentences which describe pictures representing *agent-action-object* and *agent-be-locative* relations. The question was whether semantic features of these relations would influence the order of word production. Because reversible statements such as "The boy chases the girl" pose some problems for auditory comprehension, it was thought that similarity in animacy between agent-and-object and agent-and-locative might produce word-order reversals. Pictures were presented in which both nouns were animate (*The man lifts the girl*) and both nouns were inanimate (*The ring is in the cup*). Also, pictures contained one animate and one inanimate item (*The woman lifts the rock; The mouse is in the cup*). When the nouns differed in animacy, few errors of word order were found. However, significantly more word-order errors occurred when relations were alike in animacy, and order errors occurred on one-third of the attempts with these relations. "Thus our claim is not that agrammatics have lost the capacity to produce utterances; it is, rather, that they are unable to map underlying semantic relations into the N-V-N structure" (p. 270). At least, they have trouble with this mapping occasionally.

Adaptive Strategies

A concept often can be conveyed in more than one surface structural format, and Broca's aphasics retain enough knowledge of grammatical rules to enable them to correct errors in sentences (Bliss, et al., 1976; Bliss, Tikofsky, and Guilford, 1976). Gleason, et al. (1975) looked upon the agrammatic's use of alternative surface forms as a positive response of the remaining intact system to compensate for reductions in that system. Hand, Tonkovich, and Aitchison (1979) viewed certain compensatory behaviors of one case to have been abnormal in that the result was an "ill-formed" or ambiguous sentence. Hand, et al. observed compensations in answers to questions and descriptions of a picture, a corpus in which several structures were possible; the investigators had to infer the structure that was intended or correct. Gleason, et al. were in a better position to interpret adaptive strategies because items in their Story Completion Test were designed to elicit particular structures.

Gleason, et al. (1975) observed three strategies which circumvented difficulties and still conveyed the intended message:

1. An active *search for a stressed opening word* seemed to facilitate initiation of an utterance. Initial vocatives were used, as in "Cousin, sit down"; employed more by severely impaired patients than mildly impaired patients. Also, nouns would sometimes appear at the beginning when a pronoun was expected.

2. Adverbs were used to express future tense, as in "He work again next week," and to express the comparative, as in "She is tall enough" instead of *She is taller.*

3. Concatenated phrases simplified an appropriate structure. Broca's aphasics tended to place embedded constituents into a series, as in "a large house, a white house" instead of the more efficient *large white house.* "Girl tall and boy short" was said instead of *The girl is taller than the boy.* Hand, et al. (1979) observed repetitions which appeared to convey emphasis, as in "The girl is laughing and laughing" instead of, perhaps, *The girl is laughing hysterically.* In addition, Hand's subject frequently started an utterance with "This is" or "It was" when the verb was absent, as in "This is Eddie the telephone" or "Well this is bad the cookies."

The Primary Deficit?

The dominant explanations of agrammatism discussed so far have been economy of effort, in which the patient conveys the most meaning with the fewest words, and adaptation, in which the patient uses more readily available language forms in order to convey an idea which is more typically conveyed by less available forms. However, these are explanations of adjustments made by the intact system to a deficit, rather than of the deficit itself. These features of agrammatism illustrate the holistic or organismic account of deficit introduced in Chapter 3: economy of effort and adaptation reflect "what the whole system does without a particular region." They may be signs of sparing and/or recovery of function (see Chapter 4).

PHONEMIC SUBSTITUTIONS

People with aphasia sometimes retrieve the appropriate word but substitute an incorrect phoneme for a correct phoneme, or they omit and add phonemes. These errors have been called phonemic paraphasias, or apraxia of speech, or both. Though the perceived result may be the same—a phonemic substitution, for example—the terms phonemic paraphasia and apraxia of speech are best used to refer to different primary deficits. *Phonemic paraphasia* has implied that, at a cognitive level of planning verbal production, the phonological rules of speech sound selection and combination are misrepresented. *Apraxia of speech* has implied that the cognitive representation of phonological plans is intact but that the ability to translate these plans into action, called motor programming for speech, is impaired. Treatment for apraxia of speech differs from treatment for the language disturbances of aphasia; however, no one so far has proposed a treatment for fluent phonemic paraphasias, especially in conduction aphasia. Many have held a different viewpoint, namely, that we have another situation in which different terms are used for the same disorder.

The issue is a slippery one, especially when "phonological disorder" is discussed as if it represents a single entity. Debate within clinical aphasiology surfaced when Martin (1974) concluded that apraxia of speech does not exist because phonemic substitutions follow certain patterns and occur more often in nonsense syllables than in real words. Lesser (1978) listed three orientations to phonological disorders: (1) an emphasis on neuromuscular disorders of articulation, (2) linguistic theories of disordered phonological plans at a level prior to neuromuscular processing, and (3) proposals of a central linguistic deficit of phonological organization which affects perception as well as verbal expression. These orientations need not be mutually exclusive attempts to define one deficit but can logically represent three different disorders. This section focuses on (1) and (2). Some of the apparent disagreement arises from presenting phonemic substitutions of Broca's aphasia as if they all must be explained as a single disorder, ignoring the possibility that a linguistic and a neuromuscular disorder could be present in one patient (see Blumstein, 1981).

Before sorting out the possible phonological disorders, let us consider some of the investigations of phonemic errors in aphasia. Martin and Rigrodsky (1974a, 1974b) investigated repetition by fifteen aphasics who were not identified as to site of lesion or type of aphasia. Incorrect phonemes were similar to intended phonemes, and fewer errors occurred in real words than in nonsense words. Halpern, Keith,

and Darley (1976) noted that 25 percent of thirty aphasics' errors in spontaneous speech and repetition were phonemic errors. Only two subjects in the group made such errors in spontaneous speech. Syndromes of aphasia were examined by Blumstein (1973), who found that types of phonemic errors were the same for each syndrome. However, Broca's aphasics were distinctive because of "improper control of articulatory movements" which Blumstein referred to as a "dysarthric quality." These studies leave impressions that aphasics are similar to each other in their phonological performance, but that phonological problems are rare among aphasics.

Buckingham's (1979a) incisive essay on apraxia of speech indicated that a neuromuscular disorder can be distinguished from the fluent phonemic paraphasias of posterior aphasics. The phonemic level of analysis in the studies by Martin, Halpern, and Blumstein is unable to separate the disorders, because phonetic aspects of sound production are sometimes not recorded in notations of phoneme substitution, omission, and addition. For example, posterior patients make substitution and addition errors (Burns and Canter, 1977), and so do Broca's aphasics (Trost and Canter, 1974). Errors are usually one distinctive feature away from the target phoneme (Blumstein, 1973). Yet at the phonetic or "subphonemic" level of analysis, in which neuromuscular movements of production are observed, Broca's aphasics show deviations not apparent in fluent aphasias. Blumstein and Cooper recorded a lack of synergy in voice-onset time (VOT) in Broca's aphasia which was not found in fluent aphasias (Blumstein, Cooper, Zurif, et al., 1977; Blumstein, Cooper, Goodglass, et al., 1980). Itoh, Sasanuma, and Usijima (cited in Buckingham, 1979a) found asynchronous velar movement in anterior patients. Inaccurate laryngeal and velar movements produce phonemic errors of one distinctive feature, the same outcome as in fluent aphasia but from a different level of impairment.

Buckingham's (1979a) conclusions are instructive: "The qualitative aspect of phonemic paraphasia in terms of substitution, deletion, addition, and linear switch is no different for *any* aphasic, including any patient with limb-kinetic apraxia of speech" (p. 219). He continued: "The actual situation with substitution errors is more complex, however, and we must make some finer subphonemic distinctions" (p. 210). Broca's aphasics are likely to exhibit phonetic deviations of VOT and velar function, but they may produce phonemic paraphasia without phonetic errors as well. Buckingham (1981a) advised considering the articulatory-behavioral context of utterances, such as the apraxic's "struggling attempts to initiate speech and keep it going . . . " (p. 298). This becomes part of the differentiation between apraxia of speech and phonemic paraphasia.

Refinements in distinguishing phonological impairments comes from further observations of posterior cases. Burns and Canter (1977) observed that many errors in fluent aphasia appear to accompany attempts to retrieve a word in which there are semantic and phonological confusions. Attempts to say *bag* came out as "bushel" and "basket." Various sound combinations were attempted, as for *book:* "boos, boat, bug, boot, but . . ." Successive attempts to produce a single target word appear to differentiate conduction aphasia from Broca's and Wernicke's aphasia (Joanette, Keller, and Lecours, 1980). Conduction aphasics showed a continuous progression to the target across four successive attempts, while Wernicke's aphasics showed no regular progression and actually moved farther from the target. Broca's aphasics showed no progression to the target for consonants.

While the primary deficit underlying many phonemic substitutions in Broca's aphasia is captured in the phonetic aberrations of apraxia of speech, *conduction aphasia* has been seen as an impairment of the phonemic level where linguistic errors are made in the selection of phonemes to be produced. Conduction aphasia is characterized by phonemic paraphasias without deviations of neuromuscular timing. While a deficit in short-term memory (STM) has been proposed as a basis for conduction aphasia by Shallice and Warrington (1977), they acknowledged that their subjects did not exhibit frequent paraphasias. This raises the question of whether their observed dissociation of STM can be attributed to conduction aphasia. Tzortzis and Albert (1974) and Strub and Gardner (1974) argued that the phonemic paraphasias in repetition and spontaneous speech arise from a defective phonological level of verbal formulation. In fact, phonemic paraphasias can occur to such an extent in the repetition of long and uncommon utterances that speech is unintelligible to a degree that is not seen in spontaneous speech. Repetition may place demands on phonological processing that are not as great for the conduction aphasic in spontaneous word formulation. STM weakness may contribute to this problem. As Joanette, et al. (1980) suggested, there may be a decay of phonological targets in the production process. Kertesz (1979) proposed that there are two types of conduction aphasia: an efferent variety with a more anterior lesion and less fluency, and an afferent variety with a more posterior lesion and greater fluency.

AUDITORY COMPREHENSION

The study of receptive processes in aphasia has led to the identification of possible central primary deficits which also account for expressive symptoms. These central deficits lie in the heart of Wepman's integrative levels of function, depicted in Chapter 1. Furthermore, auditory-processing capacities are crucial for communication and for the stimulation of patients in treatment. Schuell's precedents for current approaches to treatment (see Chapter 10) were founded upon her early interest in the auditory capacities of people with aphasia (Schuell, 1953a, 1953b).

Speech Perception

The speech signal is received in the primary auditory zones of both hemispheres, but perception of speech sounds is associated with the secondary auditory zone of the left hemisphere. A basic clinical and research question is whether comprehension deficits *in aphasia* can be attributed to a primary breakdown of speech perception. Wernicke's aphasia is a likely candidate for this possibility. The lesion includes the secondary auditory zone and sometimes the primary zone, and these patients have a serious comprehension problem. Some cases have auditory language test results that are lower than reading test results (Heilman, Rothi, Campanella, et al., 1979; Hier and Mohr, 1977). Luria (1966) had concluded that the primary deficit in sensory or Wernicke's aphasia lies in defective speech-sound discrimination.

However, a unilateral lesion affecting speech perception may not be sufficient to seriously impair language comprehension. In two cases of conduction aphasia, which had only subtle deficits of auditory comprehension, the right-ear response to dichotic stimulation was obliterated by left temporal lobe lesions (Damasio and Damasio, 1980). Finding the door locked in the left hemisphere, the auditory input may have taken another route to the language processor via the right hemisphere.

Speech perception requires recognition of individual phonemes and their sequences at the rapid rate in which they occur in normal speech. Temporal characteristics of stimuli such as *duration* and *sequence* appear to pose problems for people with aphasia. Brain damage in general may retard the rate at which auditory stimuli can be processed (Belmont and Handler, 1971; Van Allen, Benton, and Gordon, 1966). Recognition of the temporal sequence of nonverbal stimuli, such as pure tones and lights, is impaired after brain injury, especially from a lesion in the left hemisphere (Efron, 1963; Carmon and Nachshon, 1971; Swisher and Hirsh, 1972; Brookshire, 1975b). Aphasics are impaired in identifying duration and intensity of pure tones (Needham and Black, 1970). Left-hemisphere damage is sensitive to the time interval between stimulus pairs, as sequences of lights were reported accurately with a 12-second interval but not with a 1.5-second interval (Van Allen, et al., 1966).

The interval needed to perceive that two sounds are present was called the auditory *fusion* threshold by Lackner and Teuber (1973); aphasics had a longer fusion threshold than right-hemisphere-damaged nonaphasics who were equal to normals. Normal adults need only 20 milliseconds between two pure tones in order to report which came first, and this interval appears to be crucial for aphasics. Aphasics can discriminate stimuli at 20- to 60-millisecond intervals but have trouble perceiving their temporal order (Swisher and Hirsh, 1972). Some aphasics need as long as 400 milliseconds to achieve 75 percent accuracy (Efron, 1963). Aphasics were equal to right-hemisphere-damaged and normal controls at 428 milliseconds (almost half a second) but were the only impaired group at short intervals from 8 to 305 milliseconds (Tallal and Newcombe, 1978). Aphasics can perceive the temporal order of two sounds when there is enough time between them.

Speech perception has been tested by presenting syllable or word pairs and asking for same-different judgments, and by presenting a word and asking for a pointing response to pictures which were selected on sound similarity. Speech-perception deficits have been demonstrated with aphasic groups. Perception is better with a 200-millisecond interval between CV syllables, as opposed to the smallest possible interval (Ebbin and Edwards, 1967). Vowel sequences are perceived more readily than CV sequences (Tallal and Newcombe, 1978), and aphasics have particular difficulty when the discrimination is based on temporal cues (Carpenter and Rutherford, 1973). Some left-hemisphere-damaged patients perceive speech better when formant transitions are extended (Tallal and Newcombe, 1978). Aphasics tend to have more difficulty with discriminations based on place of articulation than on voicing (Blumstein, Baker, and Goodglass, 1977; Miceli, Caltagirone, Gainotti, et al., 1978). Broca's aphasics, while they produce phonemic substitution errors based on voicing, are able to perceive the voiced-voiceless distinction (Blumstein, et al., 1977).

The relationship between speech perception deficit and comprehension deficit has been investigated by comparing perception performance to tests of language comprehension and by comparing perception performances among different aphasia syndromes. Some patients who failed a perception test passed the comprehension test from the *Boston Diagnostic Aphasia Examination* (see Chapter 7); and others who passed the perception test failed the comprehension test (Carpenter and Rutherford, 1973). However, several investigators found a significant relationship between perception and comprehension scores, especially with the Token Test described in Chapter 8 (Ebbin and Edwards, 1967; Swisher and Hirsh, 1972; Tallal and Newcombe, 1978). Speech discrimination was not related to Token Test performance in one study (Jauhiainen and Nuutila, 1977), and no clear correspondence with word and sentence comprehension could be found in

another study (Miceli, Gainotti, Caltagirone, et al., 1980). Furthermore, speech perception deficits have not been isolated in Wernicke's aphasia (Blumstein, et al., 1977; Pizzamiglio and Parisi, 1970).

Therefore, comprehension deficit does not necessarily follow from impaired speech perception. Wernicke's aphasia is not unique among other aphasias in ability to perceive speech sounds. Cortical regions which process language semantically and syntactically can receive a clear speech signal from the right hemisphere or can discover the redundancies in a distorted auditory signal. Speech perception impairment as a primary deficit is more likely to occur when the lesion is restricted to the primary auditory zone, producing a disorder more like pure word deafness (Goldblum and Albert, 1972). It is still possible that, in a few cases of aphasia, perceptual impairment and comprehension deficit are the same problem (Carpenter and Rutherford, 1973).

Word Comprehension

Ability to derive meaning from a word is determined by having the patient listen to or read a word and then point to a picture among a few choices. Usually only the most severely impaired patients make many errors to common words at this level, but a patient with anomic aphasia occasionally fails to recognize that a retrieved word was correct. Aphasics' ability at this level is indicated by the performance of 150 subjects on pointing to objects by name in the *Porch Index of Communicative Ability* (Porch, 1967). This test has a sixteen-point scoring scale, shown in Table 7-2. Forty-five of 150 (30 percent) scored 15.00 to 15.99, and 36 (24 percent) scored 14.00 to 14.99. Only 13 aphasic patients (9 percent) averaged totally incorrect responding, 6.00 or less, while 39 percent averaged this error response level or less on naming the same objects. As in confrontation naming, common words are easier to comprehend than uncommon words (Schuell, Jenkins, and Landis, 1961).

Error analysis of picture-pointing tasks has enabled researchers to make inferences about whether word-comprehension difficulties are due to a deficit of auditory coding or of semantic coding. The procedure is to include one incorrect picture which is related phonemically to the stimulus word and another incorrect picture which is related semantically to the stimulus. Additional unrelated choices allow for observation of random incorrect responding. Schuell and Jenkins (1961b) found that aphasics made more semantic errors (59 percent) than either phonemic (21 percent) or random (10 percent) errors. The relationship between type of error and number of errors was similar to picture naming; errors were 100 percent semantic by nineteen patients making one error and 20 percent semantic by four patients making ten to twelve errors. In a similar comprehension task, the tendency to produce semantic errors corresponded with a tendency to produce semantic paraphasias (Gainotti, 1976; Gainotti, Caltagirone, and Ibba, 1975). However, there was no relationship between phonemic comprehension errors and phonemic paraphasias.

A closer look at the semantic dimension was made by Pizzamiglio and Appicciafuoco (1971). They presented three picture choices which varied according to associative strength or semantic relatedness with the correct choice. Errors tended to be the most-related pictures, indicating that patients were conceptually close to the target or were correct when comprehending a word. Also, in what has since become a consistent pattern in the ranking of severity of comprehension deficit, anomic and Broca's aphasics made fewer errors than Wernicke's aphasics. Baker and Goodglass (1979) figured that

Broca's aphasics take a normal amount of time to decode picturable nouns (approximately 200 milliseconds), while Wernicke's aphasics take an abnormally long time to decode these nouns (650 milliseconds).

There are conditions in which aphasics' word comprehension ability can be lowered. Placing a word in a neutral linguistic context at normal speaking rate, as in "You see a *cat* that is nice," makes it harder to comprehend the word *cat* than when it is presented alone (Gardner, Denes, and Weintraub, 1975). However, a word in redundant context, as in "You see a *cat* that is furry," and a word in neutral context at slower speaking rate are of equal difficulty to the word in isolation.

Aphasics' perception of semantic cues in word stress was shown to remain intact (Blumstein and Goodglass, 1972). Subjects recognized the difference between *con*vict and con*vict*, *sore*head and sore *head*, and *white*cap and white *cap*.

Meaning normally extracted from words and sentences goes beyond the direct referential meanings (denotative) depicted by pictures. A host of evaluative and emotional meanings, called "connotative meaning," surround direct referential meaning. Aphasia extends to this expanded level of interpreting linguistic input (Ammon, Moermann, and Guleac, 1977; Doehring and Swisher, 1972). Connotative deficit was correlated with denotative deficit, and anomic aphasics were more impaired in connotative judgment than Broca's and conduction aphasics (Gardner and Denes, 1973).

Short-Term Memory (STM)

Storage capacity and time in working memory (see Chapter 4) become factors in comprehension when words are sequenced into phrases, sentences, and discourse. STM was implicated by Schuell, et al. (1964) to be an impairment in all aphasics, as evidenced by reduced digit repetition and increased comprehension errors as sentences become longer. Since her observations, two basic procedures for the study of STM were developed: (1) the Peterson distractor technique is intended to measure storage *time* in working memory, and (2) free recall of word lists facilitates observation of storage *capacity* and transfer of information to LTM. The traditional clinical measure of short-term storage capacity is digit repetition.

Aphasics have consistently shown a deficit in short-term memory span for digits (DeRenzi and Nichelli, 1975; Weinberg, Diller, Gerstman, et al., 1972). Normals average around seven digits repeated in the order of presentation, called "digit span forward." While previous research has shown that aphasics are worse than right-hemisphere-damaged subjects, Black and Strub (1978) did not find this difference. Right-frontal-damaged nonaphasics were as impaired as the aphasics. Right-posterior-damaged subjects were closer to normal. Sometimes patients are asked to recall the digits in reverse order of presentation (digit span backwards), but normals do just as poorly as brain-damaged persons on this task (Black and Strub, 1978). Whether asked to recall a series of digits, letters, or words, aphasics exhibit a reduction of working memory capacity (Albert, 1976; Cermak and Moreines, 1976; Goodglass, Gleason, and Hyde, 1970; Kim, 1976).

The Peterson distractor technique (Peterson and Peterson, 1959) has demonstrated that information within STM capacity can be held for twenty to thirty seconds without rehearsal or coding applied to this information. This time is determined by having the subject recall a short series of letters or words after a brief time interval placed between the stimulus and response. Rehearsal and coding are assumed to be prohibited by filling the interval with a distracting task such as counting backwards from one hundred by threes. The Peterson procedure demon-

strated that aphasics hold auditory and visual consonant trigrams for less time than normals (Samuels, Butters, Goodglass, et al., 1971).

Some speculation has surrounded whether aphasics' expressive deficits would prohibit rehearsal of information in STM. Recall of drawings representing words which sound alike was not interfered with, as it was in a nonaphasic brain-damaged group (Goodglass, Denes, and Calderon, 1974), suggesting that inner verbal/acoustic coding is not readily available with aphasia. Locke and Deck's (1978) investigation of short-term recall in an undifferentiated group of aphasics indicated that inability to retrieve words reduced ability to maintain information in working memory. Rothi and Hutchinson (1981) employed the Peterson procedure and examined rehearsal by introducing an interval before recall which was not filled by a distractor. Whether or not there was a distractor made no difference in recall by nonfluent aphasics, indicating a failure to rehearse. Fluent aphasics in this study showed improved recall with unfilled delays, indicating an ability to rehearse.

Albert (1976) noted that, when investigating STM capacity in tests of memory span, it is important to distinguish between recall accuracy and sequencing. In pointing to a series of three or four objects out of an array of eighteen objects, aphasics were less accurate than nonaphasic brain-damaged and normal subjects by making more substitution and omission errors. Moreover, aphasics' reduction from normal increased when sequencing errors were considered. Albert considered the sequence of recall to have been impaired enough to be identified as a component of STM deficit.

As a working memory, STM applies constraints within which active processes enable a person to decode sequential linguistic input. One of these processes might be a mental "scanning" of temporal input "from left-to-right." Sternberg (1975) developed an experimental technique for making inferences about how scanning works independent of comprehension, that is, in recognition recall from a series of digits. When presented a series of digits and asked to recognize an item within that series, the subject may scan the mental representation of the stimulus series. The theoretical assumptions, methodology, and interpretation of results require some time to explain; so it is instead noted simply that STM scanning has been investigated with aphasics as a potential basis for comprehension deficit. In one study, aphasics' rate of scanning was reduced and their manner of scanning was different from normals (Swinney and Taylor, 1971). In a subsequent study, aphasics again scanned items at a slower rate than normal but their manner of scanning was not different (Warren, Hubbard, and Knox, 1977).

Because the processes of comprehension are assumed to occur in working memory, comprehension deficit ought to be related to STM deficit. However, STM has not been compared to comprehension in aphasia to the extent that perception has been, a situation which has not changed much since Flowers (1975) observed that "little experimental evidence is available to indicate the degree to which short-term recall deficit, in and of itself, can cause a communication problem" (p. 67). Aphasic immediate recall performances have been correlated significantly with tests of comprehension (Heilman, Scholes, and Watson, 1976; Lesser, 1976). Brookshire (1974, 1978b) has speculated about a few bases for comprehension disorders that are related to information decay in STM ("noise buildup"), information loss ("retention deficit"), and shrinking capacity ("information capacity deficit"). These hypothetical primary deficits have been explained with respect to possible Token Test performances. DeRenzi, Faglioni, and Previdi (1978) coupled the Peterson distractor technique with Token

Test stimuli and found that the filled delay seriously impeded aphasics' comprehension. Aphasic comprehension appears to be susceptible to decay of the mental representation of linguistic stimuli. However, STM deficit need not have a pronounced effect on auditory comprehension (Kim, 1976; Saffran and Marin, 1975).

The intimate relationship between STM and comprehension may be seen, not only as an STM deficit being the basis for a language disorder, but also as a language disorder being the basis for STM deficit. This has been suggested already with the idea that verbal formulation impairment may prohibit rehearsal. It is indicated also by STM deficit only for verbal material, while memory for nonverbal material which is difficult to label, such as abstract geometric shapes, is spared. This dissociation of verbal STM from nonverbal STM in aphasia has been demonstrated by Butters, et al. (1970) and Cermak and Tarlow (1978), and has been demonstrated with left anterior temporal lobectomy by Samuels, et al. (1972).

A few cases have been analyzed in which a dissociation of STM from long-term memory, "selective impairment of short-term memory," has been described (Saffran and Marin, 1975; Warrington and Shallice, 1969). In these cases, auditory language comprehension was only mildly impaired. In fact, these cases were described as having adequate comprehension and verbal expression but an impairment of verbal repetition. Based on this observation, STM deficit has been offered as the primary deficit underlying conduction aphasia (Shallice and Warrington, 1977). Another explanation of this disorder, phonological processing, was cited previously here. One problem with some of the evidence for the STM theory is that phonemic paraphasia, the other characteristic symptom of conduction aphasia, has been ignored in descriptions of cases. Saffran and Marin's (1975) description of repetition errors did not include this symptom. Furthermore, Broca's aphasics have shown a reduction of digit span which was equal to that in conduction aphasics, so that there is some question as to whether the latter syndrome is unique (Heilman, et al., 1976). However, a comprehensive investigation of one conduction aphasic was suggestive of limited auditory STM as being the only explanation of performances (Caramazza, Basili, Koller, et al., 1981). Caramazza, et al. concluded that auditory STM deficits account for conduction aphasia when the phonological output disorder is minimal. Also, STM deficit may be one aspect of this disorder, by way of its interaction with verbal formulation at the phonological level.

A third explanation of conduction aphasia has a more traditional tone: that it is a disconnection between auditory and motor images of words. The argument for this theory was based on a series of studies with delayed auditory feedback (DAF) during speaking (Chapin, Blumstein, Meissner, et al., 1981). Under DAF, the subject speaks or reads aloud while his own voice is heard through headphones, with a delay of a few hundred milliseconds. Normally DAF disrupts speaking considerably. Consistently, conduction aphasics have been least affected among normals and other types of aphasia.

Sentence Comprehension

Sentence comprehension is one of the most thoroughly investigated functions in clinical aphasiology. The experimenter can manipulate a wide variety of variables including rate, length, and structure. Variations in aphasic performance as a function of these manipulations are of interest to the clinician, who employs them in order to create treatment tasks which can be processed adequately by the patient (Darley, 1982). One orientation in this research is simply to study aphasics as one undifferentiated population, which permits conclusions about aphasia in general. This was satisfactory for a while because it was believed, in spite of qualitative differences in expressive symptoms, that aphasics differ among each other only in degree of comprehension deficit. However, another research orientation is now to see if the syndromes are qualitatively different in comprehension deficit.

Rate and Delayed Response. Slowing down the rate of word presentation has helped aphasics increase their sequential memory span (Cermak and Moreines, 1976; Weidner and Lasky, 1976). Also, it has resulted in better sentence comprehension (Lasky, Weidner, and Johnson, 1976; Weidner and Lasky, 1976). Pauses inserted between major constituents of a sentence have enhanced comprehension (Laskey, et al., 1976; Liles and Brookshire, 1975), but temporal expansion did not improve performance on the *Revised Token Test* (Blanchard and Prescott, 1980).

Several investigators have wondered whether delaying the patient's response would improve comprehension. It did not improve short-term recall of nonfluent aphasics but did help fluent aphasics (Rothi and Hutchinson, 1981). Undistracted delays were of no help to comprehension in studies by DeRenzi, et al. (1978) and Toppin and Brookshire (1978). Yorkston, Marshall, and Butler (1977), however, found that imposing a five-to-ten-second delay reduced anticipatory errors in following Token Test instructions. Therefore, delay may help only patients who impulsively initiate a response before the stimulus is presented completely.

Complexity. Comprehension becomes less accurate when sentences are more complex syntactically. One common method for identifying problems with particular grammatical features is the two-picture or four-picture choice. Incorrect choices are designed with respect to the feature being tested. For example, a test of understanding past tense would include the sentence *The boy swam* and two pictures, one representing the boy swimming (Parisi and Pizzamiglio, 1970). A test of passive voice, as in *The cat is chased by the dog,* would include a picture of the cat chasing the dog as well as a representation of the correct choice.

This analytical approach to sentence comprehension was prompted by the identification of syntactic rules in transformational grammar. Because the comprehension process once was thought to be shaped by transformational rules, aphasics' rank order of difficulty with different syntactic structures was considered to be indicative of the way in which their comprehension process is functioning. Although some structures were harder than others for aphasics to comprehend, the rank order of difficulty and type of errors were found to be similar to normals (Shewan and Canter, 1971; Shewan, 1976a). Also, syndromes of Broca's, Wernicke's, and anomic aphasia, while differing in degree of impairment, did not differ from each other in rank order of difficulty (Parisi and Pizzamiglio, 1970; Shewan and Canter, 1971). It was concluded that the syndromes do not differ from each other qualitatively but do differ quantitatively. Anomic aphasia possesses the best comprehension and Wernicke's aphasia the worst among these three syndromes.

In tests of sentence comprehension, aphasic patients may tend to utilize a simplified strategy which results in specific comprehension failures. Aphasics have shown difficulties comprehending past and future tense and passive sentences. Pierce (1979) concluded that patients assume a sentence is in present tense and assume that an underlying agent-action-order is represented in any noun-verb-noun surface form. Later, Pierce (1981) found that high and low-comprehending aphasics comprehend tense better when additional markers are added to the surface structure, as in "The man *has* combed his hair."

Asking subjects to decide whether a sentence is true or false relative to a picture is the procedure which was used to determine that normals possess the following order of difficulty among four basic sentence types: the easiest, simple active affirmatives (*The boy is chasing the girl*); then passive affirmatives (*The girl is chased by the boy*); then active negatives (*The boy is not chasing the girl*); and the most difficult, passive-negatives (*The girl is not chased by the boy*). Transformational complexity could not account for negatives taking longer to comprehend than passives, nor could it account for regular differences between true and false conditions. A different approach to prediction and explanation arose, called "information processing," in which the crucial parameter has been correct response latency, during which certain mental operations are assumed to occur in temporal sequence. Stimulus coding and constituent comparison were considered to be two stages of cognitive processing underlying sentence verification performance (Carpenter and Just, 1975).

Investigators have usually focused on either negative sentences or passive sentences in their studies. In the simple verification of affirmative statements such as *This is a dog,* aphasics took longer for false statements than for true statements (West, Gelfer, and Rosen, 1978). In the verification of negative statements, aphasic subjects broke down at certain stages of the coding and comparison process (Just, Davis, and Carpenter, 1977). In a study of affirmative and passive sentences, Brookshire and Nicholas (1980) analyzed aphasic processes with respect to two types of false sentence judgment. An active or passive statement could be false when, in the picture, the subject and object are reversed relative to the sentence presented; response time reflects a decision about word order. The statement could also be false relative to identity of the subject, verb, or object used in the picture; response time reflects a semantic decision regarding one constituent in the sentence. Ten aphasics with a minimum *PICA* overall percentile of 51 (four subjects above 90) exhibited the same response time pattern as normals but took much longer than normals to comprehend.

Persons with aphasia have particular difficulty comprehending negation. Using another verification paradigm, Elmore-Nicholas and Brookshire (1981) examined several variables, and negation had the strongest effect. Wilcox, Davis, and Leonard (1978) concluded that the problem lies, not necessarily in the presence of a negative marker in surface structure, but rather lies in the communicative intent of denial or negation. Negative intent does not require a negative marker in surface structure. In natural context, the affirmative *Must you bite the pen?* implies that a person should *not* bite the pen. Aphasics had distinct problems comprehending such utterances, while having little difficulty comprehending negative structures (*Won't you close the door?*) with affirmative intent. Most picture-choice and sentence-verification studies examine this feature with negative surface form and negative intent coinciding.

Differences among Syndromes. While several investigators were suggesting that syndromes differ quantitatively but not qualitatively in comprehension, Luria (1966, 1970b) had proposed that inaccurate and inefficient comprehension may be derived from different primary deficits. Comprehension problems could be due to an impairment of speech perception or to an impairment of special processes designed to handle certain grammatical relationships, such as prepositional phrases or constructions such as "father's brother." Luria looked upon the latter problem as a disruption of the "simultaneous synthe-sis" of constituents into a single idea; that is, "father's brother" means "uncle." Most of the research into distinct primary deficits, however, has focused on the dissociation between syntactic and semantic categories of receptive processing. A double dissociation has been observed in expressive symptoms, with word retrieval better than syntax in patients with anterior lesions and syntax spared in anomic aphasics with posterior lesions. Regarding comprehension, attention has centered around comprehension in agrammatic or Broca's aphasia: Can the comprehension of these patients also be characterized as agrammatic?

Several essays by Edgar Zurif, Alfonso Caramazza, and their colleagues have presented the argument that syntactic and semantic processes can be dissociated from each other in aphasia (Berndt and Caramazza, 1980, 1981; Bradley, Garrett, and Zurif, 1980; Caramazza and Berndt, 1978; Zurif, 1980; Zurif, Green, Caramazza, and Goodenough, 1976; Zurif and Caramazza, 1976). Studies have included comparisons between Broca's and posterior fluent aphasias (usually Wernicke's and conduction) or have focused solely on Broca's aphasia. Stimuli have included spoken and printed words and, therefore, have had implications for reading as well as auditory comprehension (Caramazza, Berndt, and Hart, 1981). Investigators have assumed that syntactic processes can be observed somewhat independently from semantic processes in two ways: (1) picture-choice tasks in which decisions are based on word order or semantic content, as in Brookshire and Nicholas' verification study, and (2) examination of responses to functors, or closed-class words, in comparison to substantive words, or open-class words.

Comparison of syndromes with respect to word order and semantic content started with fairly complex sentences. Five Broca's and five conduction aphasics were able to comprehend *The apple that the boy is eating is red,* in which the two subjects, *apple* and *boy,* are identified based on semantic and word-order constraints (Caramazza and Zurif, 1976). However, both types of aphasia had difficulty comprehending *The boy that the girl is chasing is tall,* in which the two subjects, *boy* and *girl,* are identified with respect to order only. This is called a *reversible* relationship, because the two subjects could be reversed and the sentence would still make sense. Both groups also dropped in performance when the picture foil represented a change in word order relative to picture foils representing a substitution of a lexical item. Five Wernicke's aphasics were impaired across all conditions. The same pattern was found by Heilman and Scholes (1976) with sentences containing direct and indirect object relations and picture-choices containing foils based on word order and lexical selection. In both of these studies, a dissociation of syntax in comprehension was found in Broca's and conduction aphasia.

Dissociation of syntax continued to be uncovered in this way with "anterior" aphasics (Samuels and Benson, 1979) and Broca's aphasics (Schwartz, Saffran, and Marin, 1980). Schwartz, et al. did not compare their five subjects with other groups, but they found that their subjects had difficulty with reversible locative statements such as *The square is on top of the circle.* Most of the errors were by far in the selection of the picture with reversal of subject and object order. Syntactic decision deficit in Broca's aphasia occurred in reading as well as in auditory comprehension, a result to be expected if aphasia indeed is a central disorder (Samuels and Benson, 1979).

Studies with reversible statements point to the notion that Broca's aphasics rely heavily on semantic and pragmatic information to understand sentences. When word order is depended upon, however, their comprehension is weakened. Deloche and Seron (1981) used reversible

sentences in a reading task to examine whether semantic/pragmatic plausibility is of assistance to the aphasic. The subjects were presented with sentences that were plausible (*The patient calls the nurse*) and sentences that were implausible (*The thief arrests the policeman*). First, plausible sentences were easier to comprehend than implausible sentences for a mixed group of forty-three aphasic subjects. Then twelve Broca's aphasics were compared with ten Wernicke's, and the Broca's were assisted by plausibility, while the Wernicke's were not. It is not clear from this analysis whether the Broca's aphasics were unique with respect to the other twenty-one aphasics studied.

Zurif (1980; Bradley, Garrett, and Zurif, 1980) was concerned that STM constraints might have confounded the results with the long and complex sentences of Caramazza and Zurif (1976) and Heilman and Scholes (1976). STM had already been minimized in studies of printed word sorting (Zurif, Caramazza, and Myerson, 1972; Von Stockert, 1972; Von Stockert and Bader, 1976; Kolk, 1978). In these studies, Broca's aphasics were unable to use functors (*a, the*) to mark constituent boundaries. They tended to group substantive words together (Zurif, et al., 1972). These studies were among the first to indicate that a central deficit of syntactic processing might be responsible for agrammatic expression and, possibly, agrammatic comprehension. Grossman (1980) broadened the notion of separation of syntax even further to include problems with a nonverbal task requiring the replication from memory of hierarchically arranged tongue depressors. Seven Broca's aphasics were unable to replicate hierarchical arrangements, while eight fluent aphasics could do so. This result was suggestive of a general cognitive deficit in a realm which coincides with the structuring of sentences.

Several studies have pointed to a problem in dealing with functors which may be unique to Broca's aphasia. In the only study so far which compared this syndrome with anomic aphasia, Goodenough created a unique paradigm to measure sensitivity to the subtle semantic nuances of articles (Goodenough, Zurif, Weintraub, et al., 1977). Subjects were shown three figures on three response buttons: for example, a white circle, a black circle, and a black square. They were given pointing instructions in which use of the article was either appropriate (*Press the white one, . . . the square one*) or inappropriate (*Press the black one, . . . the round one*). Anomics took longer to respond to the inappropriate than to the appropriate instructions, indicative of the additional processing involved in an ambiguous instruction (. . . *the black one*, when there were two black ones). Broca's aphasics showed no such response time difference. This was one of the first direct indications that Broca's aphasia involves a receptive problem with functors which corresponds to omission of these words in verbal expression.

Further investigation of functors involved measuring reaction time to recognition of closed (functors) and open (nouns, verbs)-class words (Zurif, 1980; Bradley, Garrett, and Zurif, 1980). Broca's aphasics did not exhibit a response-time distinction between closed and open-class words that had been shown with normals; also, three of four posterior aphasics displayed the normal pattern. Swinney, Zurif, and Cutler (1980) used a variation of the phoneme-monitoring technique to see if eight Broca's aphasics continued to be insensitive to functors within sentences. In psycholinguistic research, the subject is asked to listen for a phoneme in a sentence and to press a button when it is heard. Response time is indicative of processing load at the point of phoneme occurrence. In this study of aphasia, words were targets of attention instead of phonemes. Normals did not respond differently to open and closed-class words,

while Broca's aphasics responded faster to open-class words than to closed-class words.

One other aspect of verbal expression in Broca's aphasia appeared to have been reflected in comprehension (Goodglass, Blumstein, Gleason, et al., 1979). An adaptive strategy was described earlier in this chapter in which the patient tends to sequence ideas (concatenation) instead of embedding them. Twelve Broca's aphasics were compared with five Wernicke's and five conduction aphasics. Sentences such as *The man greeted by his wife was smoking a pipe* were harder to comprehend than longer sentences such as *The man was greeted by his wife and he was smoking his pipe*. However, this was a main effect across all groups; the effect was concluded to have been greater in Broca's aphasia based on "a near significant interaction" (p. 206).

A few studies indicate that Broca's aphasia may not involve a unique deficit in syntactic comprehension:

1. Twenty-two Wernicke's aphasics had the same error pattern as twenty-two Broca's aphasics in comprehending agent-action-object sentences; both groups made fewer errors to irreversible than to reversible sentences; both groups comprehended plausible sentences better than implausible ones (Heeschen, 1980).

2. In a word-sorting task, ten Broca's aphasics understood basic subject-verb-object order and the difference between articles and nouns; they had difficulty with subject-verb agreement (Gallaher, 1981).

3. Eleven Broca's aphasics were able to distinguish between " . . . Bill walking *the* dog" and " . . . Bill *the* walking dog" (Caplan, Matthei, and Gigley, 1981). These results and those of Gallaher are not necessarily contradictory to the results with black and white circles and squares and with reaction time. Insensitivity to functors may be revealed only by subtle parameters such as reaction time and in situations with minimal semantic and extralinguistic cues.

4. In a version of the Token Test in which syntactic and semantic errors could be identified, fluent and nonfluent subjects did not differ in their tendencies to make these types of error (Mack, 1981).

Like all syndromes of aphasia, Broca's aphasia includes a comprehension deficit. Zurif and Caramazza have developed ingenious methods for indicating that this comprehension deficit may be similar to agrammatic expression and, therefore, is derived from a central deficit to processes characterized as syntactic. The status of this theory is equivocal. The uniqueness of Broca's aphasia has not been supported impressively, either because other aphasics have been similar or because Broca's subjects were not compared with other syndromes in some of the studies. Caramazza, Basili, et al. (1981), however, suggested that asyntactic comprehension in conduction aphasia is due to an STM deficit because these patients do not have expressive grammatical deficits. Therefore, Broca's and conduction aphasics may make similar errors for different reasons. Direct comparison between evidence and counter-evidence is prohibited by dissimilar experimental procedures, and so the different results cannot be viewed as being contradictory. They indicate that the syntactic deficit may appear only in certain situations. Adding to the bright future for stimulating debate is a different theory, namely, that Broca's aphasia can be attributed to a centralized deficit in phonological processing (Kean, 1978, 1979, 1980).

Prepositions

Comprehension of locatives has usually been studied with a task of following instructions in which the subject places an object in a spatial relationship to another object (Smith, 1974a). Certain patients may have particular difficulty in comprehending locatives. Seron and Deloche (1981) examined the influence of "contextual bias" on following instructions with *in, on,* and *under.* That is, a movable object

such as a coin is more likely to be placed "in" a money box rather than "on" or "under" it. Experiential and perceptual/motor constraints make some spatial relationships more likely than others. Broca's aphasics were more accurate when the preposition was congruent with the contextual bias inherent in object pairs than when the preposition was incongruent with object pairs. Contextual bias had a positive influence when meaningful and specially constructed abstract objects were used. Wernicke's aphasics were helped by contextual bias only with the perceptual/motor constraints of abstract objects. Broca's aphasics, therefore, utilized the semantic cues contained in meaningful object pairs, while Wernicke's aphasics did not use these cues.

Comprehension in Context

In natural communicative situations people do not respond to words and sentences in isolation, but rather comprehend sentences amidst a linguistic context of other sentences and an extralinguistic context consisting of the perceived situation. Comprehension by aphasics is tested outside of these contexts in order to focus on the patient's problem with processing language. However, if we are to understand the impact of this disorder upon the natural use of language, we should observe more functional communication in which these contexts are present.

In order to study aphasics' use of context in the comprehension of sentences, the experimenter should create a condition in which a correct response to a sentence depends upon integration of the sentence with its context. To create this contingency, the experimenter takes advantage of the common communicative phenomenon in which what is stated is not quite what the speaker means. Metaphor is a prime example. The statement "He lost his shirt" in the context of a poker game means something other than the literal interpretation of the utterance. The interpretation "He lost all his money" is possible only with integration of context and the statement. Aphasics have demonstrated an ability to identify metaphorical interpretations of utterances by pointing to pictures (Winner and Gardner, 1977). Searle (1969) referred to two components of meaning in natural communication: (1) the literal interpretation of a proposition and (2) the illocutionary force or intent of the proposition. He considered intentions, called "speech acts," to be the basic units of communication.

Comprehension of discourse is often studied by having subjects comprehend paragraphs or text. Stachowiak, Huber, Poeck, et al. (1977) examined aphasics' comprehension of a sentence in the linguistic context of a short paragraph which was read to them. The linguistic context described a situation such as a poker game. Each paragraph contained six sentences, and the fourth sentence was an idiomatic comment such as "The others strip him right down to his shirt" which referred to prior context. The fifth sentence completed the story ("His wife gets quite annoyed"). With response based on a five-picture choice, the last sentence was "Which picture shows what happened to him?" One picture represented the correct response to the intent of the fourth statement ("They take all of his money"). Another picture represented literal interpretation of the metaphor. Half of twenty-six stories contained intended and literal interpretations that were similar, and half contained dissimilar interpretations.

Seventy-six West German aphasic subjects comprehended as well as normal controls and had the same pattern of metaphorical errors. Aphasics were able to use "verbal contextualization" or integration of sentences in order to comprehend the intent of idioms with a clearly different literal interpretation, such as "He filled his soup with pieces of bread" meaning "He got himself into a nice mess." Although Broca's and anomic aphasics comprehended more accurately than Wernicke's and global aphasics, each group exhibited the same pattern of interpretation errors. This ability to comprehend textual themes was contrasted with a distinct deficit in acontextual language comprehension with the Token Test.

Aphasics also are able to comprehend the conveyed or intended meaning of utterances by utilizing natural extralinguistic context. Wilcox, Davis, and Leonard (1978) had eighteen aphasics observe videotaped interactions between a speaker and a listener who made appropriate and inappropriate responses to the speaker's indirect requests. The speaker, waiting at a closed door with arms loaded with books, would ask "Can you open the door?" The inappropriate literal interpretation was "Yes" with no attempt to open the door. The appropriate response to the conveyed meaning relative to the situation was for the listener to open the door. Using a variety of indirect requests, Wilcox, et al. presented an equal number of inappropriate and appropriate responses, a total of eighty videotaped interactions. Subjects were to indicate by a *yes* or *no* whether the listener made the correct response. Aphasics, judged as high and low-level comprehenders based on standard language-comprehension tests, were able to identify conveyed meaning in nearly all conditions. They had difficulty in conditions where the intent was denial or negation. Experimental task scores were not correlated with scores on a standard comprehension test battery, indicating a lack of relationship between clinical performance and comprehension in natural context.

Global Aphasia

The most severely impaired patients exhibit serious limitations in even the usually least-impaired modality, namely, auditory language comprehension. Because treatment is designed to capitalize upon spared communicative abilities, the retention of comprehension capacities in global aphasia has received some attention. What do global aphasics possess buried deep within their ostensible deficits that can be used in treatment and, eventually, for improved communication?

Boller and Green (1972; Green and Boller, 1974) determined that severely impaired Wernicke's and global aphasics were able to distinguish between familiar English and meaningless speech, and could distinguish among types of requests. Though responses were rarely correct, the subjects gave appropriate kinds of responses to yes/no questions, requests for information, and commands. That is, they indicated yes or no to questions and responded to commands with body movement. Boller and Green concluded that these patients retain a rudimentary level of comprehension. The distinction between correctness and appropriateness was again employed by Boller and his colleagues to see if severely impaired patients are responsive to emotional commands, questions, and requests for information. Accuracy was low, as six of eight severely impaired subjects gave the correct response on 33 percent or less of the trials. However, emotional stimuli such as ''Are you an alcoholic?'' resulted in more appropriate responses and behavioral changes than neutral stimuli such as ''Are you an American?'' Overall scores which included correctness as a criterion were higher for emotional stimuli (Boller, Cole, Vrtunski, et al., 1979).

Word comprehension was examined by Wapner and Gardner (1979) with fourteen global aphasics who had scored below the mean for aphasia on the auditory comprehension section of the *Boston Diagnostic Aphasia Examination* (see Chapter 7). Subjects were asked to point to locations on a map of the United States and to objects in a picture of a room. High and low-frequency names were included. Additional

stimuli included words from the same semantic categories not represented in the pictures and also nonsense words. Regarding the pictured lexical items, six patients scored 50 percent correct or better on the map compared to four patients on the room, which was above chance. The map was easier across all types of lexical stimuli. Word frequency made a difference, as high-frequency names were easier. These patients also were better at rejecting inappropriate words than at identifying the pictured words. One explanation for better performance with a map was the possible use of right-hemisphere visuospatial abilities in selecting items identified by location.

Given that global aphasia involves minimal linguistic performance with which to make inferences about retention of prerequisite cognitive capacities, several investigators employed nonverbal symbol systems in order to see if these capacities remain (Baker, Berry, Gardner, et al., 1975; Gardner, Zurif, Berry, et al., 1976; Glass, Gazzaniga, and Premack, 1973). Patients were trained primarily to comprehend statements, questions, and commands constructed out of symbols arranged in syntactic order. Glass, et al. used cutout paper symbols similar to those developed by Premack for chimpanzees. Baker, Gardner, and their coworkers developed a system for aphasics called Visual Communication, or *VIC*. In both projects, global aphasics exhibited certain cognitive capacities related to natural language: (1) understanding the representational function of symbols and relations among symbols such as actor-action-object, (2) ability to answer questions and follow commands, and (3) a limited ability to express needs and feelings.

READING

In spite of the fact that reading deficit in aphasia simply reflects the central linguistic disruptions which produce auditory language problems, reading poses its own special problems. Reading can be thought of as involving transcoding a graphemic code into an auditory code as an initial step in the process. Also, reading problems of aphasics have been studied frequently by having subjects read aloud instead of by having them read for comprehension.

When Schuell and Jenkins (1961b) studied auditory word comprehension, they also looked at visual word comprehension. Errors exhibited a pattern similar to errors for auditory comprehension: 52 percent semantically related pictures, 21 percent pictures for visually similar words, and 20 percent pictures for auditorily similar words. Therefore, in comprehension, semantic confusion dominated as in the other receptive modality. However, the pattern changed for matching a printed word to a spoken word. Only 37 percent errors were semantic, while 46 percent were with visually similar words. This task appears to have tapped into a more peripheral level of processing rather than the semantic level in comprehension.

The reading aloud of words has indicated that there are three levels of paralexia (Marshall and Newcombe, 1973): *visual* (saying "bug" instead of *dug*); *surface* (saying "face" instead of phase); and *deep* (saying "eggs" instead of *hen,* "bird" instead of *robin*). Deep dyslexia is most often associated with aphasia. These semantic paralexias have been studied mostly in cases of Broca's aphasia and have been explained as an internal transcoding disorder, that is, a problem in grapheme-phoneme conversion (Patterson and Marcel, 1977; Saffran, Schwartz, and Marin, 1976; and Shallice and Warrington, 1975). The path to phonemic coding may be blocked, and the semantic error may come from intact semantic memory but lack of phonological representation to facilitate the verbal response (Saffran, et al., 1976). Deep dyslexia for reading aloud is sometimes called *phonemic dyslexia.*

Patterson (1979) explored further the deep dyslexia in two patients with agrammatism. He pointed out that patients can comprehend higher levels of graphic language than they can read aloud. Also, he emphasized the positive side of looking at reading deficits, especially relative to comprehending sentences from the "Silly Sentences Test." In this test, the patients made true-false judgments about sentences such as "Prime ministers have feathers." Although the aphasics were deficient when compared with normals, the two subjects correctly understood 85 percent and 91 percent of the sentences.

Caramazza, Berndt, and Hart (1981) argued that "receptive agrammatism" may be a more comprehensive account of reading deficit in Broca's aphasia. Anterior aphasics comprehended words better than posterior aphasics (Gardner, 1974a), but anteriors and posteriors (mostly anomic) were comparable in their sensitivity to errors in printed sentences (Gardner, Denes, and Zurif, 1975). Dissociation of syntax was shown to exist in reading and auditory comprehension (Samuels and Benson, 1979), and the word-sorting studies with Broca's aphasia involved reading. Broca's aphasics have more trouble reading aloud functors than substantive words (Andreewsky and Seron, 1975; Friederici and Schoenle, 1980). However, Wernicke's and global aphasics also have more trouble reading aloud functors (Gardner and Zurif, 1975). As noted before, Broca's aphasics were sensitive to semantic plausibility when reading reversible sentences for comprehension (Deloche and Seron, 1981).

WRITING

When hemiplegia does not keep linguistic deficits from being displayed, symptoms in aphasic writing correspond to symptoms in speech (Goodglass and Hunter, 1970; Ulatowska, Hildebrand, and Haynes, 1978). However, impaired writing is generally less complex than the pattern of verbal expression. Ulatowska, et al. concluded that aphasic writing can achieve a high level of communicative adequacy in spite of limited sentence structure. When writing descriptions of pictures, patients may exhibit in-class semantic paraphasias but intended meaning can be determined (Ulatowska, Baker, and Stern, 1979).

Aphasics make spelling errors when writing words. Wapner and Gardner (1979b) found that anterior and posterior patients differ as to type of error. The former tend to derive errors from a visual image of the word, while the latter tend to make errors based on the word's sound structure. In another study, Wernicke's aphasics were equally impaired in oral and written spelling. Some Broca's aphasics were better with oral spelling; others were better with written spelling (Friederici, Schoenle, and Goodglass, 1981).

CONCLUSIONS FOR THE CLINICIAN

We are still most confident about defining primary deficits in terms of observed functions rather than in terms of the unobservable processes underlying these functions. Deficits to be treated usually are defined as problems of auditory comprehension, reading, verbal expression, and writing. Central language deficits of aphasia are separated from modality-specific sensory and motor problems. Some further differentiation is commonly made for the aphasic patient with respect to underlying processes. Treatment programs might be addressed to speech discrimination and short-term memory capacity and sequencing. Expressive symptoms such as anomia and agrammatism are targeted for treatment. However, much of the research surveyed in this chapter has been directed toward identifying the hidden processes responsible for different symptom patterns. Someday a

patient's primary deficit may be identified as a disorganization or constriction of semantic memory, an impaired central syntactic processor, an impaired phonological system for verbal expression, and so on.

Clinical aphasiologists can find immediate application for treatment in investigations which reveal variables along which a patient's ease of processing can be manipulated. These variables include the number of surface-structure cues to semantic interpretation (Pierce, 1981), the semantic/pragmatic plausibility of sentences (Deloche and Seron, 1981), and the congruence of prepositions with the pragmatic and perceptual/motor context of objects manipulated in following instructions (Seron and Deloche, 1981).

More research needs to be done before some of the proposed cognitive bases for different symptom patterns can be used clinically for diagnosis and for planning treatment. Nevertheless, the clinician should always be suspicious of the possible existence of these primary deficits because this awareness may favorably influence treatment strategies. Research methodologies provide the means for identification and for the exercise of these processes. Current assessment procedures were born as experimental procedures. One of the directions of future theory development will be the identification of processes underlying the symptomatology which is presently categorized with linguistic labels. The possibility of a central syntactic deficit underlying Broca's aphasia is one example. Zurif (1980), who has argued for the identification of this primary deficit, has advocated some caution by noting that "... this limitation still needs to be defined in terms of the processes involved" (p. 308). Although there have been some methodological weaknesses which weaken some conclusions, the established march toward a better understanding of aphasia should be encouraged because of its potential for enhancement of services to the aphasic patient.

6 Principles of Diagnosis and Assessment

The basic purpose of diagnosis and assessment in clinical aphasiology is to plan the beginning and direction of speech and language treatment. First, the clinician decides whether the patient is a candidate for treatment. If treatment is appropriate, the clinician then decides on the approach to treatment. The clinician may decide that some symptoms warrant specific speech or language treatment, while other symptoms warrant a referral to where the most appropriate management can be provided. Other objectives include predicting the amount and rate of recovery and measuring recovery with repeated formal examination. Results of regular testing, moreover, may signal the need for modification of treatment plans. Thus diagnosis and assessment are an integral part of the treatment process and, in effect, comprise the first step of treatment.

Diagnosis and assessment are somewhat different shades of the decision-making process for meeting these objectives. *Diagnosis* pertains to identification of the presence of a disorder and of the type of disorder that is present. Identifying type of disorder involves considering differences among similar possible disorders, called differential diagnosis. *Assessment,* also called appraisal, becomes paramount once the disorder has been identified. The several components of aphasia should be identified and the various levels of deficit determined. Assessment is directed primarily toward preparing a plan of treatment.

SOURCES OF INFORMATION

In addition to observation of the language deficit, information about medical history and current etiology is applied to differential diagnosis and assessment.

Personal History

Personal history includes educational and occupational background, avocational interests, premorbid personality, and family structure and history. In most clinical settings this information is obtained from the patient and family members. When the clinician has access to medical records in the hospital or nursing facility, some of this information may be available from reports by a social worker. Information needed for diagnosis and assessment should be obtained first. Informal assessment is facilitated when the clinician possesses correct background about age, address, family names, and occupation, so that the clinician can check on the patient's accuracy in talking about these topics or in responding to questions about them.

Educational, occupational, and recreational interests can be a gross indication of level, modes, and frequency of language usage prior to onset of aphasia. Individual style of language use can be inferred from spared language and from level of frustration relative to degree of impairment. That is, high frustration with a mild impairment suggests that a great deal of importance was attached to premorbid language skills, and minimal frustration with a mild impairment suggests that linguistic precision may not have been of much concern. Also, levels and styles of language can be inferred from observing the spouse and asking him or her about the patient's talking preferences.

Medical Information

Medical history and current medical information are obtained from the medical records where the patient was hospitalized during the acute phase of his aphasia or from the records of the patient's personal physician. When working in a hospital, the clinician may read reports regarding the current hospitalization in the *medical chart,* which may be kept on a transportable rack in the nurses' station of the patient's ward. Previous medical history sometimes is kept in the nurses' station, filed separately in a cabinet. In a hospital the clinician has easy access to complete medical information. Several sources of medical information are used for diagnosis, prognosis, treatment planning, and monitoring performance during treatment. These include the medical history, results of neurological examination and laboratory tests, nursing notes, doctor's orders, and doctor's progress notes.

The *medical history,* which may be summarized in the current chart and is detailed in filed records, is helpful for prob-

lem identification and prognosis. For problem identification, the patient may exhibit symptoms which may be accounted for by etiologies which occurred prior to the current reason for hospitalization. A patient may have suffered more than one stroke, with the most recent stroke producing aphasia and a previous stroke having produced disorientation. Prognosis for recovery of language might be less encouraging because of the complicating condition produced by the previous stroke, and the existence of multiple strokes increases the likelihood that the patient may suffer still another stroke. A valuable source of information concerning prior conditions is the discharge summaries from previous hospitalizations.

With evidence of more than one neurological insult occurring at different times, the clinician should attempt to sort out which symptoms originate from which insult. Speech or language deficits resulting from the most recent cause might have a better chance for recovery than speech or language deficits resulting from prior damage. This sorting process is done by reviewing records of clinical evaluation and management subsequent to previous damage and by interviewing the patient, if possible, and family members concerning when symptoms were observed for the first time.

Complicating conditions may interfere with recovery by reducing the ability of the central nervous system to adjust to the most recent damage and by reducing the patient's ability to undergo the rigors of standard speech or language treatment. These conditions include heart disease, arteriosclerosis, diabetes, arthritis, alcoholism, and neurosis or psychosis. The elderly population is especially susceptible to these illnesses.

Description and results of the *neurological examination* and *laboratory tests* indicate the existence of neurological impairments in addition to aphasia and provide evidence for the type, location, and size of the lesion. EEG, angiography, brain scan, and CT scan were introduced in Chapter 3. Whenever applicable, the clinician should also look for *surgical reports* which indicate location of lesion and, in the case of removing a tumor, prognosis based on success in getting to malignant tissue. Complete assessment of the range of possible cognitive and emotional deficits is available from the report of a neuropsychological examination. Evidence of type, location, and extent of etiology is useful for anticipating the pattern of aphasia and for prognosis. Date of onset, especially with CVAs, traumatic injuries, and surgery, is also important for prognosis.

The *doctor's orders* generally appear near the front of the current medical chart. They are an outline of the primary care physician's plan of treatment. The physician lists the medications and therapeutic services which the patient is to receive in the hospital. Referrals are prepared based on this list.

Nursing notes, doctor's progress notes, and notes from other hospital services provide much descriptive information concerning the patient's medical status and progress, emotional state, and general behavior. Nursing notes indicate how the patient is functioning in the hospital environment and may provide some idea of how well the patient is communicating outside of the speech-language clinic. There may be a note that the patient does not follow instructions. Sometimes a judgment is attached to this observation which the clinician may need to confirm or clarify. For example, the patient may be seen by a nurse as being uncooperative when, rather, the patient merely cannot respond because of aphasia. Notes concerning meals may be an indication that the patient has dysarthria in that drooling and swallowing difficulties would be described. Also, observations are directed toward monitoring the effects of medication.

FORMAL ASSESSMENT OF LANGUAGE

Medical histories and current medical reports are not always available to the speech-language pathologist, especially in settings where this information must be requested from elsewhere. The clinician depends on careful observation of behavior in order to determine whether the patient has aphasia. Formal test procedures enable the clinician to be systematic in making a comprehensive assessment of the behaviors which are pertinent for identification. Attention to qualitative features of patient behavior are helpful in distinguishing aphasia from other disorders which interfere with communication; attention to number of errors leading to a quantitative assessment provides an indication of severity of deficit. Treatment plans are based primarily on these behavioral observations. Every effort should be made, however, to obtain medical records in order to develop a more complete understanding of the origin and evolution of a patient's impairments.

The Valid Aphasia Test

The most important characteristic of a test is that it be valid. Validity refers to whether the test measures what it is intended to measure. A test possesses *content validity* when it measures the domain of behaviors which are pertinent to the problem being examined. An aphasia test is constructed from our knowledge of the defining features of this disorder.

Aphasia, by definition, is a disorder of language which leaves the processes of reasoning and storage of conceptual knowledge basically intact. Therefore, test content is developed so that *it measures basic language ability and minimizes the influence of intelligence and educational experience.* Performance on the language tasks should not be subject to individual variations in reasoning skill or knowledge of the world.

Asking a patient "Who is President of the United States?" is a test of knowledge and orientation as well as of language comprehension. Content should be within the knowledge base of all persons and be homogenized in this way throughout. Ideally, we want errors to indicate that the person has aphasia rather than minimal formal education, a culturally different education, or a disorder of memory, orientation, and reasoning.

Examination of language function also entails *minimizing the influence of extralinguistic context.* Tasks involving environmental cues, for example, permit the aphasic patient to perform based on cognitive processes which are not impaired. As a result, the disorder is not measured as precisely as it could be. However, if the examiner's intent is to measure communication, which relies on environmental context, then an influence of extralinguistic context on performance is desirable.

As a central disorder of language processing, aphasia is manifested in all relevant modalities. Therefore, *all four major language modalities are tested.* Tests are constructed so that each modality can be examined with minimal interference from other modalities. There are subtests of auditory comprehension, reading, verbal expression, and writing.

Aphasia is identified more clearly when it can be distinguished from modality-specific nonverbal problems such as the agnosias, apraxias, and muscle weaknesses. To facilitate these differentiations, an aphasia test *includes tasks in which both stimuli and responses are nonverbal.* Visual recognition, for example, is assessed by a task of picture or shape-matching; and visuomotor disturbances (constructional apraxia) are tested with picture or shape copying. Simple copying exposes the influence of muscle weakness on any writing task.

An aphasia test should accommodate the variations in aphasia, between and within patients. One variation is in the severity of involvement in each modality. Therefore, tests *measure degree of involvement, whether it be mild, moderate or severe.* To do this, a test contains subtests of language which vary in difficulty; and levels of task difficulty are usually defined with respect to the linguistic levels of word, sentence, and paragraph. Task difficulty is also defined with respect to levels of language use. These levels include nonpropositional deployment of words such as in counting, saying the days of the week, or reciting a previously memorized verse; tasks of replication, such as repeating and copying; and tasks of transcoding, such as reading aloud and writing to dictation.

Another way in which aphasic persons vary is along the dimensions which define the different syndromes of aphasia. Functions which are crucial for syndrome identification include auditory language comprehension, repetition, and spontaneous verbal expression. Building a measure of verbal fluency parameters into test construction requires attention to qualitative aspects of expressive language such as its completeness and the use of paraphasias. These considerations may be built into the test's scoring system.

Now we have a fairly complete outline of a valid test structure (Table 6–1). These subtest categories permit the detection of degree of deficit in each modality and the comparison of behaviors which differentiate among syndromes. Repetition and copying are used to detect and measure motor speech and writing impairments. Because the tasks of replication and transcoding involve language input and output, the mode of input for these tasks is specified in the receptive sections of Table 6–1.

Test procedures can be illustrated with subtests for auditory comprehension. This language function is tested in relatively pure form by the examiner's presenting an auditory language stimulus and the pa-

TABLE 6-1. Structure of a valid aphasia test representing four sections and levels of tasks within each section.

Auditory	Visual	Speech	Writing
Perception	Perception		
Recognition	Recognition		
		Nonpropositional use	Nonpropositional use
(Input)		Repetition	Writing to dictation
	(Input)	Reading aloud	Copying
		Propositional language:	Propositional language:
Word	Word	Word	Word
Sentence	Sentence	Sentence	Sentence
Discourse	Paragraph	Discourse	Paragraph

tient's making a nonlinguistic response which indicates that the meaning of the stimulus was comprehended. Variations in degree of comprehension deficit are identified by increasing the length and complexity of verbal stimuli while maintaining the nonverbal requirements of the response as much as possible. At the level of sentence-length input, three types of responses are generally used: (1) pointing to a picture or object within a set of pictures or objects, (2) manipulating objects in response to instructions, and (3) indicating a *yes* or *no* response to simple questions.

Expression is tested in pure form by presenting nonverbal stimuli and requesting a verbal response. At the word level, a picture of an object is shown and the patient is asked to retrieve its name. At the sentence level, a picture of an event might be presented and the patient must describe it. The retrieval of language for expression is tested in a variety of circumstances, namely, in response to a variety of inputs which are often auditory-linguistic. The patient may be asked to complete a sentence, to answer a question with more than just a ''yes'' or ''no,'' or to define a word. Because auditory comprehension usually is tested first, the examiner is aware of its possible contribution to performance on these expressive tasks.

Certain statistical procedures are used to demonstrate the validity of a test. *Construct validity* (or factorial construct validity) refers to whether the psychological components measured by a test are consistent with the theory underlying the test. A common statistical method is factor analysis, which identifies interrelationships among subtest scores (see Chapter 4). *Criterion-related validity* refers to how closely the test relates to another measure which is ideally a more direct representation of what the test is intended to measure. Usually, scores from an aphasia test are compared with scores from another aphasia test which itself may have unknown validity (Spreen and Risser, 1981). The statistical measure of the relationship between two sets of scores is a correlation. A correlation between two aphasia tests is considered to be only an indirect indication of validity.

The Reliable Aphasia Test

Reliability refers to the consistency or stability of test scores in spite of variation with respect to factors unrelated to what is being measured. There are several types of reliability. The consistency of a test within a single patient is determined by a measure of *test-retest reliability*. A correlation is obtained between the first and second administrations of the test to several patients. To see if scores are stable in spite of differences among clinicians, *interexaminer reliability* is obtained. Test scores from at least two examiners are compared from the same group of patients. A high reliability coefficient means that different examiners would obtain the same results on any given administration of a test. *Intraexaminer reliability* is a measure of the clinician's consistency in scoring. A clinician scores the same performance a second time, usually from a video recording. Brookshire (1978b) noted that a high reliability coefficient means only that there is a relationship between two sets of scores, and does not confirm that the scores are stable or are essentially equivalent. He suggested that a percentage of agreement is a better measure of reliability. High reliability is important for measuring recovery because the clinician wants to be confident that a change in test scores is due to a true change in the patient, and not due to sources of random variability unrelated to the functions being tested.

One other source of variability is the test itself. A patient's performance on a subtest might have been different if a different set of items had been used in that subtest. The internal consistency of test items is indicated by measures of *content reliability*. When a test has two forms, the two versions are compared, using a correlation. When a test is not constructed in two forms, internal consistency is measured by deriving one score from half of the test's items and another score from the other half. Usually every other item is used for a score reflecting half of the test. The two scores are compared with a special correlation formula which provides what is called the split-half reliability coefficient.

The influence of minute-to-minute or day-to-day variability in the patient is minimized by *including a sufficient number of items per subtest* so that the patient's general capability for a task is measured accur-

ately. An extreme example would be to use one item to measure current naming ability. The patient may be unable to name the item in one moment and, minutes later, be able to name it readily. Depending on which moment the test was given, the patient would be identified as having 0 percent naming ability or 100 percent naming ability. Therefore, a function generally is tested with around ten items so that random variability in either direction is counterbalanced. With a sufficient number of items per subtest, a performance of 50 percent, for example, is a more consistent indication of function than responses to particular items.

Test-retest reliability is maximized by another feature of test construction, namely, the *standardization of administration and scoring procedures.* Standardization is found in the instructions for administration and scoring provided in the test's manual. It is intended to reduce the influence of external variability that can occur from changes in one examiner, differences between two examiners, and differences in the environment. It maximizes the likelihood that the test is given in the same way each time it is administered so that the patient's performance is assessed according to the same criteria each time. Standardization is achieved by making the instructions explicit and comprehensive and by the examiner's faithful following of these instructions. Clinicians sometimes adjust their presentation of auditory stimuli for comprehension tasks in response to the patient's performance. Salvatore, Strait, and Brookshire (1978) found that experienced clinicians reduce rate of presentation after an error or for more severely impaired patients. They recommended audio tape presentation of stimuli in order to maintain consistency.

Finally, internal consistency is achieved when *subtest items are equivalent samples of the domain of behaviors and content being tested.* If the goal were to measure ability to name common objects, the subtest would include ten or twenty varied objects that are equivalent in familiarity.

ADMINISTERING THE FORMAL TEST

While test manuals include general instructions and guidelines unique to the particular test, some additional tips might be helpful in approaching the situation. Middle-aged and elderly adults are not accustomed to being tested, and so the mere idea of a "test" can be anxiety provoking. The clinician should spend some time getting to know the patient before a formal test is presented; this gives the patient time to become familiar with the setting and the clinician. Furthermore, adults may associate a test with "getting a grade," and not with planning treatment or measuring recovery. The purpose and general characteristics of testing should be explained, especially prior to the first examination after onset. Most adult patients are very understanding of the test situation.

From the responses of fifty aphasic patients to a questionnaire, Skelly (1975) found that they had been offended by testers who were either "bellicose or indifferent." Skelly elaborated:

> Questions were hurled at the aphasic person in a voice that somewhat frightened him or were presented so blandly as to extinguish motivation for cooperation. One patient said that a questioner "barked at me as if I were a dog. I thought he might hit me if I answered." The reverse effect obtained with another aphasic person: "I felt he couldn't care less and probably wouldn't listen even if I did say something." (p. 1141)

Skelly suggested that some difficulties on a test could be a reaction to the clinician.

Patients' irritation with testing comes partly from their awareness that the situation provokes much more frustration and failure than what they are used to in treatment sessions. Administration should not be changed to make the test easier for the patient. Apologies are not warranted. Rather, the clinician should pace administration and provide empathic encouragement in a way that defuses frustration. Some frustration is inevitable and appropriate; and, therefore, it should be allowed and acknowledged as being natural.

Encouragement should be general and not informative as to manner of success or failure on specific items in a task. The test is intended to provide information about the patient's current level of function and is not intended to be therapeutic. Patients look for clues about their performance by watching the clinician score responses. The score sheet should be hidden from view and a notation should be made for each response, if only a $(+)$ and $(-)$. If only errors are recorded, the patient may become unnecessarily attentive to the frequency of this differential response by the clinician.

The idea is to obtain the maximum amount of information in the shortest time. With tests in which the clinician's feedback is not specified, there can be an occasional urge to see if an error can be corrected with a little help. These efforts can turn into several minutes of trial-and-error, postponing completion of the test. The clinician can figure out correction strategies after the test is completed. Schuell (1966) described a strategy for abbreviating a long test. For some patients, certain subtests will result in such obvious total failure or total success that administering them in their entirety will not be informative.

Results should be reported to the patient and interested family members as soon after the test as possible. Not being informative during the test enhances validity and reliability of results. Being informative afterward contributes to a realistic perception of the disorder and can be encouraging. Also, the patient has a right to know. Results should be explained in terminology that the patient and family understand and not necessarily with the terminology of the test or of clinical aphasiology.

DIFFERENTIAL DIAGNOSIS

Adults may exhibit a great variety of deviations in language behavior, and the clinician is often faced with deciding whether the language pattern represents aphasia or another disorder. Traditionally, the identification of aphasia coincides with the identification of patients to be treated for language impairment by the speech-language pathologist. Other language disorders are secondary symptoms of primary disorders which require remediation by a specialist in the primary disorder. For example, schizophrenic language patterns are secondary symptoms of a primary disorder of thought processes. A psychiatrist treats the primary disorder, looking for changes in language patterns as one indication that treatment is effective. The speech-language pathologist treats a language impairment when it is the primary disorder, as is the case with aphasia. The basic problem for the speech-language pathologist in differential diagnosis is deciding whether the patient's language behavior represents a primary or secondary deficit.

The analysis of informal and formal behavioral observations is directed toward answering some basic questions: (1) Does the patient possess a speech or language impairment? (2) Is this impairment an aphasia? (3) If the primary disorder is aphasia, what is its type and severity? (4) What is the prognosis for recovery, with and without treatment? (5) What is the plan for treatment? The present section is addressed to questions (1), (2), and (3). Answers come from consideration of several factors including etiology, location of lesion, nature of onset, progression of the disorder, mental competence, language behavior, level of awareness, and affect and personality. The speech-language pathologist attends primarily to the distinctive qualitative features of language behavior. The final diagnosis is often a team effort after assessment of all aspects of the problem.

Secondary Language Impairments

Secondary language impairments can be divided between those due to brain damage and those without known brain damage. The latter include mainly the psychoses, which by themselves are not generally confronted by speech-language pathologists. However, psychotic reactions to brain damage may be seen in a few patients.

The Schizophrenias and Malingering. The language behavior of schizophrenias, the largest group of psychoses, has been of considerable interest (Vetter, 1968), with some attention to comparisons between schizophrenic language and the jargon of Wernicke's aphasia. In contrast to aphasia, schizophrenia has a gradual onset in most institutionalized cases, while the onset of aphasia is sudden; schizophrenia begins at a relatively young age, while Wernicke's aphasia occurs especially in older adults; there is no known neurological cause of schizophrenia, while aphasia is the direct result of a focal brain lesion; and schizophrenia is regressive, while some recovery occurs with aphasia.

The primary deficit in schizophrenia is a breakdown of thought processes which is inferred from the patient's verbal expression (Fromkin, 1975). One characteristic disturbance is *loose associations,* in which expressed ideas have no apparent connection. In milder forms the loose connections of thought may not become apparent until ten or fifteen minutes into a conversation, when the individual switches topics. Rochester, Martin, and Thurson (1977) studied interviews of forty schizophrenics with an average age of twenty-five, and they offered the following example:

> I've got to find myself a little woman who is my equal, who'd like to who knows how to embroider jeans preferably another Cancer, cause I am a Cancer. It's my horoscope in the zodiac. In other words, they give me a needle on the Queen's birthday image.... (p. 100)

Another characteristic is *overinclusion,* in which thinking is cluttered with irrelevant ideas. This is a failure to exclude competing irrelevant or contradictory thoughts. The patient may also suffer from *hallucination,* a false perception occurring without external stimulation ("I see snakes in my bed"), or *delusion,* a false belief in spite of overwhelming evidence to the contrary ("My doctor wants to kill me").

One's thought patterns are revealed in verbal expression. The unusual language in schizophrenia has received the attention of linguists and neurologists. Chaika (1974) considered it to be a special linguistic phenomenon called "schizophrenic language," and Lecours and Vanier-Clement (1976) called it "schizophasia." Chaika found that it is difficult to pin this language down to a single characterization, probably because schizophrenia comprises many different forms, from the fluent, incoherent speech of the hebephrenic to the withdrawal and muteness of the catatonic. Lecours and Vanier-Clement noted that schizophasia is found in only a few schizophrenics. DiSimoni, Darley, and Aronson (1977) administered some aphasia tests, including parts of Schuell's short test of aphasia (see Chapter 7) and the Token Test (Chapter 8), to twenty-seven chronic schizophrenics. They found normal naming ability, syntax, and adequacy of response, which was defined as number of

errors and degree of elaboration. Also, schizophrenic responses tended to be irrelevant while aphasic responses were relevant. The degree of deficit in listening, reading, and writing in schizophrenia was less than that found in aphasia.

Because one could characterize schizophrenic utterances as containing verbal paraphasias and neologisms, this psychotic use of language has been compared with the jargon in Wernicke's aphasia. Among her six characteristics of schizophrenic language, Chaika (1974) suggested that neologisms and a failure to self-monitor are similar to Wernicke's aphasia. Lecours and Vanier-Clement (1976) added that some errors of syntax and the production of utterances according to previously uttered phonological features are found in both schizophrenic language and the jargon of aphasia. They suggested, however, that schizophrenics are more aware of their linguistic deviations than the Wernicke's aphasic. Fromkin (1975) cautioned that some of Chaika's characteristics of schizophrenic language are similar to normal slips of the tongue and, therefore, are neither necessarily derived from pathological processes nor distinguishing characteristics of schizophasia. Fromkin was critical of any attempt to deal with schizophrenia as a language disorder.

Lecours and Vanier-Clement (1976) sorted through their own observations and those of Chaika and Fromkin, and identified several differences between schizophasia and jargonaphasia. Schizophrenia is singularly characterized by frequent morphemic paraphasias and recurrence of words from the same semantic field. "Glossomania," which is the selection of words based on their phonological similarity, is more frequent in schizophasia. There is some intentionality and awareness in this language. Wernicke's aphasia is more likely to consist of frequent unintentional neologisms and lack of awareness of jargon in its early stages.

"Ordinary speakers think and talk standard; jargonaphasic speakers think standard and talk deviant; schizophasic speakers think quaint and talk accordingly" (Lecours and Vanier-Clement, 1976, p. 557).

In order to obtain compensation for an injury, a person may pretend to have aphasia, which is called "malingering." Porch and Porec (1977; Porec and Porch, 1977) identified certain characteristics of simulated aphasia. The pattern of simulated aphasia on the *Porch Index of Communicative Ability* (see Chapter 7) is almost the "opposite" of aphasia, namely, a larger degree of deficit on easy tasks than on the difficult tasks. Malingerers tend to make the same mistakes on all tasks. Simulated aphasia may involve the following: agrammatism and motor speech impairment without expected hemiparesis; childlike word selection, grammatical forms, and articulation; inconsistent behaviors such as changing strategies in the middle of testing; or overdoing a single aphasic symptom.

Dementias. Language impairment is a secondary symptom of a vast array of *organic brain syndromes* (OBS) in which the primary impairment is dementia caused by brain damage. Just as we could refer to the language *of* schizophrenia, Wertz (1978) referred to these language disorders as the "language of generalized intellectual impairment." Language behavior in these disorders is qualitatively different from aphasia, so that "aphasia in dementia" is an inappropriate concept. In their presentation of diffuse and focal organic brain syndromes, neurologists Strub and Black (1981) wrote of the speech-language pathologist's role: "All such patients will not be treatment candidates, but by means of a thorough language evaluation, the speech pathologist will be able to determine appropriate candidates for rehabilitation and provide other services to those patients and their families that are not selected for treatment" (p. 79).

Dementia refers to a large number of brain diseases in which there is slowly progressive deterioration of cognition, personality, and social behavior. The four classic categories of cognitive impairment include memory loss, disorientation as to time and place, intellectual decline, and faulty judgment. The patient may also have reduced awareness of surroundings and fluctuation of mood or emotion. There is not necessarily a general reduction in all of these areas; the different dementias display different patterns of impairment. Language disturbance is always included, but varies from muteness in one patient to streams of fluent speech ("logorrhea") in others (Obler and Albert, 1981).

Any comprehensive review of the dementias is a labyrinth of similar or overlapping disorders categorized in various ways. The dementias are differentiated relative to etiology (diffuse and multifocal), site of lesion (cortical and subcortical), speed of onset (acute and chronic), and progression (irreversible and reversible). Alzheimer's dementia arises from diffuse deterioration of the brain, while arteriosclerotic dementia consists of multiple small infarcts. Dementia is found from subcortical damage, as in Parkinson's disease. It may appear suddenly after multiple head injuries or may arise insidiously over a long period of time, as in Alzheimer's disease. Most dementias are progressive conditions which are irreversible (no improvement is possible) or reversible (improvement is possible with medical and behavioral treatment). Some irreversible dementias are treatable in that treatment can slow down or arrest progression. Treatable syndromes are produced by metabolic diseases (thyroid or pituitary), vitamin deficiency, drug intoxication, or multiple strokes, tumors, and traumas. Depression can masquerade as dementia, with problems of memory and concentration due to a lack of motivation (Strub and Black, 1981). Many true dementias are treated with behavioral techniques and environmental manipulations aimed at improving orientation and minimizing confusion (Barns, Sac, and Shore, 1973).

The most common cause of dementia after age fifty is *Alzheimer's disease.* Alzheimer's dementia is not an inevitable endpoint of aging, though it is caused by changes in the brain that are seen in the "normal" aging brain. Aging may be accompanied by mild changes in cognition and personality, which cannot be termed dementia but which are considered in the assessment of aphasia in elderly patients. Furthermore, the increased likelihood of multiple infarcts in the elderly may lead to cognitive deficits prior to the occurrence of a lesion which produces aphasia. Alzheimer's disease, on the other hand, produces a language disturbance which, in its advanced stage, is similar to Wernicke's aphasia (Obler and Albert, 1981). This dementia traditionally has been equated with presenile dementia (onset before age sixty-five). However, because presenile and senile dementias represent the same pathologies, the age-related division is now considered to be unnecessary. Valenstein (1981) wrote: "Although it is still debated whether or not there is a separate presenile form of Alzheimer's disease, it has become common practice to use the term Alzheimer's disease to refer to any dementia that has the characteristic clinical and pathological findings, regardless of the age of the patient" (p. 94).

The language in Alzheimer's dementia was described by Obler and Albert (1981).

Early stages: The patient responds appropriately in basic comprehension tests but gives vague interpretations of proverbs. He or she can repeat long sentences with high transitional probabilities, contrary to Wernicke's aphasia. Verbal expression is personalized, repetitious, and vague.

Intermediate stages: Comprehension is reduced with errors in answering yes-no questions. Repetition begins to break down on long high-probability sentences. Patients are verbose when asked to name objects. Verbal expression contains verbal paraphasias and some jargon.

Later stages: The patient becomes mute except for occasional jargon. Objects may be named correctly amidst some jargon, but the patient is not aware of it.

The patient is distinguished from the aphasic primarily with respect to the pragmatics of communication. "For example, eye contact is diminished in later stages of Alzheimer's disease. Also, the dementing patient will touch the test objects more than is appropriate" (Obler and Albert, 1981, p. 392). When asked what kind of work he did, a seventy-three-year-old man with moderately advanced Alzheimer's dementia replied: "Oh, when I first laughed along, I lived, uh, worked in Boston. When I second I worked the whole crew, I worked together" (p. 393).

Results of language testing have been reported with unspecified dementias. Halpern, Darley, and Brown (1973) administered portions of Schuell's Minnesota test to ten persons with chronic brain syndrome; Porch (1971a, 1981a) provided language profiles with the *Porch Index of Communicative Ability* (PICA) on one hundred patients with bilateral brain damage. Others have presented additional *PICA* profiles of patients with dementia (see Chapter 7). Halpern, et al. (1973) showed mild-to-moderate reduction of language function in all categories tested. Verbal fluency was within the normal range and syntax was "almost unimpaired." However, Porch has demonstrated a wider range of verbal impairment including patients who are totally unresponsive to the test items.

Specific symptoms of aphasia such as paraphasia and jargon have been described in the language of patients with dementia. This is not surprising because diffuse brain damage would certainly include the language zone of the left hemisphere. Hecaen and Albert (1978) noted: "Sentences are started and not finished; perseveration is intense. In spontaneous or responsive speech the features of dementia may mix with paraphasias and verbal amnesia to the point of total jargon aphasia and to such an extent that it becomes impossible to distinguish the two orders of impairment" (p. 75).

Studies of picture-naming behavior after bilateral damage have shown qualitative differences between aphasic naming errors and naming behavior in dementia (Weinstein and Keller, 1963; Rochford, 1971). The naming errors of dementia were referred to as "non-aphasic misnaming" by Geschwind (1967). Errors appear particularly in relation to the hospital and illness. Geschwind (1967) noted that the patient "may call the hospital a 'hotel,' the doctors 'bell boys,' and the nurses 'chambermaids,' and will not accept correction." Nonaphasic misnaming arises from disorientation, memory loss, and perceptual difficulty. Picture-naming errors may come from misrecognition of the object; the error represents an object that looks like the pictured object. These errors are rare with unilateral left-hemisphere damage (Newcombe, Oldfield, Ratcliff, et al., 1971).

Confabulation has been reported in patients with Alzheimer's dementia and dementia from chronic alcoholism (Mercer, Wapner, Gardner, et al., 1977). Confabulation is the production of statements that are false and that may include bizarre or fantastic features. It usually appears when there is a lapse of memory. When asked about a recent medical examination, a resident of a nursing home said, "Yes, Dr. Joyce Brothers examined me. She came to my room and said I would be going home in a couple of days."

Schwartz, Marin, and Saffran (1979) conducted a detailed linguistic study of a case of presenile dementia (age sixty-two). Language difficulties were concentrated in fluent but vacuous verbal expression and frequently incorrect confrontation naming. However, the patient comprehended sentences containing comparative adjectives and spatial prepositions and had no problem reading aloud. Therefore, language impairment did not cut across all modalities and did not affect use of syntax. Careful study indicated a marked impairment of semantic memory.

Confusion. The acute confusional state is differentiated from dementia. It is an abrupt change of behavior usually due to a metabolic imbalance, adverse drug reaction, head trauma, alcohol or drug withdrawal, or a combination of these. It is "characterized by a clouding of consciousness, incoherence in the train of thought, and difficulty with attention and concentration" (Strub and Black, 1981, p. 90). Confused patients may become very disoriented, incoherent, and hallucinatory. Acute confusional states are caused by a primary medical disorder and are usually completely reversible. When this condition lasts for weeks or months, it can be mistaken as Alzheimer's dementia. Fluctuations in level of consciousness distinguish the confusional state from dementia. Confusion is seen during the posttraumatic amnesia period following closed head injury (Levin, 1981; see Chapter 2).

Wertz (1978) discussed the "language of confusion" as a secondary symptom of the confused mental state. Of ten cases studied by Halpern, et al. (1973), eight had rapid onset. Five were due to trauma, and three were caused by hemorrhage. The location of damage producing language of confusion was bilateral or multifocal. Wertz added that confusion which follows a focal or unilateral lesion is likely to be temporary.

Wertz pointed out that confused patients do well on standard language tasks by exhibiting vocabulary (comprehension and retrieval) and syntax within normal limits. These tasks require the patient to converge on a single response, as in object naming. However, these patients produce irrelevancies and confabulation in more open-ended language situations, such as when asked to define a word or respond to an open-ended question. Halpern, et al. (1973) found that a principal problem of confused patients was in the relevancy of their responses in language tasks, while patients with dementia were generally relevant. This appears to have been the only clear distinction between confusion and dementia in the language study by Halpern; however, other investigators have described confabulation and irrelevancies in patients with dementia.

Focal Deficits. Other disorders are more similar to aphasia in terms of etiology and less similar in terms of symptoms. That is, certain disorders result from focal lesions confined to one cerebral hemisphere and are produced by the typical causes of aphasia such as CVA, tumor, or trauma. Their course involves some degree of recovery instead of progressive deterioration. However, because of their location, these lesions result in specific impairments of cognition which do not necessarily include language function (see Table 3–3). Language usage may be modified, nevertheless, when the primary deficit interacts with language function.

A focal lesion in the left or language hemisphere, which would tend not to result in aphasia, would be located in the posterior portions supplied by the posterior cerebral artery or the anterior portions supplied by the anterior cerebral artery. Modality-specific disorders of reading and writing, alexia and agraphia, were mentioned in Chapter 1. Pure alexia with agraphia is associated with damage to the angular gyrus of the left parietal lobe; pure alexia occurs from a lesion in the left occipital lobe. Damage to the left frontal lobe, anterior to the motor speech region,

has been discussed minimally in this text. Actually, the anteriormost regions of the frontal lobe often are not differentiated clearly between left and right hemispheres in terms of impaired function. Hecaen and Albert (1978) noted that clinical evidence has made it difficult to be specific about functional regions of the anterior frontal lobes. "It is premature, we believe, to attempt to correlate specific behavioral deficits in human beings with specific regions within the frontal lobes" (p. 367).

Nevertheless, Hecaen and Albert cited a few categories of impairment associated with frontal lobe damage, none of which include language impairment. A commonly observed result of frontal damage is personality disorder. There is the well-known case of Phineas Gage, who in 1848 suffered a construction accident in Vermont. An explosion sent a 3½ foot rod through his skull and into the right front of his brain. He sat up and soon asked, "Where's my rod?" Though he lived for another twelve years, his personality was transformed. "In place of the softspoken, reliable foreman he had been, there now stood a loud-mouthed, obnoxious soul who cursed continuously; exhibited little sense of purpose, and wandered aimlessly until his death in San Francisco in 1860" (Gardner, 1974b, p. 267). The frontal lobe personality is euphoric, with a lack of concern for the present and future. The euphoria may be only apparent, as these patients will state that they are not happy, and euphoric periods may alternate with periods of apparent depression. There is occasional loss of impulse control, with erotic behavior, sexual exhibitionism, and lewd remarks. Other characteristics of frontal lobe pathology include reduced initiative or spontaneity of motor activity and disorders of attention and memory.

Latent aphasia is a concept of language disorder with which Boller (1968) described language difficulties observed in patients with left-hemisphere lesions but without clinical evidence of aphasia. Prior to Boller's use of the term, latent aphasia referred to subtle language difficulties in patients without aphasia, especially those with right-hemisphere lesions (Pichot, 1955; Eisenson, 1959). Boller and Vignolo (1966) had identified an auditory comprehension deficit with the Token Test (see Chapter 8) in nonaphasic left-hemisphere-damaged subjects. Later, left-hemisphere-damaged nonaphasics also showed a deficit in producing animal names in one minute, averaging 14.7 while normals averaged 19.9 (Boller, 1968). They were not deficient, however, in naming objects with low-frequency words.

The nonverbal deficits of patients with focal lesions in the **right hemisphere** (RH) were surveyed in Chapter 3. These patients perform worse on nonverbal, largely visual-spatial sections of intelligence tests than on the verbal sections. On the *Wechsler Adult Intelligence Scale* (WAIS), commonly given by neuropsychologists, patients with right parietal lobe damage are impaired on replicating block designs, object assembly, picture arrangement, and memory for designs (McFie, 1975). Patients with right frontal or temporal lobe damage have their principal difficulty with picture arrangement and memory for designs. They are often disoriented as to time and place. RH patients are also noted for disorders of affective or emotional behavior. Gardner, Ling, Flamm, et al. (1975) compared RH subjects to LH subjects with aphasia in their understanding of humor in cartoons. Reactions of RH subjects ranged from no smiles or laughter at all by some to inappropriate hilarity by others. LH aphasics exhibited more normal reactions to the cartoons. Gardner, et al. (1975) stated that their observations supported a well-established suggestion that "patients with minor hemisphere pathology may well behave in ways less appropriate to a given affective situation than those with lesions

of comparable size in the dominant hemisphere'' (p. 409).

Neurologists and neuropsychologists frequently diagnose the RH patient as displaying no clinical sign of language impairment. These patients have been shown to make few object-naming errors (Weinstein and Keller, 1963; Boller, 1968; Newcombe, Oldfield, Ratcliff, et al., 1971). In spite of finding slower-than-normal response times, Newcombe, et al. (1971) concluded that their RH subjects were essentially unimpaired in naming. RH subjects have also been equivalent to normal subjects on auditory sentence comprehension (Boller and Vignolo, 1966; DeRenzi, 1979; Parisi and Pizzamiglio, 1970). However, this finding has been contradicted to some degree when RH patients were below normals but better than aphasics with the *Revised Token Test* (McNeil and Prescott, 1978).

RH-damaged patients are impaired in recognizing certain types of symbols (Wapner and Gardner, 1981). In this study, discussed in Chapter 1, aphasics were impaired in recognizing "relatively linguistic symbol systems," while RH-damaged subjects were equivalent to normal controls. However, RH-damaged subjects were impaired in recognizing "relatively nonlinguistic symbols" in pictured object recognition, recognition of correct placement for symbols such as dollar or addition signs, and recognition of the correct context for traffic signs. Aphasics were not impaired on these tasks.

A statistically significant difference from normal performance on simple language tasks can be demonstrated in RH-damaged patients. Gainotti, Caltagirone, Miceli, et al. (1981) compared fifty of these subjects with thirty-nine normals on a word-comprehension task in which picture foils were semantically related to the correct choice. Although the RH-damaged group averaged only 1.35 errors out of twenty items, it was a statistically significant difference from normal. This difference may not be considered to be clinically significant, however. RH-damaged patients have had difficulty comprehending passive sentences (Hier and Kaplan, 1980), especially in making decisions about agent-action-object order (Heeschen, 1980).

Areas of comprehension deficit in RH patients have begun to appear in studies which tap into the interrelationship between language processing and nonverbal functions associated with the right hemisphere. RH patients make errors in recognizing the emotion expressed in the intonation pattern of utterances (Schlanger, et al., 1976). This reduction of emotional sensitivity occurs with nonverbal and verbal stimuli (Cicone, et al., 1980; DeKosky, et al., 1980).

The RH specializes in simultaneous spatial processing (Chapter 3). When this processing style is normally utilized in a language task, a RH-damaged person may run into difficulty. This was shown in solving two-term series problems such as "John is taller than Bill, who is shorter?" in which the adjectives of the two parts of the problem do not match (Caramazza, Gordon, Zurif, et al., 1976). The RH-impaired subjects did not differ from normals when the two adjectives were congruent. Read (1981) found the same difficulty with incongruence in three-term series problems; but his patients with more focal, right temporal lobe lesions comprehended these more complex problems very well. Caramazza, et al. (1976) suggested that the RH-coding strategy of spatial imagery is involved particularly in the incongruent condition.

In understanding discourse, an RH-damaged patient may have problems integrating elements into a single coherent theme. He or she may have trouble getting the point. This difficulty may stem from impaired use of context to perceive the intent of an utterance, a communicative skill that is present in many cases of aphasia. RH-impaired patients are as likely to point to the literal interpretation of an utterance as point to the metaphorical interpretation, while aphasics tend to select the metaphorical interpretation (Winner and Gardner, 1977; see Chapter 5). Focal RH damage creates problems in interpreting proverbs (Hier and Kaplan, 1980) with a tendency to be literal when telling the moral of a story (Wapner, Hamby, and Gardner, 1981). Also, there is difficulty in selecting the punch line of a joke (Wapner, et al., 1981).

RH patients also exhibit peculiar deviations of expression, which are beginning to be thought of as a communication disorder. RH norms for the *PICA* (see Table 7-4) from 111 subjects were developed by Deal, Deal, Wertz, et al. (1979a); a discriminant analysis on eighty-six subjects showed that 62 percent of the RH profiles were similar to aphasia. Expressive deficit from RH lesions was suggested in Boller's (1968) study where these patients, like the LH nonaphasics, retrieved fewer animal names in one minute (13.65) than the normals (19.9). Boller did not consider this deficit to be latent "aphasia" but rather it was considered to be a sensitivity of one language function to any brain damage. RH-damaged subjects were impaired in telling complete stories and in guessing a word from linguistic context (Rivers and Love, 1980).

Myers (1979) identified some specific deviations in interviews and picture descriptions from twenty RH patients; these deviations were similar to the story retelling of subjects in Wapner, et al.'s (1981) study. When communication problems occurred they tended to consist of irrelevant and often excessive information, of missed implications of questions and, therefore, of literal treatment of questions and events. They lacked "(1) the ability to integrate discrete items of information into a whole; and (2) the ability to provide an interpretation of events or situations'' (Myers, 1979, p. 38). Myers provided the following example of an answer to "What happened to you and why are you in the hospital":

> Wife and I were taking—were visiting Labor Day weekend . . . We arrive Saturday afternoon. Visit my in-laws. Saturday evening—after evening I had dinner with my in-laws. Saturday night my wife and I slept in separate rooms . . . Sunday morning when I awoke, my wife gave me breakfast. She gave me toast. (p. 38)

This focus on details and somewhat delayed route to the point of the question prompted the examiner to remind the patient of the question:

> I had breakfast, toast and egg beaters, which I like. Margarine—Fleischman's margarine . . . supposed to be low in cholesterol. My wife went in kitchen . . . I was calling her. Apparently my voice sounded different. She looked. She said, "Ohh! John has a stroke." She was upset, so upset. (p. 38)

Along with some unusual word selection and some wandering off from the point, this patient expressed literal details instead of a synthesized answer containing the implication of what happened Sunday morning. Myers found that eight RH patients were deficient in the number of interpretive concepts used to describe the cookie-theft picture from the *Boston Diagnostic Aphasia Examination* (see Chapter 7) and were deficient on a test of visual integration. She suggested that both deficits may be due to a primary deficit of information integration which underlies visual perceptual function and intrudes upon verbal expression.

As consideration of the role of the right hemisphere in language function continues (Myers, 1980), the speech-language pathologist may assume a new role in the rehabilitation of patients with RH damage. This role awaits further delineation of their communication deficits. If their language behavior is secondary to deficits of emotion, imagery, and synthesis, the neuropsychologist may become the primary provider of treatment.

Meanwhile, patients with secondary language deficits have generally not been thought of as candidates for speech-language treatment. In Brookshire's (1978b) chapter on test interpretation and treatment decisions, a case of focal damage in a nonlanguage region of the left hemisphere and a case of RH damage were presented to illustrate instances in which speech-language treatment was not recommended. The former case displayed a memory problem instead of a language deficit, and the latter case "did not possess any significant impairments specific to speech and language processes" (p. 115). Confusion and dementia have been treated behaviorally with reality orientation therapy and other similar regimens conducted by the staffs of long-term care facilities (Folsom, 1968; Barns, et al., 1973). These therapies are directed toward the problems of disorientation and faulty memory. Regular training of language processes and instruction in communicative strategies can be difficult to carry out with disoriented and confused patients. Without an escort service in a long-term care facility these patients may not arrive for treatment on time or may have difficulty finding the clinic, and the more severely impaired patients may not remember the goals of treatment or the clinician from one session to the next. The purely aphasic patient does not have these problems.

Primary Disturbances of Speech and Language

The neurogenic disorders traditionally treated by the speech-language pathologist are the dysarthrias, apraxia of speech (verbal apraxia), and the aphasias. In this section, the essential characteristics which distinguish these disorders are reviewed.

Differential Diagnosis. Etiological characteristics separate the dysarthrias from apraxia of speech and aphasia. While apraxia of speech and aphasia are caused by focal lesions in the left cerebral cortex, the dysarthrias may result from these causes and a variety of diseases which affect the central and peripheral nervous systems below the level of the cortex (Darley, Aronson, and Brown, 1975; Rosenbek and LaPointe, 1978; Wertz, 1978). Within the cortex, damage to a premotor region of the frontal lobe (Broca's area) produces apraxia, while damage to frontal and posterior regions produce aphasia (see Chapter 3). Apraxia and aphasia usually have sudden onset, while dysarthrias may appear suddenly or gradually depending on the etiology. Also, some etiologies of dysarthrias, such as multiple sclerosis and amyotrophic lateral sclerosis, involve progressive deterioration of the central nervous system.

The presence or absence of muscle weakness has several implications for the symptomatology of these disorders. Dysarthria is the manifestation of muscle weakness in the speech mechanism, disrupting respiration, phonation, resonance, and articulation. Any oral muscle movement is impaired, and the speech symptoms in conversation appear also in more automatic production such as counting or recitation. Apraxia of speech and aphasia, on the other hand, are disorders which do not involve paralysis of speech musculature. Performance varies according to linguistic level in both disorders. Neither disorder involves impairment of vegetative functions such as chewing or swallowing.

Distinguishing among these three disorders in terms of speech symptoms has been subject to some debate and inconsistency of definition. Dysarthrias and apraxia of speech have been differentiated on the basis of the volition of movement and consistency of articulatory errors (Johns and LaPointe, 1976). Dysarthrias are impairments of volitional and nonvolitional movement, while apraxia is an impairment primarily of volitional movement. Most dysarthric errors are consistent among levels of volition and upon repetition of a response, while apraxic errors are inconsistent among these levels and upon repetition. The main diagnostic problem with respect to aphasia is between sound substitutions in aphasia and those in apraxia of speech (see Chapter 5). The articulatory problems of Broca's aphasia are usually the product of an accompanying apraxia of speech.

Differential diagnosis among the aphasias is given much attention in other chapters of this book. A dichotomy of the aphasias has been established with respect to fluency of verbal output and general location of the lesion. This dichotomy is differentiated further in Figure 6–1. In this depiction of the aphasias, the syndromes are identified with respect to three criteria: fluency of spontaneous verbal expression, level of auditory comprehension, and level of verbal repetition. The objective criteria in these categories were developed by Kertesz (1979; Kertesz and Poole, 1974) in order to use performance on the *Western Aphasia Battery* for classifying aphasic patients. On the basis of test scores, eight aphasias can be divided into two groups of four based on Kertesz's rating of verbal fluency. Nonfluent and fluent aphasias can be subdivided into groups of two based on level of auditory comprehension. Finally, the relative abilities of patients to repeat permit us to define the eight syndromes of aphasia.

Identification with Test Scores. It is tempting to conclude that a person has aphasia and to recommend language treatment simply because a person makes errors on a test of aphasia. Can we use test scores to identify aphasia? We are wary

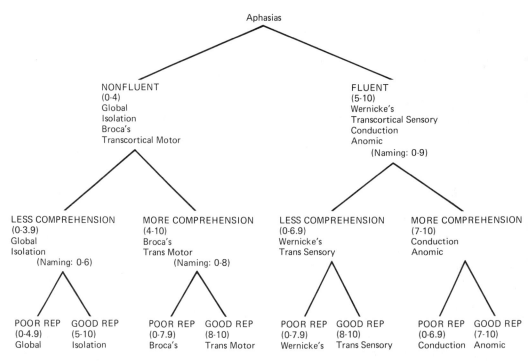

Figure 6-1. One guideline to differential diagnosis of the aphasias is levels of function according to fluency, auditory comprehension, and repetition. Kertesz's (1979) criteria from the *Western Aphasia Battery* provide fairly neat distinctions represented in this decision matrix (see Chapter 7, Table 7–5).

about using the mere occurrence of errors as an indication of aphasia. Normal adult performance on comprehensive tests, as shown in the next chapter, includes errors on certain sections of these tests. Non-brain-injured persons may be fatigued and have a momentary lapse of attention; level of intelligence may interact with language function in high-level testing no matter how hard the test's author had tried to eliminate its influence; and literacy would certainly influence reading and writing performance. Also, test scores may signify only the presence of pathological language function whether it be a primary or secondary deficit. A deficit usually is identified with respect to a standard for what is normal, which might be 100 percent correct test performance and/or a delineation of how nonbrain-injured adults perform on a test of language functions. Therefore,

if a test is to provide an objective basis for identifying aphasia, the test-maker provides an analytical aid for the clinician. Two devices are commonly used to facilitate the identification of aphasia with test results: (1) data indicating nonaphasic and aphasic performances on the test or (2) a "cutoff score." Both are derived from normative samples representing nonaphasic and aphasic language ability.

Test manuals should provide an indication of how normal adults would perform on the test. Usually scores derived from a sample of the nonbrain-injured population are provided. For example, on the *Auditory Comprehension Test for Sentences* (Shewan, 1979) normals scored an average 20.07 out of 21 possible points. They were minimally variable with a standard deviation of 1.17. Therefore, a score of 18 could be considered to represent language pathology. The clinician still cannot be certain that an 18 is necessarily an aphasic performance because there is no information in the test manual about how nonaphasic brain-damaged persons would do. On this comprehension test the least impaired group of aphasics, those with anomic aphasia, averaged 14.83 with a standard deviation of 4.02. The information from such norms indicates that test scores can distinguish easily between normal performance and aphasic language pathology.

Some tests are accompanied by guidelines for differentiating aphasia from secondary language deviations and for differentiating among the syndromes of aphasia. These guidelines are established with reference to expected patterns of deficit among language modalities or among specific language functions such as repetition and word retrieval. Charts for summarizing degrees of deficit in each of these areas are provided to facilitate recognition of these patterns (see Chapter 7).

A cutoff score represents the lowest level of normal performance on a test. Any score below it on a valid test of language would be indicative of a language disorder. Only a few aphasia test manuals provide a cutoff score. DeRenzi (1979) derived a cutoff for a short version of the Token Test of auditory language comprehension. He determined the interval around the mean score of 90 percent of 215 nonbrain-injured subjects. The lowest end of the interval was the cutoff. This score was discriminative between normal function and pathology in that 7 percent of 200 aphasics were at or above the score. On the other hand, 84 percent of RH patients were at or above the cutoff. Some amount of overlap would seem to be reasonable, because a few mildly impaired aphasics would be expected to be functionally "normal" in auditory comprehension. Holland (1980a) suggested that error in diagnosis from the cutoff should be in the direction of calling aphasics "normal" rather than

calling some normals "aphasic," because a few aphasics can be within functionally normal limits on a test.

Certain legal questions arise which call for objective identification of aphasia and for determining the degree of aphasia and its impact on certain functions (Udell, Sullivan, and Schlanger, 1980). One question is of *competency* which involves whether the patient is able to function in the best interest of himself or of those for whom he is responsible (Porch and Porec, 1977). Common competency issues include the capacity to stand trial, to assume parental activities, to live independently, to conduct business and personal affairs, and to drive. The ability to understand one's will, called testamentary capacity, is indicated by assessment of receptive language (see Morse, 1968). A second question deals with *compensation,* which involves determining how much impairment the patient has sustained. The clinician may assess a patient who is seeking compensation from an employer or the government or who is suing a physician or hospital because of an accident during surgery.

Summary and Comment

The language disorders have been differentiated between primary and secondary language impairments. Aphasia is the one primary language disorder. Most of the disorders in this section are summarized in Table 6-2. This table serves to emphasize the variety of information needed in order to recommend treatment based on the best possible identification of the disorder.

Without medical information, the clinical aphasiologist becomes suspicious of the presence of dementia when the patient is unresponsive, detached, and disoriented. Also, the family often reports a condition that has developed gradually. The confusion that comes from head trauma may accompany an anomic aphasia, and Levin (1981) indicated that the speech-language

TABLE 6-2. Distinguishing characteristics of primary and secondary language disorders.

	Differential Diagnosis					
	Schizophrenia	Dementia	Confusion	Focal Deficit (RH)	APHASIA	Verbal Apraxia
Onset	Sudden/gradual Early adulthood	Sudden/gradual Any age	Usually sudden Any age	Usually sudden Any age	Usually sudden Any age	Sudden Any age
Brain Damage	None evident	Diffuse Multifocal	Diffuse Multifocal	Focal	Focal	Focal
Progression	Brief to irreversible	Often progressive deterioration	Usually temporary	Spontaneous recovery	Spontaneous recovery	Spontaneous recovery
Awareness		Reduced in some cases	Reduction is a primary deficit		Unimpaired	Unimpaired
Mental Competence	Impaired: disorganized thinking	Impaired memory orientation, intellect, judgment	Impaired	Impaired orientation, judgment, visuo-spatial functions	Relatively unimpaired	Unimpaired
Language	Secondary deficit	Secondary deficit: Confabulation Muteness or jargon	Secondary deficit: Confabulation	Clinically unimpaired Secondary deficit related to processing style of RH	Primary deficit: Comprehension Paraphasias Agrammatism	Unimpaired
Personality and Behavior	Bizarre or muted	Fluctuates Restless		Muted emotions Bizarre socially	Unimpaired Natural reaction to loss	Unimpaired

clinician may develop a role in treating the patient's failure to monitor language deviations and the patient's memory problems. The language of focal RH damage is suspected when the patient appears to talk normally and may even have left hemiparesis. The linguistic level of discourse analysis may provide a framework for identifying the linguistic wanderings resulting from RH injury. Finally, one more diagnostic issue remains which has not been defined clearly by research.

The elderly aphasic, a patient of sixty-five years and older, may have an aging component within the language deficit. Therefore, we are faced with the question of how much of the language deficit is due to normal aging. Psycholinguistic investigation of normal aging is in its infancy, and so we can only guess that aging may play a small role in the symptomatology of certain patients (Davis, Forthcoming). This component of the deficit would not be amenable to treatment in the way that the aphasic component is usually responsive to stimulation. Aging has minimal effect on short-term memory capacity but may slow down the rate of scanning in STM. Comprehension is affected at the paragraph level tested by question-answering after hearing or reading the paragraph. Memory of the paragraph may be a pertinent factor. Slowing down of word retrieval may be a function of reduced perceptual-motor efficiency and of familiarity with the tested lexicon. The precise role of aging in language function has not been determined. We might suspect that its greatest impact on aphasia is with the mildly impaired elderly patient in whom aging would take up a higher percentage of deficit than in other aphasic patients.

ASSESSMENT

Assessment emerges in the forefront of concern once the disorder has been identified. Once we know the patient has aphasia, for example, we pay attention to certain decisions which lead to a plan for treatment of the linguistic problem. These decisions involve coming to an understanding of the patient's primary aphasic deficit or combination of deficits, and then coming up with an inventory of the patient's specific strengths and weaknesses in the use of language. Assessment of language is complete when clinical performance is compared with functional performance.

Primary Deficits

Knowing what to look for as a possible primary deficit has been restricted by our limited knowledge of the components of language processing and, therefore, of the possible primary breakdowns underlying a pattern of secondary symptoms. To a considerable degree, we still define primary deficits in the general terms of language modalities, especially when analyzing receptive problems. Concerning auditory comprehension, components such as short-term memory and speech sound perception have been identified as parts of the system that could be impaired. Expressively, we can isolate components such as word retrieval or syntactic formulation. Word retrieval appears to be a multistage process, and a primary breakdown can be identified with one of the stages if we can be confident about our understanding of what these stages are and of how to expose them for analysis. As indicated in the previous chapter, object sorting may become part of testing in order to determine whether an entangled semantic memory is the basis for word-finding errors.

For now let us consider how we analyze test results for the purpose of identifying deficits toward which our treatment is directed.

Modality Comparisons. Sometimes the primary source of an aphasic patient's secondary symptoms is an additional disorder such as hearing loss, an agnosia, apraxia of speech, or another one of the disorders surveyed in Chapter 1. Modality-specific deficits combined with aphasia are indicated when levels of performance are compared among the four language modalities. Figure 6-2 shows patterns indicative of aphasia and of aphasia complicated by an auditory perception deficit, visual or special reading deficiency, or a speech disorder such as apraxia or dysarthria. An overlaid auditory deficit is shown by an auditory level which is below the reading level, as can sometimes occur in Wernicke's aphasia caused by a lesion which intrudes upon the primary auditory zone of the left temporal lobe. Illiteracy can produce a pattern in which reading and writing are well below levels of auditory and oral language functions. A motor speech disorder is indicated when the speech modality is well below the writing modality.

Task Comparisons. The strategy for finding a primary deficit in test results includes comparison of performances among different tasks. As a general rule, no single task performance is necessarily definitive as to the nature of a primary deficit. That is, pointing to pictures or repetition do not define the problems of an aphasic patient. Deficient performances on such tasks merely are indicative that a primary deficit exists and should be considered to be secondary symptoms. Something caused pointing to pictures to be faulty or repetition to be reduced. As Goodglass and Kaplan (1972) suggested, a single task is one "window" through which to observe the outcome of a process.

Figure 6-2. Comparisons among levels of performance in the four language modalities are indicative of different primary deficits. (a) Aphasia pattern. (b) Aphasia with an auditory perception deficit. (c) Aphasia in an illiterate patient. (d) Aphasia with a motor speech disorder, such as apraxia of speech.

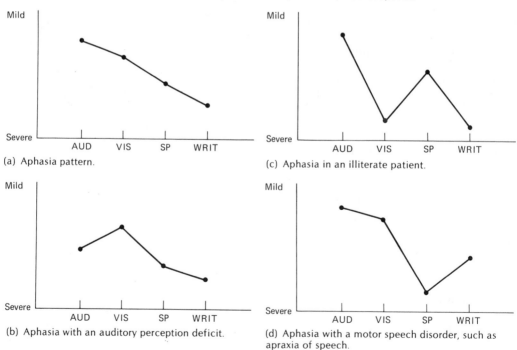

(a) Aphasia pattern.

(b) Aphasia with an auditory perception deficit.

(c) Aphasia in an illiterate patient.

(d) Aphasia with a motor speech disorder, such as apraxia of speech.

Looking through several different windows achieves a full view of the process. Therefore, defining a patient's deficits in terms of a specific task on a test, a kind of "pure task blindness," provides an incomplete definition of the patient's problems.

Many aphasia tests are not designed so that tasks can be compared with the same linguistic content. Sidman, Stoddard, Mohr, et al. (1971) advised that some testing be done with systematic stimulus/response control:

> Different stimuli, responses, and stimulus-response relations may be affected by different variables, and in quantitatively different ways by the same variables. To clarify the factors responsible for such variability, tests must hold modulating variables constant, maintain stimulus constancy while varying responses required of the patient, and response constancy while varying stimuli. To compare stimulus-response relations that differ in their stimuli *and* responses is contrary to elementary scientific good sense. (p. 121)

The more general scientific principle here is that *comparison is facilitated by changing one variable at a time.* Two tasks may differ by changing the input modality and keeping the response constant: (1) presenting a spoken word and requiring a pointing response and (2) presenting a printed word and requiring a pointing response. Comparison of performance between these tasks permits the following possible problem identifications: (1) if the first task is deficient but not the second, the problem is specific to auditory function; (2) if the second task is deficient but not the first, the problem is specific to visual function or reading; or (3) if both tasks are deficient, the problem may be with verbal material in both modalities which is indicative of aphasia.

The test performance of each patient should be carefully analyzed in the search for primary deficits, regardless of whether the patient might appear to fit a syndrome category. When a patient is a clear-cut case of Broca's or Wernicke's aphasia, we cannot assume that the only primary deficit lies in syntactic processing, speech perception, or semantic memory. The objective is to *find a "common thread" underlying various deficient performances.*

In order to get an idea of task comparison strategy for a case of aphasia, let us consider comparing performances on four tasks of replication involving the same linguistic content (Table 6-3). In this example, we still are comparing the status of modalities, and we are thinking in terms of a score on each task rather than in terms of qualitative aspects of behavior. The secondary symptoms of three hypothetical cases are represented by a good score (+) and a poor score (−). In each case we look for what the deficient performances have in common. Case *A* is impaired in repetition and reading aloud, and the common feature of these symptoms is the speech modality. Therefore, we would suspect

TABLE 6-3. Tasks of replication with three hypothetical cases are shown to illustrate task comparison strategy for interpreting test results. (+) refers to strength and (−) refers to weakness rather than to absolute success or failure on each task.

Task	Stimulus	Response	Secondary Symptoms		
			A	B	C
Repetition	Audition	Speech	−	+	+
Reading aloud	Vision	Speech	−	−	+
Writing to dictation	Audition	Writing	+	−	−
Copying	Vision	Writing	+	+	+

that a primary deficit would be restricted to the speech modality, especially because the other three modalities are used well in writing to dictation and copying. This patient would be treated for a speech disorder, not a repetition disorder (and, perhaps, not even for aphasia). Case *B* has a problem with two tasks which utilize all four modalities and does well with the other two tasks using all four modalities. Therefore, the primary deficit is not modality-specific, and we must consider another basis for deciding on the common thread underlying the deficient tasks. In this example, the common thread is that reading aloud and writing to dictation involve transcoding, the translation of a graphemic code into a phonemic code and vice versa. The primary deficit is transcoding. In case C, the deficit is more specific, namely, transcoding from a phonemic code to a graphemic code. In each case, the hypothetical primary deficit is defined according to *a characteristic shared by the impaired functions which is not present in the spared functions*. When a patient is especially impaired on one task, we pay attention to what is unique about that task.

Now, let us examine three tasks of auditory comprehension and attempt the same comparison strategy. Table 6–4 represents three symptom patterns relative to good (+) and poor (−) scores on forced choice pointing to pictures, following instructions, and answering yes-no questions. Case *A* is a typical aphasic, with problems on all three tasks. The common

thread is sentence-level auditory input indicating a primary deficit of sentence comprehension. Further comparison between prepositions and other structures may isolate a primary difficulty in comprehending spatial relationships. Case *B* has a particular problem with following instructions but does well comprehending statements and questions. Therefore, the patient does comprehend the preposition. The feature of the impaired task which is not shared by the other tasks is the requirement to sequence motor acts in the response. The primary deficit may not be comprehension per se but, rather, may be a limb apraxia which influences the response mode. If only instructions were used to test comprehension, we might have an erroneous impression of this patient's deficit. The response mode also may be the culprit in case *C*, because it is a distinguishing feature of the task. Some aphasics are unable to generate a consistently accurate "Yes" or "No," in spite of being able to comprehend the linguistic level of input. Such comparisons of performance often are carried out after formal testing, because existing formal tests do not allow for such meticulous examination.

Primary expressive deficits also are revealed in comparisons among a variety of circumstances. Agrammatism is seen in repetition and reading aloud as well as in spontaneous verbal expression and picture description. The patient's problem to be treated is not defined as a repetition deficit

TABLE 6-4. Three hypothetical cases illustrate task comparison within auditory language comprehension. Let us assume that each stimulus involves comprehension of a spatial relationship, such as "The hat is under the table" (Statement), "Put the hat under the table" (Instruction), and "Is the hat under the table?" (Question).

Task	Stimulus	Response	A	B	C
Auditory comprehension	Statement	Pointing	−	+	+
Auditory comprehension	Instruction	Manipulation	−	−	+
Auditory comprehension	Question	"Yes"/"No"	−	+	−

but, instead, is defined as an agrammatism which is revealed through the window of repetition. Similarly, word retrieval deficits are revealed most clearly with divergent tasks as well as with the more traditional convergent tasks. Divergent language behavior was described in Chapter 5.

As indicated previously, task comparison can be a strategy for distinguishing a modality-specific deficit from aphasia. Visual agnosia, for example, could contribute to the appearance of auditory comprehension deficit, when tested by pointing to objects, or to the appearance of naming deficit, when tested by naming a visually presented stimulus. Brookshire (1978b) listed several other factors which should be eliminated when agnosia is thought to be present: (1) sensory deficit, which is excluded when the patient can match objects in the suspect modality; (2) comprehension deficit, which is excluded when the patient can identify the object presented in another modality; (3) expressive deficit, which is excluded if the patient can name the object when presented in another modality; (4) unfamiliarity with the test stimulus, which is excluded when the item is recognized through another modality. All of these decisions can be accomplished through task comparison, when one component of the task—the stimulus, response, or material (verbal or nonverbal)—is varied, and the others are kept constant.

The outcome of assessment is a list of problems or primary deficits on which treatment is focused. A patient with Broca's aphasia may have the following problem list: (1) mild auditory comprehension deficit, primarily with prepositional phrases, (2) moderate reading deficit, (3) moderate agrammatism, (4) delays in word retrieval, (5) apraxia of speech, (6) right hemiplegia, (7) severe agrammatism in writing with the left hand. The problems are translated into specific goals for treatment. The research reviewed in

Chapter 5 indicates that when a syndrome can be identified clearly, we might assume that there is a single primary deficit upon which treatment can be focused. The patient with Broca's aphasia may have a single problem defined broadly as a central impairment of syntactic processes. This deficit would be responsible for reductions in all four modalities. The patient with Wernicke's aphasia may have a primary deficit in semantic organization. Such notions mean that defining problems with respect to modalities is a secondary consideration leading to a varied attack on the primary deficit in treatment.

Item Comparison. Item comparison is considered *within a task* when a patient makes errors on some items but not others. Generally, each item within a task is selected by the test's author to be homogeneous, and a few errors are considered indicative of level of function. However, especially when different sentences are used as input, there may be some subtle differences among items which are creating special problems for an individual patient. There may be differences in familiarity with vocabulary among the items or subtle differences in sentence structure to which the patient is sensitive. The clinician tries to determine whether there is a characteristic of the missed items which distinguishes these from the correct items. For example, a patient with minimal education may not be familiar with certain vocabulary. If such a distinctive characteristic in the missed items can be identified, then the clinician may conclude that the primary deficit in this task is not auditory sentence comprehension per se but, rather, is an educational deficit contributing to comprehension ability. If the distinctive characteristic is a syntactic structure, then the primary deficit is defined as a specific kind of auditory language comprehension problem with respect to a certain syntactic structure. In either case, the characteristic of the item should be tested repeatedly to determine whether the item truly represents a peculiar problem.

Positive and Negative Symptoms

The British neurologist Hughlings Jackson (1879) advised that a complete clinical examination of someone with aphasia, an "affection of speech" as he called it, includes identification of the positive symptoms as well as the negative ones. Negative symptoms reflect a deficient component of the language function and include both primary and secondary symptoms. Positive symptoms, on the other hand, are indicative of intact or spared components of the language function. Negative symptoms are found particularly in the propositional use of language, while positive symptoms are found usually, but not exclusively, in the non-propositional use of language. Positive symptoms include circumlocution in anomic aphasia and the adaptive strategies of Broca's aphasia described in Chapter 5.

This distinction can be expanded with attention to the patient's linguistic strengths and weaknesses and, even more generally, to the patient's communicative strengths and weaknesses. The common clinical strategy of recording strengths and weaknesses includes attending to various levels of ability within a deficient function as well as attending to spared versus disturbed functions. As a result, when auditory language comprehension is impaired, a retained ability to comprehend at least a word in isolation is considered to be a linguistic asset. Comprehension of a word when some helpful context is added is considered to be a communicative asset. As Holland (1977b) suggested, the clinician should be looking for what is right about a patient as well as for what is wrong. Therefore, a complete assessment produces an inventory of an aphasic person's strengths and weaknesses among a variety of language functions.

Level of impairment often is judged by comparing a patient's test scores with a range of performance exhibited by a large sample of aphasics used as a normative group when the test was developed. The *PICA* (Porch, 1981a) and the *BDAE* (Goodglass and Kaplan, 1972) provide methods for identifying degree of deficit in this way (see Chapter 7). With other tests, degree of deficit is indicated with respect to 100 percent performance on the test. Degree of deficit often is labeled with terms like mild, moderate, marked, or severe; however, these terms may be used without a specific reference to what they mean. As general indicators, they are helpful for summarizing a patient's pattern of deficits.

Tests involve two basic approaches to measuring the degree of deficit within each language modality. One approach is to include several subtests within a modality which vary in their level of difficulty. Receptive tasks vary with respect to the length and linguistic complexity of input, and expressive tasks vary with respect to the length and complexity of language required in the patient's response. Severity of impairment is judged relative to the level of successful performance achieved among subtests. Another approach relies less on a task hierarchy and more on the sensitivity of the scoring system to variations in the patient's response. Few subtests are administered in a single modality, but the patient's score can have a wide range based on dimensions of correct and incorrect responses. Both approaches are valuable, not only for identifying amount of impairment, but also for measuring amount of recovery by a patient.

A traditional limitation of aphasia test batteries has been their ability to identify strengths and weaknesses of patients who are at either end of the severity continuum. Brookshire (1978b) discussed thoroughly the problem of testing low-level (severely impaired) and high-level (mildly impaired) patients. Test batteries adequately reveal the weaknesses of low-level patients, but they often are not sufficiently easy to reveal the patient's strengths. These batteries adequately reveal the spared language abilities of high-level patients, but they often are not sufficiently difficult to reveal the patient's deficits. This limitation takes on an additional dimension regarding mildly impaired aphasics, because tests contain a ceiling level of performance which prohibits a substantial range of improvement to be measured for these patients. Special tests have been developed to provide measurements of mild deficits. Mild deficits are most consistently revealed in the patient's writing (Keenan, 1971). Another valuable approach to assessing mild aphasia simply is to ask the patient to describe problems with language and the situations in which these problems occur. The clinician should devise supplemental methods for uncovering and measuring areas of ability in low-level patients. These methods should follow criteria for validity and reliability. Low-level aphasics are more likely to display language in nonpropositional usage than in propositional usage.

Clinical and Functional Performance

Linguistic performance can appear to differ between the contexts of clinical examination and natural settings. Natural settings are rich in familiar contextual cues which interact with linguistic input to aid comprehension and to supplement verbal expression. The aphasic patient at home or in familiar social settings often converses with someone who shares knowledge with the patient of a range of subjects, and the listener can use this knowledge to interpret incomplete aphasic utterances. Agrammatic omissions and phonemic paraphasias may sometimes seem insignificant to a listener who is more concerned about the patient's message than about linguistic virtuosity. These factors create an atmosphere for linguistic performance which differs from the clinical examination.

The clinical assessment of aphasic language, especially in the formal test situation, has been designed primarily to afford a clear view of linguistic ability without the aid of extralinguistic context. Tests of language are intended to assess what might be impaired in aphasia and not what usually remains intact. Therefore, the circumstances presented to patients are sometimes quite estranged from what the patient might deal with in natural environments. To examine auditory language comprehension, one test requires the patient to "put the bell between the penny and the spoon" (Schuell, 1965b) and another instructs, "Tap each shoulder twice with two fingers keeping your eyes shut" (Goodglass and Kaplan, 1972). Such tasks are created so that a correct response must be based on sufficient analysis of the linguistic input rather than on cues to conceptual knowledge derived from the situation. If the task is more true to life, such as presenting a hammer, nail, and board to the patient and asking the patient to "pound the nail into the wood," the patient can respond appropriately based on recognition of the nonverbal context. The linguistic input can pass by without notice. In test situations which minimize extralinguistic influences, the patient may comprehend less than he or she appears to comprehend in natural settings (Wilcox, et al., 1978). When a deficit found with a test is observed in natural settings, the impact of the deficit on natural communication can be determined.

Also, the patient may simply use language less efficiently in clinical circumstances. Whitbourne (1976) found that older adults exhibit more test anxiety than younger adults. Older people are not as accustomed to being tested as younger people, and their concern may reduce their performance more than would be seen in more relaxing and familiar settings. Wepman (1976) observed that some patients tend to verbalize less effectively when asked to make a specific linguistic response. Conversation about familiar topics sometimes frees them to retrieve their own words and thereby exhibit a more efficient word-finding ability. A complete assessment of primary and secondary negative symptoms includes observation in clinical and natural settings, and positive symptoms should be observed in both circumstances.

REVIEW OF DECISIONS

This chapter introduced the clinician to the information and decision strategies that are applied to diagnosis and assessment of aphasia and related disorders. The chapter should be applicable no matter what published test or spontaneously created test is used to gather behavioral observations of a patient. When the patient is first seen, important decisions include whether he or she has a language impairment and whether the language impairment is aphasia (and, therefore, is treatable by traditional language methods). Much of the information obtained is used to make a prediction about recovery; this decision is a topic of Chapter 9. Assessment is directed toward planning treatment which develops out of accurate identification of each patient's problems. Assessment strategies are incorporated continuously in the analysis of behavior during treatment. Chapters 4 and 9 address reasons for waiting three weeks to a month after onset before administering a comprehensive examination in order to plan long-term treatment. At this time most patients begin to present a clear picture of primary deficits and spared functions.

7 Comprehensive Tests of Language Function

This chapter is concerned with tests which are designed to facilitate the clinician's comprehensive examination of the four language modalities, as well as related functions. The next chapter will include supplemental tests of functional communication and several special measurements of one modality or another, facilitating more thorough assessment, for example, of auditory language comprehension. Both chapters are intended to familiarize the reader, not only with the tests themselves, but also with literature addressed to these procedures.

Most attention is given to three test batteries: the *Minnesota Test for Differential Diagnosis of Aphasia* (Schuell, 1965b), the *Porch Index of Communicative Ability* (Porch, 1967), and the *Boston Diagnostic Aphasia Examination* (Goodglass and Kaplan, 1972). These have been noted to be the most popular or widely used aphasia batteries (Emerick and Hatten, 1979; Kertesz, 1979). They differ in their orientation with respect to the three major goals of testing stated by Goodglass and Kaplan (1972) and, therefore, provide representative illustrations of how each goal can be achieved. These objectives are (1) "comprehensive assessment of the assets and liabilities of the patient in all language areas as a guide to therapy," (2) "measurement of the level of performance over a wide range, for both initial determination and detection of change over time," and (3) "diagnosis of presence and type of aphasic syndrome, leading to inferences concerning cerebral localization" (p. 1).

MINNESOTA TEST FOR DIFFERENTIAL DIAGNOSIS OF APHASIA (MTDDA)

This may be the archetypical test for aphasia. Though other examination procedures had been reported before its inception (Halstead and Wepman, 1949; Head, 1926; Robbins, 1939), Hildred Schuell's *MTDDA*, sometimes referred to as "the Schuell test," was the first comprehensive test for adult aphasia and anticipated the structure and content of most subsequent test batteries.

Purpose

Of the three goals of examination, the *MTDDA* is oriented most toward the comprehensive assessment of the patient's strengths and weaknesses in all language modalities as a guide to planning treatment. Additional aims include differential diagnosis and prediction of recovery. Differential diagnosis, in this case, refers to whether the patient has aphasia or aphasia plus perceptual disorders, apraxia, dysarthria, or some other result of brain damage. It does not refer to differentiating aphasia from chronic brain syndrome, for example, or to differentiating among the syndromes of aphasia.

Development

The *MTDDA* evolved from seven revisions made over seventeen years, beginning with the first form in the summer of 1948 (Schuell, 1965a). Brown and Schuell (1950) described the different levels of language performance in each modality that were considered in constructing the first form. After five revisions, form 6 was made available in 1955 on a limited basis for experimental use. At the Minneapolis Veterans Administration Hospital, this research edition was administered to 155 neurologically stable aphasic patients and 50 nonaphasic patients between 1955 and 1958. Data on test-retest performance and for a factor analysis were gathered during this period. The 1965 version was the eighth form, and included only minor changes from forms 6 and 7. After Schuell's death in 1970, the test and the interpretation manual were revised only slightly by Sefer (Schuell, 1973). The *MTDDA* has been used extensively by speech-language pathologists, and Thompson and Enderby (1979) wrote that " . . . it is still the most widely used aphasia assessment in Britain" (p. 195).

Description of the MTDDA

The *MTDDA* is the most comprehensive of the tests for aphasia; it takes two to six hours to administer, three hours on the average. It consists of forty-six subtests divided among five sections: auditory disturbances, visual and reading disturb-

ances, speech and language disturbances, visuomotor and writing disturbances, and disturbances of numerical relations and arithmetic processes. Within each of the four language modality sections the subtests are graded in difficulty, from easy to difficult. The test is supplemented with clinical rating scales for each modality which serve as a guide for communicating test findings to others and direct attention to functional communication goals for the patient.

The section assessing *auditory disturbances* contains nine subtests, including common word recognition, serial word recognition, answering yes/no questions, following instructions, and understanding a paragraph. Two additional subtests, digit and sentence repetition, are intended to examine auditory short-term memory, but instructions are for the patient to say the digits and sentences. Expressive deficits confound any inference about short-term memory from a repetition task. Also, there is a test of speech-sound discrimination.

Visual and reading disturbances are assessed with eight subtests and a provision for scoring reading rate during one of these subtests. Therefore, nine scores are obtained in this section of the test. Perceptual abilities are observed with subtests of form and letter matching. Visual language is assessed with word, sentence, and paragraph comprehension. Speech is required from the patient with two subtests of oral reading (reading aloud).

Speech and language disturbances are examined with fifteen tasks. Speech function receives attention with tests of oral movement, rapid alternating movements for speech sounds, and repetition of words and phrases selected and organized according to particular speech sounds. Nonpropositional, automatic verbal expression is tested by having the patient count to twenty, say the days of the week, and complete sentences. Propositional language is assessed in a variety of circumstances such as picture naming, answering questions, using a word in a sentence, describing a picture, defining words, and retelling a paragraph.

Visuomotor and writing disturbances are observed with ten subtests. Visuomotor ability is checked by having the patient copy Greek letters, a wheel, and English letters. Propositional language is tapped with tests of word, sentence, and paragraph writing.

Numerical relations and arithmetic processes are assessed with four subtests including making change, setting a clock, and two levels of basic addition, subtraction, multiplication, and division.

The subtests vary as to the number of items tested. The auditory word-recognition subtest contains eighteen items, and the visual word-recognition task contains thirty-two items. The patient attempts to complete eight sentences and attempts to name twenty pictures. The number of items in the *MTDDA* totals 537; while, in contrast, the *Porch Index of Communicative Ability* contains 180 items.

Administration and Scoring

Formal test materials include an interpretation manual, an administrative manual, a record booklet, and two packs of visual stimulus cards. The administration manual includes instructions to be given to the patient and instructions for the clinician in administering and scoring each task. Overall pattern of performance can be seen quickly with a summary of test scores on the cover page of the record booklet.

Schuell recommended that, because of its length, the *MTDDA* should be given in more than one session. The clinician should stop testing when the patient is fatigued or uncomfortable. Assessment with this test may take an especially long time if the clinician is in a setting, such as a nursing home, where patients may be scheduled for half-hour sessions. For a quicker general assessment of all language modalities in such settings, the clinician may choose to use a shorter test or a carefully selected sample of subtests and items from the *MTDDA* (Schuell, 1966). In discussing Schuell's test, Thompson and Enderby (1979) noted that clinicians "... tend to avoid any procedure which is cumbersome or seems redundant." They added: "Over many test administrations they eventually learn which items seem useful to them. However, because this is done on an intuitive basis, and looks like a lazy approach to a 'scientific' test, clinicians are often embarrassed by the fact that they do not give the full test" (p. 196). Thompson and Enderby took a systematic approach to developing a short form of Schuell's test with only five items per subtest.

The method of scoring varies somewhat among the different subtests; however, most subtests involve plus-minus scoring. Two of the speech and language subtests are scored based on a scale, and one subtest in this section permits a half point for partially correct responses. Notes about the patient's behavior may be recorded in the record booklet.

Standardization

Norms. The research edition of the *MTDDA* was administered to aphasic and nonbrain-injured patients who were described in detail by Schuell, Jenkins, and Jimenez-Pabon (1964). The average number of errors and standard deviations for each subtest are available in the interpretation manual. Mean correct scores for each modality are presented in Schuell's text (Schuell, et al., 1964). Only a few subtests were given to 157 aphasic patients; thirty-eight of the forty-seven subtest means were obtained from 75 patients. In the interpretation manual, mean errors on individual subtests are reported for each of Schuell's diagnostic categories from the group of seventy-five aphasic patients. The sizes of these diagnostic groups range from six to twenty-six. The size of the group with simple aphasia uncomplicated by additional problems is twelve for most of the subtests. In considering what is represented by average scores per modality, the clinician should realize that the auditory section does contain two subtests involving repetition and that the reading section contains two subtests involving reading aloud. Therefore, the mean scores for each of these modalities does not represent purely receptive functions.

The test was administered to fifty nonaphasic hospital patients. The determination of whether a patient has a language deficit is made, in part, based on whether the patient has difficulties on this test. Therefore, it is assumed that nonaphasic persons would have no difficulty. This was demonstrated with respect to most of the subtests (Schuell, 1965a, 1973). However, on the paragraph reading subtest 74 percent of the nonaphasic group made an average of 1.86 errors. Averages of around 1.5 errors were made by the nonaphasics on written and oral spelling although, in this case, only 36 percent and 26 percent of the group respectively made any errors. These difficulties may have been related to the educational background of some of these subjects.

Validity and Reliability. The question of whether the *MTDDA* truly meets its objectives was based on content and construct validity. Schuell believed that language function is a single process underlying varied forms of language behavior, which is the unidimensional view of aphasia described in Chapter 4. Aphasia was considered to vary only in degree of deficit in the four language modalities. The content of the *MTDDA* was developed based on these assumptions. A factor analysis of the test provided support for these assumptions and served as an indication of

construct validity (Schuell, Jenkins, and Carroll, 1962). A cluster-analysis by Powell, Clark, and Bailey (1979) yielded four groups of patients aligned according to severity. Criterion-related validity was not investigated by Schuell. Also, reliability of Schuell's test has not been investigated. The test-retest series reported by Schuell, et al. (1964) involved retesting upon termination of treatment with test-retest intervals ranging from one to thirteen months. The purpose of this series was to measure recovery, not to examine stability of the measurement device.

Interpretation

Differential Diagnosis. The *MTDDA* was not designed to facilitate identification of aphasia syndromes, since Schuell did not recognize such differences within the category of aphasia. However, by knowing what to look for the clinican can use performance in the picture description, comprehension, and repetition tasks as evidence for identification of syndromes.

The Minnesota test is intended to differentiate aphasia from normal levels of language function with the aid of the normative data in the interpretation manual. An adaptation of the short version (Schuell, 1957) was used by Halpern, et al. (1973) to differentiate among aphasia, apraxia of speech, confused language, and generalized intellectual impairment or the dementia of chronic brain syndrome. This adaptation and additional tests were employed later to differentiate these disorders from chronic schizophrenia (DiSimoni, et al., 1977). Interpretation guidelines are primarily provided in the test manual to differentiate among the categories of communication disorders defined by Schuell.

Schuell's classification of neurogenic communication disorders has undergone at least two revisions. In the revised interpretation manual (Schuell, 1973), Sefer simply reorganized the categories from five major and two minor categories to seven major categories. These categories were not tied clearly to any particular site of lesion, partly because localizing technology was not very sophisticated in the 1950s. *Simple aphasia* (Schuell's Group 1) represented reduced language function in all modalities without complicating conditions. *Aphasia with visual involvement* (Schuell's Group 2) consisted of simple aphasia with more severely reduced reading and writing functions. *Mild aphasia with persisting dysfluency* (Schuell's Minor Syndrome B) was simple aphasia with articulatory problems that Schuell described as a mild dysarthria. *Aphasia with scattered findings compatible with generalized brain damage* (Schuell's Group 4) was described by Schuell as aphasia with visual and motor involvement. Sixty-eight percent of this group showed impaired mental status. There was evidence of regressive behavioral changes and bilateral brain damage (Schuell et al., 1964). This group could be questioned as being truly aphasic (Porch, 1979). *Aphasia with sensorimotor involvement* (Schuell's Group 3) resembled aphasia with what may have been apraxia of speech. Ninety-four percent of this group had hemiplegia or hemiparesis which is suggestive of nonfluent aphasia or Broca's aphasia with apraxia. *Aphasia with intermittent auditory imperception* (Schuell's Minor Syndrome A) was used for patients who behaved as if they were deaf. Descriptions of this group are consistent with mild forms of Wernicke's aphasia or pure word deafness. *Irreversible aphasic syndrome* (Schuell's Group 5) was used for almost complete loss of language function in all modalities; a global aphasia.

Prognosis and Recovery. Prediction of recovery is contingent upon identification of Schuell's categories. Average amount of recovery in each test modality is displayed graphically in Schuell's text for each of the five major groups (Schuell, et al., 1964). General conclusions about

amount and pattern of recovery are given for the seven categories in the interpretation manual (Schuell, 1973). Amount of recovery is described as either excellent, limited but functional, or poor. Categories with excellent recovery in all modalities include simple aphasia, aphasia with visual involvement, and mild aphasia with persisting dysfluency. With visual involvement, reading and writing improve more slowly than speech. With persisting dysfluency, normal articulation patterns can be acquired when the patient establishes conscious control of speech movements. Limited recovery of language is attributed to aphasia with generalized brain damage, aphasia with sensorimotor involvement, and aphasia with intermittent auditory imperception. With generalized brain damage, the patient is " . . . usually incapable of persistent self-directed effort" (Schuell, 1973, p. 13). With sensorimotor involvement, the speech modality recovers more than the others, but the final level of recovery is still below that of simple aphasia. The irreversible syndrome has a poor prognosis. Though auditory comprehension may become functional, the other language modalities do not.

The *MTDDA*'s value as a measure of recovery, especially during the acute phase, has not been demonstrated clearly. Its use in this regard would be contingent on its reliability and its sensitivity to small changes in the patient's language functions. This capability can be questioned because of its unproved reliability and its plus-minus scoring system. The Minnesota test's ability to reflect levels of language function is based primarily on its range of task difficulty within each modality and the large number of items in certain subtests. Therefore, in terms of the patient's proportion of successes on individual tasks and of ability to progress up the task hierarchy, recovery of language function can be measured to some extent. Hagen (1973) used this test to measure changes in treated and untreated patients

with three and six-month intervals between administrations. Its length prohibits
more frequent retesting unless selected
portions are used especially during spontaneous recovery, when changes occur
more rapidly.

Treatment Planning. Any test is a
guide to treatment planning when a clinician applies certain common principles to
the interpretation of test performance. If a
test assists in the identification of a disorder, this narrows the options for direction of treatment. If a test assists in the
identification of primary deficits underlying test performance, then the clinician
can direct treatment even more accurately
to the appropriate problems. Simply because of its comprehensiveness, the
MTDDA provides many circumstances for
task and item comparisons so that the
clinician can make inferences about the
basic problem or problems to be treated.

There are no guidelines in the test
manual for translating test results into
treatment plans. However, common principles of treatment design (see Chapter 10)
can be applied to interpretation. Three
principles in combination can be an aid to
making such decisions from test performance: (1) select an adequate stimulus,
(2) elicit responses instead of forcing them,
and (3) select a task that is challenging but
successful for the patient. The *MTDDA*
provides a wide sampling of potentially
adequate types of stimuli, of situations in
which responses can be elicited, and of the
kinds of circumstances in which a patient
can use language successfully.

PORCH INDEX
OF COMMUNICATIVE ABILITY (*PICA*)

While not as comprehensive in number of
tasks and items as the Minnesota test,
Bruce Porch's *PICA* is the most completely
standardized aphasia test. It took some
time for many experienced clinicians to
adjust to the unique features of this test.
Yet, with the expanding realization that
treatment methods should stand on a scientific base and that clinicians are ac-
countable for demonstrating recovery,
no matter how small, sensitivity to principles behind the *PICA* and use of this test
have expanded. Nevertheless, Emerick
and Hatten (1979) felt the need to advise
that the *PICA* " . . . is not, however, the
Holy Grail of aphasiology that some overly
zealous diagnosticians impugn it to be"
(p. 290). Porch (1967) did indicate that it
would be scientifically advantageous if one
test with appropriate characteristics were
generally accepted, but he added that a
standard test " . . . would not solve all the
problems of aphasia testing, but would
serve as a starting point for improving
communication between researchers and
serve as a spring-board for the development of better methods . . . " (p. 3). The
PICA has been deified and vilified; it has
been the most scrutinized of comprehensive aphasia tests; it has had an enormous
influence on clinical aphasiology.

Purpose and Development

The *PICA* is oriented most toward the
second of the three aims of testing by providing a sensitive and reliable measurement of degree of deficit and amount of
recovery. Measurement of change is based
on a multidimensional scoring system
which is intended to be sensitive to subtle
differences among aphasic behaviors. Because the *PICA* is designed to measure
recovery, it has been employed for making
predictions of amount of recovery in terms
of test scores.

From "what was to be a nine-month
study of certain aspects of aphasia"
(Porch, 1967, p. iii), the basic battery and
multidimensional scoring system were
developed during a six-year period beginning in 1959. The test manual was published in two volumes in 1967. Volume II,
Administration, Scoring and Interpretation, was

revised in 1971 and again in 1981. The newest manual includes additions to the scoring procedure and revised subtest categories for summarizing results (Porch, 1981a).

Description of the PICA

The *PICA* consists of eighteen subtests of the four language modalities and of object manipulation, visual matching, and copying abstract forms. The order of subtest administration differs from other batteries (Table 7-1). The basis for this organization is discussed in the next paragraph. For summarizing performance patterns, the subtests since 1967 were categorized only according to the modality of responses, not according to both language input and output. The eighteen subtests, therefore, were labeled as *gestural, verbal,* and *graphic.* In 1981 Porch adjusted subtest categories according to function, as shown in Table 7-1.

Two principles guided construction of the test battery. First, internal consistency among subtests is enhanced to facilitate comparison of performance among subtests. Each subtest consists of ten items involving ten objects which are used throughout the eighteen subtests. These objects are a toothbrush, cigarette, pen, knife, fork, quarter, pencil, matches, key, and comb. Consistency is maintained further by use of the same scoring system for each subtest. Second, because the same objects are used throughout the battery, responses based on recall of recent linguistic information are minimized by the way in which the tasks are ordered. Minimal linguistic information about the objects is given by the examiner early in the test, with maximum information deferred until later in the test. As a result, the

TABLE 7-1. Order of administering *PICA* subtests. *(Adapted by permission from Porch, B. E., Porch Index of Communicative Ability: Theory and Development, Volume 1. Palo Alto, Calif.: Consulting Psychologists Press, 1967).*

Test	Output (1967)	Function (1981)	Task
I	Verbal		Describes function of object
II	Gestural	Pantomime	Demonstrates function of object
III	Gestural	Pantomime	Demonstrates function in order
IV	Verbal		Names objects
V	Gestural	Reading	Reads function and position
VI	Gestural	Auditory	Points to object, given its function
VII	Gestural	Reading	Reads name and position
VIII	Gestural	Visual	Matches picture to object
IX	Verbal		Completes sentence with object name
X	Gestural	Auditory	Points to object, given its name
XI	Gestural	Visual	Matches object to object
XII	Verbal		Repeats name of object
A	Graphic	Writing	Writes function of object
B	Graphic	Writing	Writes name of object
C	Graphic	Writing	Writes name to dictation
D	Graphic	Writing	Writes name when spelled
E	Graphic	Copying	Copies name of object
F	Graphic	Copying	Copies geometric forms

order of subtests also tends to present the patient with more difficult subtests prior to easier ones.

DiSimoni, Keith, Holt, et al. (1975) investigated whether a short version would be capable of providing the same information as the complete version. In addition to the scores obtained from each subtest and the average score for each of the three response modalities, a single *overall* score is derived. DiSimoni and his colleagues questioned whether an abbreviated version would result in the same overall score as the complete test. Using a step-wise regression analysis of 222 administrations of the complete *PICA,* they determined that only ten subtests and five objects are needed to achieve the same overall score that would be obtained from a complete test. Two other short versions produced similar results (DiSimoni, Keith, and Darley, 1980). Phillips and Halpin (1978) described a version shortened by using five objects, and it was reliable but had less sensitivity to recovery over four weeks than the complete *PICA* (Lincoln and Ells, 1980).

Administration and Scoring

Test materials include two manuals, a guide to test format and instructions, the ten objects in duplicate, a score sheet, and other forms for administering the graphic subtests and for various ways of summarizing and analyzing results. Porch found that it takes an average of about 61 minutes to give this test, with a range of 22 to 143 minutes.

Administration is restricted to some fairly explicit guidelines prescribed in the manuals in order to maximize the likelihood that the patient is assessed in the same way each time the test is repeated. These prescriptions include exactly what the clinician is to say to the patient in the administration of each task. Standard test conditions include a test room free of distractions, a prescribed seating arrangement, a particular arrangement of the objects, and procedures specified for each task. The order of task presentation must be consistent, and completing the battery in one session is preferred.

The most unique feature of the *PICA* is its scoring system. A multidimensional system of 16 scale points was conceived so that the many dimensions of aphasic responding could be quantified. The scale was designed to be descriptive and yet manageable, and to be applicable for each of the subtests.

The *PICA's* multidimensional scoring system reflects the degrees of correctness and incorrectness in aphasic behavior and, therefore, provides more information quantitatively than a plus-minus scoring procedure. It is based on five dimensions of patients' responses: *accuracy* (correctness), *responsiveness* (amount of information needed by the patient to complete the task), *completeness* of the response, *promptness* (time to respond), and *efficiency* (motoric facility). These dimensions are combined into a rank order of response adequacy shown in Table 7–2, where 16 represents the most adequate response and 1 represents the least adequate response. Responses between 16 and 8 would represent correct responses with a plus-minus system, while 7 through 1 would be incorrect. Each of the patient's 180 responses is assigned one of these numbers during administration. In the most recent revision, Porch (1981a) did not change scoring, but did add diacritical markings so that a patient's behavior could be recorded more precisely.

Though this scale is used for each subtest, the individual levels have subtle variations of meaning when applied to different tasks. In order to maximize consistent application of this scale on retest and by different clinicians, detailed definitions and examples of the scale points are given for each subtest in the scoring manual.

TABLE 7-2. Multidimensional scoring system of the *PICA. (Adapted by permission from Porch, B. E.,* Porch Index of Communicative Ability: Theory and Development, Volume 1. *Palo Alto, Calif.: Consulting Psychologists Press, 1967).*

Score	Level	Description of Response
16	Complex	Accurate, complex, and elaborate
15	Complete	Accurate and complete
14	Distorted	Accurate, complete, but with reduced facility
13	Complete-delayed	Accurate, complete, but slow or delayed
12	Incomplete	Accurate but incomplete
11	Incomplete-delayed	Accurate, incomplete, slow or delayed
10	Corrected	Accurate after self-correction of error
9	Repetition	Accurate after repetition of instruction
8	Cued	Accurate after cue or other information
7	Related	Inaccurate but related to correct response
6	Error	Inaccurate
5	Intelligible	Intelligible but not related to test item
4	Unintelligible	Unintelligible, differentiated
3	Minimal	Unintelligible, not differentiated
2	Attention	Attention to item but no response
1	No response	No awareness of test item

Also, Porch recommended at least forty hours of training, including extensive scoring practice, prior to the clinical application of the *PICA.* Such training has become widely available to clinicians through workshops conducted by clinicians who have extensive experience with this test.

The numbers assigned to each response are averaged at different levels, and these means are recorded on the score sheet. The mean scores are used for determining degree of deficit, summarizing patterns of deficit, and figuring predictions of subsequent performance. The ten responses for each task are averaged to provide a mean response level for each subtest. With the 1967 version, subtest means have been averaged to provide mean response levels in the gestural, verbal, and graphic categories. The 1981 revision permits interpretation with the seven categories shown in Table 7-1. A single mean response level is derived to reflect overall level of communicative ability.

Standardization

The *PICA* is especially noted for its norms and reliability, which were determined during development of the test. Several measures suggestive of its validity have accumulated since the test was published, and these measures have been obtained by different investigators.

Norms. Interpretation of test performance is aided by translating raw scores into percentiles which indicate the degree of deficit with respect to a large sample of left-hemisphere-damaged aphasic subjects (280 in 1971, 357 in 1981). The translation of raw scores into percentile scores is accomplished with tables provided in the administration and interpretation manual. Porch's sampling of the aphasic population was designed to reflect the typical age, race, sex, education, occupation, and etiology of aphasic patients. Stroke was the dominant etiology of the group, reflecting the predominance of stroke in the typical clinical caseload of the period of test development. Also, a percentile table is given based on a sample of one hundred bilaterally brain-damaged subjects (Porch, 1971a, 1981a). Volume II includes several typical profiles of aphasia representing different degrees of deficit and a few profiles reflecting motor speech disorders. Pannbacker (1979) was concerned that the representativeness of Porch's original sample was diluted with the inclusion of bilingual speakers and a few patients with bilateral or diffuse brain damage. Porch (1979) responded by noting that the few bilinguals in the sample had been educated in the United States and that the bilaterally damaged subjects were separated from the aphasic sample in the revised manual of 1971. Pannbacker's concerns had been addressed to the sample of 150 used for the first interpretation manual.

Duffy, Keith, Shane, et al. (1976) administered the *PICA* to 130 normal subjects. While it takes an average of one hour for an aphasic patient to complete the *PICA*, most of the normal subjects breezed through it in about half that time. A score of 15 is generally considered to be the most typical best performance on the 16-point scale. These normal subjects showed some difficulty in areas influenced by education that are similar to areas of difficulty shown by the 50 normals who had been given the

MTDDA. Ninety-five percent of Duffy, et al.'s sample averaged 12.95 on the graphic subtests, with an average of 9.63 on writing sentences (subtest A). Moreover, in demonstrating the function of objects, these subjects averaged 11.52 (subtest II) and 12.79 (subtest III). Also, 95 percent of the normal sample averaged 12.05 on the first verbal subtest, which requires a spoken description of object function. This finding indicates that the criterion for a score of 15 on subtest I is seldom met by the normal population. Nevertheless, this does not invalidate the interpretation devices of the *PICA*, which are based on how 357 aphasic persons did on the test, not on how well normals might perform on it. Because data from normal adults is absent from the *PICA* manual, a small portion of Duffy, et al.'s (1976) data is presented in Table 7–3.

Percentile tables based on mean response scores were developed from 111 right-hemisphere-damaged patients by Deal, Deal, Wertz, et al. (1979a). Table 7–3 includes a sample of these results. Patients with right-hemisphere damage, assumed to be largely nonaphasic, are shown to have some reduction of *PICA* performance, especially in the graphic section. A more detailed comparison between left-hemisphere aphasic (LH) performance and right-hemisphere (RH) perform-

TABLE 7-3. Mean response level performance on the *PICA* is compared among normal adults (Duffy, et al., 1976), right-hemisphere-damaged adults (Deal, et al., 1979), and aphasic adults (Porch, 1971a). To approximate comparison with the average scores of normal adults, the 50th percentile scores are drawn from the studies of brain-damaged patients.

	Overall	Gestural	Verbal	Graphic
Normal Adults				
Range	13.40-14.99	13.73-15.00	13.48-15.03	11.18-15.03
Average	14.46	14.66	14.55	14.12
Right Hemisphere				
50th Percentile	13.31	14.07	13.90	12.32
Left Hemisphere (Aphasia)				
50th Percentile	10.64	12.73	11.20	7.50

ance is shown in Table 7-4. As aphasia increases in severity from the 90th to the 25th percentile, the difference between aphasia and right hemisphere damage increases. The difference shows up first (90th percentile) in the graphic modality. With increased severity the verbal problems of aphasia become more dramatic.

Validity. The *PICA* was intended to be a measure of communicative ability, and its validity should be considered with respect to the distinction between language and communication made in previous chapters of this book. An analysis of content validity indicates that, because most of the eighteen subtests examine language function outside of communicative contexts, the *PICA* is a test of language function but not of communication in the broad sense. Martin (1977) argued that this test has weak validity as a measure of communicative ability, in that it may be a measure of aphasic language deficit but not of communicative deficit.

Construct validity was examined by Clark, Crockett, and Klonoff (1979) to determine whether the *PICA* measures the particular dimensions of communicative function that were intended. Several factor analytic statistical procedures were applied to Porch's correlation matrix of subtest means derived from the original sample of 150 patients (Porch, 1967). One analysis revealed three factors which did not correspond precisely to the three output categories of gestural, verbal, and graphic. A general factor was found by using a different factor analysis. These results support the notion that the *PICA* measures three dimensions of communication and a general dimension of language related to the test's overall score.

Criterion-related validity has been assessed somewhat indirectly, generally as a result of other investigators' using the *PICA* as a criterion for validating other tests. It correlated at 0.93 with the *Aphasia Language Performance Scales* (Keenan and Brassell, 1975), at 0.89 with Kertesz's *Western Aphasia Battery* (Sanders and Davis, 1978), and at 0.93 with the *Communicative Abilities in Daily Living* (Holland, 1980a). The high correlation with Holland's *CADL* is of interest because it measures communicative adequacy instead of linguistic adequacy (see Chapter 8). Holland also developed a measure of aphasic patients' communication in their natural environments and used this measure as a criterion to compare with the *CADL* and the *PICA*. The *PICA* correlated at 0.55 with this measure of natural communication. Therefore, the *PICA* has strong criterion-related validity with respect to other tests of aphasia but may fall short of

TABLE 7-4. Percentile scores from 111 right-hemisphere-damaged patients *(Deal, et al., 1979)* are compared with percentile scores from 280 left-hemisphere-damaged aphasic patients *(Porch, 1971a).*

Percentile		Overall	Gestural	Verbal	Graphic
90th	*RH*	14.53	14.66	14.85	14.40
	LH	13.77	14.30	14.45	12.60
75th	*RH*	14.00	14.48	14.57	13.52
	LH	12.56	13.75	13.75	10.17
50th	*RH*	13.31	14.07	13.90	12.32
	LH	10.64	12.73	11.20	7.50
25th	*RH*	12.23	13.56	13.55	10.10
	LH	7.84	10.73	5.00	5.90

equivalent validity with respect to natural communicative function in daily life.

Validity of the *PICA*'s multidimensional scoring system has been investigated with respect to whether this scale truly represents a hierarchy of behavior, namely, whether it is truly an ordinal scale. As explained by Duffy and Dale (1977), ordinality means that a 12 is better than an 11 and a 6; but a 12 is not necessarily twice as good as a 6, and the distance between and 12 and 11 is not necessarily the same as the distance between a 6 and a 5. Studies by McNeil, Prescott, and Chang (1978) and by Duffy and Dale (1977) suggested that the scale indeed represents different levels of communicative accuracy and efficiency, but that the nature of the scale's ordinality may not correspond in certain respects to other ways of ranking the acceptability of communicative behaviors. In these two studies, students not familiar with the *PICA* were asked to develop their own rankings of the scale-point definitions comprising the *PICA* scale. These rankings were based on students' judgments about the functional communicative adequacy of the behaviors. The rankings were derived in different ways, but both studies showed that repeats (9) and self-corrections (10) were considered to be better than incomplete responses (12). In this respect, therefore, the *PICA*'s multidimensional scale may not entirely reflect what people consider to be more or less adequate communicative behaviors. Furthermore, McNeil, et al. found students' rankings of *PICA* scale definitions to vary among subtests, suggesting that the true ordinality of these behavioral levels depends on the situation. A test with several 16-point scoring systems which are most appropriate for the subtests would be unwieldy at best; however, borrowing the *PICA* scale for research should be done with caution because its application in certain circumstances may not be as valid as a modified scale.

Reliability. Prescribed administration procedures and carefully defined scale-point definitions for scoring contribute to the *PICA*'s demonstrated high reliability. Porch (1967) reported inter-examiner and test-retest reliability. Agreement among three trained scorers of thirty patients was shown, with correlations of 0.93 or better for subtests and 0.97 or better for response categories. Stability of forty patients' performance was assessed with a retest two weeks or less after their first test. Correlations between tests were 0.90 or better for all but five subtests. All shifts from the first to second testing were in a positive direction with an average shift of 0.39 on the sixteen-point scale. Test-retest correlations for the response categories were 0.98 overall, 0.96 gestural, 0.99 verbal, and 0.96 graphic. These correlations indicate that this test is very reliable when the scorer has had at least forty hours of training in administration and scoring.

Interpretation

The mean response level scores for each subtest, for the function categories, and for overall performance are the starting points in using the *PICA* for differential diagnosis, prognosis, and treatment planning.

Differential Diagnosis. Mean scores reflect general degrees of deficit in various language functions, and the pattern of these deficits can be indicative of different disorders. Recognizing the pattern of deficit is facilitated by plotting mean response levels on forms provided with the test. These forms have changed between the original subtest classification of 1967 and the new classification of 1981. The *modality response summary,* which has been displayed prominently (see Wertz, 1978), was not retained in the 1981 revision.

Some effort has gone into determining whether profiles from the *PICA* might reflect different syndromes of aphasia, especially because syndromes are identified partly according to degree of comprehension deficit. Porch (1971a) presented a profile for "aphasia with impaired verbal monitoring." His description of this impairment corresponds to Wernicke's aphasia. The profile shows the low verbal scores which would be obtained with fluent jargon. Later, Porch (1978; 1981a) proposed hypothetical relationships between the functions isolated in specific subtests and the different regions of the left hemisphere responsible for these functions. If these functions are differentiated in this way, then patterns of deficit from the *PICA* might be related to locations of brain damage. Six patterns were proposed and related to six regions of the brain. Porch (1978) presented single case illustrations of patterns related to damage in four of these regions. He considered these proposals to be tentative and merely indicative of an approach to detecting site of lesion.

PICA profiles have been used to distinguish among aphasia, apraxia of speech, and dysarthria (Porch, 1971a; Wertz, 1978). Pure apraxia, which is relatively rare, and dysarthria would be indicated by near-normal receptive language, and verbal scores much lower than graphic scores. Apraxia of speech usually occurs with Broca's aphasia, and the administration manual contains an example of "aphasia with severe formulation difficulty." The apraxia would push verbal scores downward so that they would be equal to or below the graphic scores (see Figure 6–2). An impairment of receptive language in the gestural category and an impairment of graphics would reflect the aphasic component of this combined disorder (see Wertz, Rosenbek, and Collins, 1978).

There has been a belief that "*PICA* profiles are virtually insensitive to differential diagnosis" (Pannbacker, 1979, p. 248). Porch (1979) replied that several studies have shown the *PICA* to be sensitive to

nonaphasic disorders in addition to the motor speech disorders already mentioned here. Profiles from patients with diffuse bilateral brain damage are available (Porch, 1971a, 1978; Watson and Records, 1978; Wertz, 1978). One commonly mentioned telltale sign of right-hemisphere or bilateral brain damage is an impairment on the object-matching tasks (VIII, XI) which falls below auditory comprehension (VI, X). Also, bilaterally damaged patients generally do less well on the easiest subtests than aphasic patients; and, with repeated testing, bilateral patients are likely to show a progressive regression of function instead of the recovery which is typical of aphasia.

Porch has pointed out that the objective identification of aphasic and nonaphasic disorders is important, not only for appropriateness of rehabilitation, but also for legal disputes pertaining to decisions about competency and compensation (see Chapter 6). He has investigated use of the *PICA* in identifying cases of neurosis and psychosis in which there is no brain damage and cases of malingering where aphasia is feigned (Porch and Porec, 1977; Porec and Porch, 1977). In the administration manual, Porch (1971a) presented an "aberrant pattern" illustrating poor performance on the easy tasks, a random pattern of up-and-down response levels. Subjects instructed to mimic aphasia, including speech pathology students and bartenders, produced a profile which was in the opposite direction of the typical aphasia profile (Porch and Porec, 1977).

Prognosis and Recovery. The *PICA* has been used extensively as an objective measure of recovery (see Chapter 9). It provides a single summarizing score which can be treated statistically to represent changes in single subtest-related functions, response categories, and overall language function. Mean scores are used as the basis for predicting later levels of function. The overall score, in particular, is a single indicator as to the amount of recovery made by an aphasic patient; and, because it reflects performance on all 180 items of the test, the overall score is the most reliable of the mean scores. Reliability is not as strong at the level of certain subtest means. Several types of analysis have been suggested for predicting recovery.

Averages of the nine highest subtest scores and nine lowest subtest scores are considered in prediction. The difference between the high and low percentiles, called the "High-Low gap," is indicative of what Porch referred to as the *dynamic range* of a patient's pattern of performance at any time in his or her recovery. The dynamic range is a theoretical range of functional ability in which *the high percentile represents the patient's potential for overall recovery;* it is a basic concept used by Porch in developing methods for predicting a patient's recovery. That is, the patient's best performance soon after onset is considered to be an indication of potential for maximum overall recovery at least five or six months later. Also, the patient's reaching that potential would be an indication that dismissal from treatment should be considered. A critical analysis of the High-Low gap was made by Wertz, Deal, and Deal (1981). Porch has recommended three methods of prediction.

The *High Overall Prediction* method or HOAP method (Porch, 1971a) involves use of a table of high and low-score percentiles in the administration manual (also, see Wertz, Deal, and Deal, 1980; Darley, 1982). Basically, the overall score at one month postonset is translated into its corresponding high score in the table. That high score is used to derive the predicted overall score at six months postonset. This method is consistent with the theory that the initial high scores represent the upper limit of the dynamic range.

A simpler method is called the *Short Direct or HOAP Slope* method (Porch, 1981a). With this method, the predicted overall score at six months postonset is found directly on a graph. However, in a study of eighty-five patients, Wertz, et al. (1980) concluded that both of the HOAP methods are woefully inadequate as predictors. There was a high frequency of predictions which were a great distance from their targets. Porch and Callaghan (1981) suggested that variation in recovery around a prediction should be expected. They redefined the problem relative to a correction factor that might be added to the predicted score.

The third suggestion is the *peak-mean difference* (PMD), another measure of variance reflecting a dynamic range. The PMD is derived with a formula utilizing the differences between the highest score and the mean score of each subtest (Porch, 1981a). In a study of twenty-four aphasic patients, Aten and Lyon (1978) concluded that the PMD, as well as other measures of variance on the *PICA,* was incapable of adequate prediction. Porch and Callaghan (1981) countered with the observation that anterior and posterior patients differ in PMD changes over time; therefore, pooled data would show disappointing results. As Porch, Collins, Wertz, et al. (1980) suggested, test scores may need to be supplemented with data concerning other factors in order to maximize statistical prediction of recovery.

Treatment Planning. As was indicated with respect to the *MTDDA,* the general principles for deciding where to begin in treatment apply to the results of any aphasia battery. Performance patterns from the *PICA* indicate the areas of language function which are successful but challenging for the patient. Brookshire (1978b) recommended that treatment be carried out with tasks producing 10 to 13-level responses from the patient; Porch (1981a) recommended treatment to be within the 9 to 15 range.

Porch (1981b) explained how the *PICA* can be used to plan treatment. His reference points were three levels of function exhibited in test results. The first is fully operational processing, represented by subtests on which the patient scores 15's. The second is a mid-range of responding in which the patient is accurate, but only after delays, self-correction, repeats, or cues, all of which are within scores of 8 to 13. The third reference point is beyond the patient's capacity, represented by subtests producing inaccurate responses; scores of 7 or below. The second level or midrange was referred to as the "fulcrum" of a hypothetical sigmoidal function curve. Porch stated that the tasks on the fulcrum lead to treatment.

Issues Surrounding the *PICA*

Although certain issues pertaining to this test have been mentioned, other debates found in the literature have been reserved until now, for the reader's convenience.

Order of Subtests.   One of Emerick and Hatten's (1979) opinions about the *PICA* was that starting out with the most difficult task often overwhelms patients and disturbs subsequent performance. The test does begin with the most difficult verbal subtest, but the next two tasks of object manipulation can be relatively easy for some patients. In terms of objective performance by Porch's standardization sample of patients, some subtests are preceded by more difficult tasks and others by easier tasks. Though the problem posed by Emerick and Hatten should be recognized, a sensitive examiner can minimize potential early frustration and continue to follow the guidelines for administration. Dumond, Hardy, and Van Demark (1978) used *PICA* subtests to investigate a general question about the effect of order of task difficulty on aphasic patients' performance. They found no difference in level of performance between hard-to-easy and easy-to-hard-ordered tasks. However,

they used five objects per subtest instead of ten, since their aim was not to evaluate the *PICA* per se. Although the effect of task order on performance with the *PICA* is an unanswered question, the test has been administered frequently enough to suggest that its impact on the patient's ability to take the test is minimal in most cases.

Formality of Administration.   Keenan and Brassell (1975) commented on aphasia batteries in general by feeling that they are too time-consuming, too restricted as to where they can be given, and too formal in standardization of administration. Standard tests, they said, " . . . have been so formal that they have served to break down the rapport which clinicians spend so much time and effort to establish" (p. 2). Emerick and Hatten (1979) perceived the *PICA* as being rigid enough, especially as to what appeared to be "mechanical" responding to the patient, to break down the clinician-client relationship.

Naturalness of interaction is sacrificed to some degree in order to achieve consistency, and therefore reliability. However, a client's reaction to any test is related as much to the clinician's handling of the situation as it might be to the test itself.

Patients can be advised about the general nature of the *PICA* prior to taking it for the first time. Nonspecific reassurance can be given by the clinician during and between subtests without breaking the rules of administration. Task instructions and stimuli can be presented warmly and calmly, without the coolness and pressure implied by the mechanical image of the *PICA*. Also, the sixty minutes that the *PICA* usually takes need not be harmful to a relationship that develops during several weeks of circumstances that are different from testing. The potential hazards of formal testing may not be eliminated, but they can be minimized and their existence should be only temporary.

Statistical Application of Mean Scores. There has been some question as to what a mean score from the *PICA* represents. Silverman (1974) cautioned that a subtest mean does not necessarily describe the patient's performance on a task. A mean of 10.0 could be obtained from a performance on one subtest in which the ten responses were 10, 10, 11, 10, 9, 10, 10, 9, 10, 11. In this case, the mean score is identical to most of the responses and close to the others and, therefore, is representative of the patient's actual behavior. On the other hand, a mean of 10.0 could be obtained from scores of 15, 5, 13, 14, 6, 15, 7, 6, 5, 14. In this case, the mean is not representative of the patient's actual behaviors on the task. A mode, the most frequent response, might be more descriptive than a mean.

Porch (1974) responded that a single mode can be rather difficult to obtain. In the second example above, there would be four modes for one task. Most important, however, is that the mean scores were not intended to be descriptive but were intended to be convenient single quantifications of level of performance with certain statistical advantages, one advantage being that they are single summarizing scores. Van Demark (1974) added that the clinician can be somewhat descriptive with the *PICA* by using the individual item scores. Modes can be used when description is the purpose for using the numbers, such as in clinical report writing. Also, the diacritical markings recommended in the lastest revision of the manual enable the clinician to describe behavior more precisely (Porch, 1981a).

Even for the purpose of having a single representative score to use statistically, the mean was criticized by Silverman (1974) because it is most technically appropriate when derived from an interval or ratio scale, not from an ordinal scale. Though Porch (1974) listed disadvantages to using the mode statistically, and he and Van Demark (1974) cited advantages for using a mean, Duffy and Dale (1977) provided the most supportive basis for using a mean derived from an ordinal scale. Porch viewed the mean as a necessary compromise to achieve certain statistical advantages. Duffy and Dale, however, compared Porch's ordinal scale with an interval scale derived from the sixteen levels of behavior in the *PICA* scale. From the test results of fifty patients, correlations between the ordinal *PICA* scale and the derived interval scale were above 0.99 for all eighteen subtest means and all summary means. Duffy and Dale concluded that the scoring system of the *PICA* functions as an interval scale and, therefore, the means can be used statistically with confidence.

BOSTON DIAGNOSTIC APHASIA EXAMINATION (BDAE)

In the 1960's, several studies by Harold Goodglass and his colleagues included a basis for classification called the "Boston V.A. Diagnostic Aphasia Test" (Goodglass, Quadfasel, and Timberlake, 1964) or the "Boston VA Hospital Aphasia Test" (Barton, Maruszewski, and Urrea, 1969). Hints about the contents of the test appeared in articles by Goodglass, et al. (1964) and Goodglass, Klein, Carey, et al. (1966). The "Boston Exam" was made available to the general clinical community in 1972. Albert, et al. (1981) provided a recent account of this assessment strategy.

Purpose and Development

The Boston Exam is oriented most toward diagnosis of the presence and type of aphasia, leading to inferences concerning the location of brain damage (Goodglass and Kaplan, 1972). As an aid to planning treatment, it is a relatively comprehensive battery which contains twenty-seven subtests. The *BDAE* is primarily designed for the sampling of language behaviors which have been demonstrated to be discriminative in the identification of aphasic syndromes. These behaviors include auditory comprehension, self-initiated and conversational speech, word retrieval, and repetition. When a symptom pattern indicative of a syndrome is apparent from test results, the probable site of brain lesion may be inferred. The researcher who wishes to group or describe subjects according to syndrome may use the *BDAE* as an objective basis for such categorizing.

The literature reveals early development of some of the unique features of the Boston Exam. Distinguishing features of aphasic spontaneous speech were studied by Goodglass, et al. (1964), who presented a rating scale profile of speech characteristics which later appeared in the *BDAE*. The subtests of auditory comprehension and the severity rating scale were also described in this report. Other portions of the Boston Exam, which are designed to assess certain peculiarities of auditory word comprehension and naming, were introduced by Goodglass, et al. (1966). They exposed occasional clinical phenomena such as (1) reduction of object naming without impairment of letter naming or number naming; (2) reduction of auditory comprehension for body part names but not for object names; and (3) reduction of color naming without other naming difficulties, as in pure alexia.

Description of the BDAE

The first section assesses *conversational and expository speech*. Conversational speech is elicited with questions suggestive of an initial interview and with open-ended conversation about familiar topics. Then a picture, called the ''Cookie Theft,'' is presented for the patient to describe. The clinician must record each utterance verbatim, with the aid of a tape recorder when necessary.

The *auditory comprehension* section consists of four subtests. There are two subtests of word recognition. The first involves having the patient identify objects, actions, letters, numbers, colors, and shapes by pointing to these items on stimulus cards. The drawings are smaller than on most cards and the items are somewhat crowded. Occasionally, therefore, visual problems may interfere with this task. The other word-recognition subtest involves pointing to body parts. Right-left discrimination problems, which may result from left parietal lobe damage, are investigated within this task. Two additional subtests in this section involve following commands and then answering yes-no questions, some after short paragraphs are read to the patient.

The *oral expression* section contains subtests for oral and verbal apraxia, non-propositional speech, repetition, and word retrieval. The tests of nonpropositional speech include reciting days, months, and the alphabet, counting, reciting previously memorized verses, and singing. A unique feature of the *BDAE* is its thorough assessment of repetition. The patient must attempt to repeat phrases and sentences which increase in length and which alternate between high and low probability of usage. Word retrieval is assessed under three stimulus conditions, or as Goodglass and Kaplan (1972) put it, through three ''windows'' to the central word-retrieval function. Patients respond with single words to questions spoken by the clinician. Confrontation naming of visual stimuli is examined with the same stimulus cards used for the auditory comprehension section. Therefore, comprehension and naming within the six previously mentioned categories can be compared. Also, divergent word retrieval is assessed by instructing the patient to produce as many animal names as possible in a specified amount of time. Word and sentence reading aloud is assessed here as well.

The *understanding written language* section consists of five subtests of word recognition, comprehension of spelling, word comprehension, and sentence and paragraph comprehension. The *writing* section contains seven subtests in which writing mechanics, nonpropositional writing, writing to dictation, written spelling and word retrieval, and sentence writing are assessed.

The manual contains several suggestions for supplementary testing of verbal and nonverbal functions. The tests of nonverbal functions include those functions which might be impaired along with language, especially in cases suffering damage to the parietal lobe. The parietal-lobe battery includes tests for constructional apraxia and finger agnosia. Constructional apraxia is examined with subtests of drawing and block design replication. Finger agnosia is assessed with subtests of finger recognition and naming. Although these subtests were standardized and included in the formal test summary, materials for administration have not been provided with purchase of the test.

Administration and Scoring

Test materials include a set of stimulus cards containing pictures and reading items, an examination booklet, and an administration and interpretation manual. The examination booklet is convenient in that it contains task instructions and is used for recording scores and behavioral observations. The *MTDDA,* on the other hand, involves one booklet with task instructions and another booklet for recording performance. The *BDAE* manual contains general guidelines for administration and scoring, and these guidelines also appear to some extent in the protocol booklet. Administration of this test is similar to giving the Minnesota test because guidelines leave room for a little flexibility by the clinician and, therefore, are not as rigid as with the *PICA.* The *BDAE* takes one to four hours to administer.

The main purpose of the conversational and expository speech section is the description and assessment of somewhat natural oral language, with reference to the telltale signs of aphasic syndromes. Scoring is accomplished with an *aphasia severity rating scale* and a *profile of speech characteristics,* shown in Figure 7–1. The severity rating is based partly on the degree of burden placed on the normal listener for the exchange of messages in a conversation with an aphasic person. The speech profile is based on six dimensions of oral expression, similar to other scales used to rate fluency (Benson, 1967; Kerschensteiner, et al., 1972), and on the degree of auditory-comprehension deficit revealed in the auditory comprehension section of the battery. The seven parameters together are discriminative among types of aphasia. Figure 7–1 illustrates a typical profile of Broca's aphasia.

Scoring of the auditory, oral, reading, and writing sections differs among subtests with plus-minus scoring, four point scales, and counts of the number of paraphasias in most of the oral expression subtests. The total possible score varies among subtests from 8 or 10 points on some subtests to 105 points on confrontation naming. Therefore, reporting of subtest scores should be in terms of a ratio. Test performance can be summarized on the profile form shown in Figure 7–2.

Verbal expression in subtests of automatic speech, repetition, and word retrieval is described by noting the frequency of motor speech difficulty, paraphasias, and jargon. Speech-language pathologists are surprised by a category of articulation impairment called "stiff," a term not normally used by these professionals and therefore difficult to interpret. Three major categories of paraphasias—phonemic, verbal, and neologistic—are employed. A count of these errors comprises one part of the z-score profile shown in Figure 7–2. The term literal paraphasia is used instead of phonemic

Patient's Name _____J.M._____ Date of rating __2 – 26 – 70_____

Rated by __H.G._____

APHASIA SEVERITY RATING SCALE

0. No usable speech or auditory comprehension.

(1.) All communication is through fragmentary expression; great need for inference, questioning and guessing by the listener. The range of information which can be exchanged is limited, and the listener carries the burden of communication.

2. Conversation about familiar subjects is possible with help from the listener. There are frequent failures to convey the idea, but patient shares the burden of communication with the examiner.

3. The patient can discuss <u>almost all everyday problems</u> with little or no assistance. However, reduction of speech and/or comprehension make conversation about certain material difficult or impossible.

4. Some obvious loss of fluency in speech or facility of comprehension, without significant limitation on ideas expressed or form of expression.

5. Minimal discernible speech handicaps; patient may have subjective difficulties which are not apparent to listener.

RATING SCALE PROFILE OF SPEECH CHARACTERISTICS

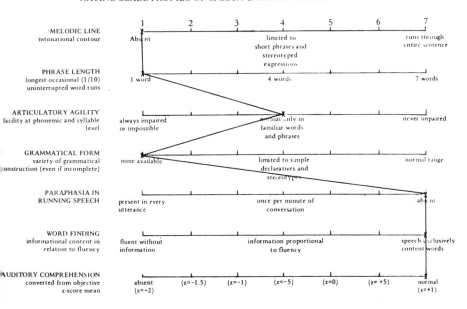

Figure 7-1. A subjective severity rating scale indicates general communicative ability. A rating scale profile of speech characteristics is one means by which different syndromes are characterized. Here, fluency and auditory comprehension are the main criteria (see Figure 6-1). An example of Broca's aphasia is shown. *Reprinted by permission of the publisher. From Goodglass, H., and Kaplan, E., The Assessment of Aphasia and Related Disorders. Philadelphia, Pa.: Lea & Febiger, 1972)*

173

Z-SCORE PROFILE OF APHASIA SUBSCORES

NAME: **J.M.**　　　　　　　　　　　　　　　　DATE OF EXAM: **12-9-68**

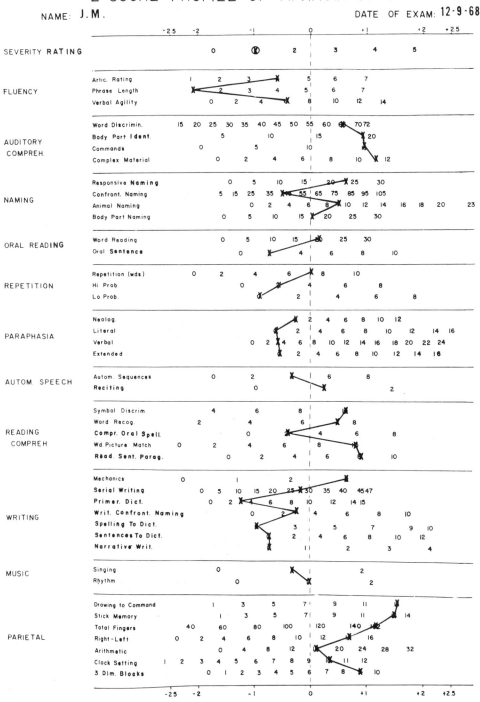

paraphasia, and neologisms are distinguished from phonemic paraphasias based on whether more or less than half of the error differs from the sound structure of the required word. Some of the errors often are difficult to classify with respect to the three major categories. Much of the difficulty lies with paraphasias that sound like the required word but possess attributes of either verbal paraphasias (an error that is a semantically unrelated dictionary word, such as saying "name" instead of *main*) or neologisms (a nondictionary word, such as saying "tipe" instead of *pipe*). The former example could be either a phonemic or verbal paraphasia; the latter example is simply indicative of a fine line between phonemic and neologistic paraphasia, both of which may possibly reflect an impairment of the same process. Classification of paraphasias for purposes of clinical description may involve considering a patient's general tendency with unambiguous errors in order to decide how to classify the ambiguous errors.

Standardization

Norms. The test manual reports mean scores, ranges, and standard deviations on thirty-eight measures from a sample of 207 aphasic patients. Details concerning age, etiology, education level, and so forth are not reported. Scores were not obtained from each patient in the sample for each measure. The sample size per measure ranges from 147 to 195, except the subtest of body-part naming, which is represented by a sample size of 50. For thirty-three of the thirty-eight measures, the sample size ranges from 180 to 195.

In order to relate a patient's subtest performance to the standard sample of aphasic patients, Goodglass and Kaplan provide a z-score frame of reference on the test performance summary shown in Figure 7-2. The z-score scale at the top of the profile represents standard deviations from the mean, which is designated at *0* on the scale. A score on the 0-line can be considered to be a "50th-percentile" level of performance with respect to an aphasic population. The z-score enables subtest scores to be interpreted with respect to a normative distribution of aphasic performance. Therefore, performance between -1 and $+1$ z-scores represents about 68 percent of the aphasic population, 34 percent on each side of the mean. Performance between -2 and $+2$ z-scores represents about 95 percent of the aphasic population. In the literature, performance on the Boston Exam is often presented in terms of z-score severity levels, which are obtained simply by visually locating an approximate z-score equivalent to the test score on the profile form.

Borod, Goodglass, and Kaplan (1980) presented data on the *BDAE* from a sample of 147 normal adults. This information includes average scores, ranges, and cutoff scores for each subtest. In general, the cutoff scores were derived from the lowest score in the range.

Validity. The Boston Exam has been assessed as a measure of communicative ability, as a tool for the identification of syndromes, and, as such, as a predictor of site of lesion.

Criterion-related validity as a measure of aphasic communicative ability was investigated by Holland (1980a) and Ula-

---

Figure 7–2. The z-score profile summarizes subtest scores from the *Boston Diagnostic Aphasia Examination.* An example of Broca's aphasia is shown. In research, subjects often are described according to their z-score level of performance. *(Reprinted by permission of the publisher. From Goodglass, H., and Kaplan, E., The Assessment of Aphasia and Related Disorders. Philadelphia, Pa.: Lea & Febiger, 1972)*

towska, Macaluso-Haynes, and Mendel-Richardson (1976). Holland found that the *BDAE* correlated at 0.84 with her *Communicative Abilities in Daily Living* (CADL) and at 0.49 with her criterion measure of communication in real-life circumstances. Ulatowska and her colleagues compared the *BDAE* to an assessment of functional communication skills at patients' homes with role-playing tasks and a modified *PICA* scoring scale. They found no significant correlation between *BDAE* scores and the home-visit scores with twelve aphasic subjects. Again, we find a strong relationship between formal tests but not between a formal test and naturalistic measurement.

Construct validity for identifying syndromes was evaluated with a factor analysis of test performances by 189 aphasic subjects. The factor analysis was to determine whether test performance is based on a limited number of independent underlying factors which are discriminative among types of aphasia. These factors might include auditory comprehension and speech fluency, as noted in previous discussions of syndromes. Aphasic subjects were selected who " . . . have each symptom in *relatively isolated* (not necessarily pure) form, or show some selectivity in the sparing of certain language functions" (Goodglass and Kaplan, 1972, p. 15). Though these investigators recognized the apparent circular reasoning and data manipulation associated with this strategy of subject selection, their intent was to use subjects who would exhibit syndromes and then to identify the nature of the factors underlying the Boston Exam. They found five factors: (I) reading and writing, (II) a "spatial-quantitative-somatognosic group" reflecting parietal lobe functions, (III) articulatory and grammatical fluency, (IV) auditory comprehension, and (V) paraphasia. Factors III, IV, and V represent aspects of language function which have been related to different areas of the brain and have defined aphasic syndromes. Reading and writing were iden-

tified as a dimension which can vary independently from auditory-oral language function, especially in patients with occipital lobe damage. Therefore, the *BDAE* measures language functions which are associated with different areas of the left cerebral hemisphere and which are differently affected among the syndromes of aphasia.

Finally, it is of interest to see how well the Boston Exam is able to predict the site of brain lesion based on patterns of test performance. Chapters 1 and 3 contain references to studies establishing that nonfluent aphasia is related to anterior cortical damage and that fluent aphasia is related to posterior cortical damage. Kertesz (1979), with a test which is similar to the *BDAE*, demonstrated relationships between the aphasia syndromes and site of lesion. Naeser and Hayward (1978) presented CT-scan data from nineteen patients who had been given the Boston Exam. Readers of their article are advised that the lateral composite drawings of lesion sites in the left hemisphere for the subjects with Broca's and Wernicke's aphasia are reversed in the publication. At first glance, therefore, these drawings appear inconsistent with their conclusions. Nevertheless, their drawings of lesion sites are consistent with expectations from Broca's, Wernicke's, conduction, transcortical motor, and global aphasias which had been identified independently with *BDAE* patterns.

Reliability. Of the indicants of test-retest reliability, only interexaminer reliability of the Profile of Speech Characteristics (Figure 7–1) is reported in the test manual. Three judges listened to tape recorded conversations of ninety-nine aphasic patients. Their agreement as to rating the six dimensions of oral language is as follows: melodic line (0.85), phrase length (0.90), articulatory agility (0.90), grammatical form (0.90), paraphasia in running speech (0.79), and word finding (0.78). Interjudge reliability of this rating was reported by Goodglass, et al. (1964). They also reported the degree of agreement among three independent judges with the severity rating (Figure 7–1). With fifty-three cases of aphasia there was full agreement on 38 percent of the cases; on 57 percent of the cases two judges agreed within one point. Ulatowska, et al. (1976) investigated interexaminer reliability with twelve of the *BDAE* subtests and two of the speech-rating parameters. She found complete agreement by three examiners on 76 percent of the test items and a one-point discrepancy in scoring on 22 percent of the items. Goodglass and Kaplan (1972) investigated the internal consistency of *BDAE* test items with thirty-four aphasic subjects. Correlations for twenty of the twenty-one subjects studied ranged from 0.80 to 0.98, with fourteen being 0.90 or higher. Items within the body-part identification subtest were relatively inconsistent, with a reliability coefficient of 0.68.

Interpretation

Differential Diagnosis. The *BDAE* provides an objective basis for the identification of aphasic syndromes and for pinpointing the deviations from these syndromes in patients who do not quite fit the classification molds. Furthermore, it facilitates the identification of specific deficits which have been associated with particular sites of damage, such as color-naming problems associated with occipital lobe damage. The manual provides patterns of spontaneous speech associated with these syndromes (see Figure 7–1). These include profiles of a prototypical case and of the range of performance for Broca's, Wernicke's, and anomic aphasias. A typical case is provided for conduction and transcortical sensory aphasia. In addition, prototypical z-score profiles from individual cases are provided in the manual. The clinician should assume that some variability exists within the syndromes and, therefore, should not feel compelled to find a precise match between

a patient's performance and the examples in order to label a patient with some confidence. The pattern of deficits, not absolute scores, is important for classification.

In addition, Obler and Albert (1981) provided descriptions of the Cookie Theft picture obtained from patients with Alzheimer's dementia. Their summary of language symptoms is based on performances with certain subtests of the *BDAE*.

Prognosis and Recovery. The *BDAE* does not contain a formalized basis for making predictions about recovery. However, the different syndromes have been shown to possess different characteristics of recovery. In that the *BDAE* facilitates identification of the syndromes, it can be used as a basis for predicting amounts and patterns of recovery. The characteristics of recovery associated with each syndrome are presented in Chapter 9. Use of the *BDAE* for measuring recovery has little documentation in the literature. Sparks, Helm, and Albert (1974) reported changes in certain functions measured by this test with patients who had received Melodic Intonation Therapy. One reason for exclusion of the *BDAE* from such studies is that it does not provide a single score for overall language function. A single score is easier to deal with statistically than a complex pattern of scores from the z-profile. Also, many of the subtests in the *BDAE* contain few items and/or only a few scale points for scoring, which would tend to decrease the sensitivity of these subtests to small changes of language functions. The *Western Aphasia Battery*, described later in this chapter, was developed as a modification of the *BDAE* in a way that would provide a measure of recovery.

SHORT APHASIA TESTS

The "short" tests usually contain fewer subtests per modality, fewer items per subtest, and simpler scoring methods. They were designed in part to take no more than one hour to arrive at an assessment of the four language modalities.

Halstead-Wepman-Reitan Aphasia Screening Tests

Halstead and Wepman (1949) described a test of agnosias and aphasia which was developed originally by Halstead in 1935 as a convenient instrument for neurologists to present standard stimuli to their patients. Two hundred tests were distributed to military neurologists and neurosurgeons during World War II. The original test is no longer available, but a pocket-sized version of the stimuli and record form developed in 1955 is available from the University of Chicago. This miniature, Form M, was reviewed by Tikofsky (1979). Another version with fewer items was developed by Reitan (see DeMyer, 1974) and is used by some neuropsychologists for diagnosis.

A Short Examination

An abbreviated version of the 1955 research edition of the *MTDDA* was intended to take only thirty to thirty-five minutes to administer (Schuell, 1957). Later, Schuell (1966) considered any short test to be inadequate for a complete description or incisive interpretation of aphasic behavior. In order to reduce testing time, she recommended establishing a baseline and ceiling within each modality, using the complete *MTDDA*. For each modality, the clinician should start with a subtest on which the patient should make a maximum of one error (baseline) and should stop testing on the subtest producing 90 percent failure (ceiling).

British investigators Thompson and Enderby (1979) asked, "Is all your Schuell really necessary?" They suggested that a much shorter *MTDDA* would discriminate among aphasic persons as well as the complete version. They determined which subtests and items of the *MTDDA* were too

easy or too difficult for aphasic patients in order to arrive at a short version. A score sheet and marking scale for the revised Minnesota test are available from the authors. Another short form was developed by Powell, Bailey, and Clark (1980).

Sklar Aphasia Scale

The *SAS* first appeared in 1966 and was revised in 1973, primarily with a more refined scoring system consisting of a five-point scale which replaced the earlier three-point scale (Sklar, 1973). The purpose of this test is to provide a measure of degree of impairment of language function after brain damage in the four language modalities. It is easy to administer and score, and yields a breadth of information in a relatively short period of time.

Administration time with the *SAS* ranges from fifteen minutes to one hour. Each modality is sampled in sections for auditory decoding, visual decoding, oral encoding, and graphic encoding. Each section contains five subtests and each subtest consists of five items, for a total of one hundred test items. The kit includes an administration and interpretation manual, a protocol and scoring booklet, a set of stimulus cards, and some objects used in the auditory and speech sections. The five-point scoring system includes zero points for a normal response and four points for an incorrect response. Therefore, a higher score represents greater impairment. Performance is summarized in terms of percent of impairment within each modality, and a total impairment score is derived by averaging the scores from each modality.

The degree of impairment is measured relative to maximum possible test performance instead of relative to a standard sampling of aphasic performance, as with the *PICA* and *BDAE*. Normative data was not provided; however, Sklar (1973) reported that a sample of twenty adults indicated that the *SAS* is " . . . within the ability of average adults with eighth grade educations'' (p. 12). Concurrent criterion-related validity studies demonstrated that the *SAS* measures the same functions as Eisenson's *Examining for Aphasia*, the *Halstead-Wepman Aphasia Screening Test,* and Schuell's *Short Examination for Aphasia.* A German version of the *SAS* discriminated among aphasic subjects, normal subjects, brain-damaged patients without aphasia, and patients with chronic schizophrenia (Cohen, Engel, Kelter, et al., 1977). Reliability was not reported in the manual.

Aphasia Language Performance Scales

Keenan and Brassell (1975) developed the *ALPS* out of a dissatisfaction with the tests available in 1970. Keenan and Brassell constructed a test that would not be time-consuming, would not be limited by space and environmental restrictions, and would not be so formal as to interfere with natural interaction between the clinician and patient. The *ALPS* can be administered in twenty to thirty minutes, enables the four language modalities to be measured conveniently at bedside, and is given informally to elicit the patient's best response. This test does not consist of multiple subtests within each modality, but rather of a series of items increasing in complexity within each modality. The informality of the test is reflected in the labels of *Listening, Talking, Reading,* and *Writing* for the four sections, called ''scales.'' Each scale contains ten items, for a total of forty items.

The *ALPS* consists of an administration manual, a set of cards for the reading scale, and a score sheet. Other materials to be added by the clinician include a stopwatch and certain objects which can be carried easily in a pocket. The manual includes specific instructions for presenting and scoring each item, and the examiner is encouraged to present these items in a relaxed and personable manner. Four scores are derived, a possible ten points for

each scale. Several reliability and validity studies are reported in the manual. Retest reliability with twenty-two aphasic subjects was 0.83 for listening, 0.94 for talking, 0.88 for reading, and 0.94 for writing. The higher consistency for the expressive scales may be due partly to more thorough testing of some items in these two sections. One study of validity involved a comparison with the *PICA,* using fifty aphasic subjects. A correlation of 0.93 was found between the *ALPS* total score and the *PICA* overall score.

Interpretation guidelines include a translation of scores for each scale into a rating of severity of impairment. A chart is provided on which the clinician can record repeated administration of these scales, resulting in a graph of recovery. Keenan and Brassell also provide some case studies in which results are related to goals for treatment.

OTHER COMPREHENSIVE TESTS

In addition to the *MTDDA, PICA,* and *BDAE,* several other relatively comprehensive tests have been developed. The aphasia tests in this section are recognized widely in aphasiology; but they are not used widely, as evidenced by their infrequent appearance in the literature as a basis for describing subjects or as a means of measuring recovery. One of these tests, the *Western Aphasia Battery,* has been used extensively by Kertesz and his coworkers to classify aphasias and to measure recovery; but it is a relatively new test.

Examining for Aphasia

Jon Eisenson's (1954) test is of historical significance as one of the first commercially available assessments of aphasia and related disorders. It is organized into receptive and expressive sections. The receptive section includes subtests for agnosias and receptive aphasias; word comprehension is tested in the agnosia section, and sentence level material is in the aphasia section. The expressive section includes subtests for apraxias and expressive aphasias. There is minimal use of scoring, and administration and interpretation of this test are best left to an experienced clinician.

Language Modalities Test for Aphasia (LMTA)

In constructing the tasks in the *LMTA*, Wepman and Jones (1961) gave special attention to defining input and output relationships. Pictured and linguistic inputs are paired with verbal and nonverbal responses, resulting in tasks which require identifying a semantic relationship between input and output, and tasks of imitation (repeating, copying) and transcoding (reading aloud, writing to dictation). Many of the items are similar to those found in the Halstead-Wepman-Reitan screening batteries. The test has not been revised since 1961.

The *LMTA* was produced in two equivalent forms, Form I and II. Each form contains an initial set of eleven items which can be used for a twenty-minute screening and forty-six additional items divided into two "cycles." These divisions are to facilitate breaking up administration into two or three sessions if the patient should fatigue easily. The test should take one to three hours to administer. A unique feature of test construction is that all visual inputs are presented with a 35-mm. film strip, and the projector is not included with purchase. Scoring is either plus-minus for input matching items or a six-point scale for verbal and graphic responses. The scale reflects identification of phonemic, syntactic, or semantic errors and jargon behavior. Longhand notation is encouraged.

Standardization is dealt with minimally in the instruction manual. An earlier version was given to 168 aphasic subjects, and the current revised version was given to 50 subjects. Performance of these subjects is not presented in the manual. Two validation studies were reported in the literature. Construct validity was assessed with a factor analysis reported by Jones and Wepman (1961) using the original large group of patients. Criterion-related validity was addressed by Spiegel, Jones, and Wepman (1965) with the group of 50. In this study, a relationship was found between test performance and the independent grouping of these patients according to their different patterns of spontaneous speech. Interjudge reliability of the *LMTA* was 0.88 and higher for the different measures in the test.

Interpretation of results as to severity of disorder is hampered without any reference to performance of a standard aphasia population, and without a clear indication of test performance by persons without brain damage. Identification of type of aphasia is discussed in the manual according to Wepman's unique classification system which includes syntactic, semantic, pragmatic, and jargon aphasias.

Neurosensory Center Comprehensive Examination for Aphasia (NCCEA)

The *NCCEA* is the first of two comprehensive batteries described here that were developed in Canada (Spreen and Benton, 1969; revision, 1977). Before it was made available from the neuropsychology laboratory at the University of Victoria in 1969, it was being developed as an international test for aphasia (Benton, 1967). The need for an international test was recognized at a meeting in 1966 of the Research Group on Aphasiology of the World Federation of Neurology. Benton had suggested to this group that the *NCCEA* could satisfy the need for "a battery consisting of functionally equivalent versions to be applied in different language communities" (Benton, 1969, p. 39). At that time, Spreen and Benton were working on an American version, and De Renzi and Vignolo were working on an Italian version in Milan. Benton (1969) reported on developments since 1966 which included arrangements for standardizing the tests in clinics and school systems in the United States, France, Germany, and Italy. Benton and Hamsher (1978) continued this effort with an English version of the *Multilingual Aphasia Examination* (MAE).

The *NCCEA* consists of twenty subtests for aphasia and motor speech disorders and four control tests for certain patients to determine whether errors on some of the language tasks might be due to modality-specific sensory or perceptual problems. The aphasia battery includes typical subtests for auditory comprehension, reading, speech, and writing. However, certain unique features include an auditory comprehension subtest consisting of a shortened version of the Token Test, a reading comprehension subtest consisting of twelve written commands from the Token Test, and two tactile naming subtests, one for each hand, in which an object hidden from view is handled and named. Control tests, for example, include two tasks intended to determine whether tactile naming errors might be due to tactile agnosia instead of a word-retrieval deficit. Objects to be identified are hidden from view, and the patient must select an object which matches an object presented to the visual modality. Of course, word-retrieval deficit is implied also from errors in naming the same objects presented to other modalities.

Administration of the *NCCEA* includes the use of thirty-two objects arranged on four trays for several of the tasks. A duplicate set is needed for three of the control tests. Some auditory stimuli are presented with a tape recorder. Scoring is plus-minus for most subtests, and a five-point scale is used for naming subtests. It may take one to three hours to administer.

For normative information, the test was administered to a large group of aphasic subjects, to brain-damaged nonaphasics, and to nonbrain-injured controls. The data from these studies are not reported in the manual, but the data resulted in percentile scales for each group to assist in ranking an individual's test performance. Studies of validity and reliability are not reported in the manual. However, in a study similar in purpose to Spiegel, et al.'s (1965) investigation of the *LMTA*, Crockett (1977) compared *NCCEA* performances of fifty-seven aphasic patients to their scores on a seventeen-item verbal rating of natural language use. He found that four distinct aphasic patterns derived from the rating scale were similar to four groups derived from a multivariate analysis of test performance. The four aphasic groups could be characterized with reference to typical parameters of fluency and severity. This study serves as an indication of the *NCCEA*'s construct and criterion-related validity.

Interpretation of test performance is aided with a profile sheet on which the pattern of deficit is recorded. Severity relative to a standard aphasia population is indicated by test scores shown on this profile sheet relative to percentile levels. The control tests assist in differentiating aphasia from tactile agnosia and visual perceptual disorders. Further interpretation of patterns is influenced by the experience of the examiner. The *NCCEA* has been used in studies of recovery (see Chapter 9).

Western Aphasia Battery (WAB)

The *WAB* also was developed in Canada at the University of Western Ontario (Kertesz and Poole, 1974). Its publication is planned for 1982 by Grune and Stratton. It is a modification of the *Boston Diagnostic Aphasia Examination* and is similar in purpose; namely, to identify the syndromes of aphasia. The *WAB* possesses some differences from the *BDAE* in structure and content, but the main difference lies in the *WAB*'s increased reliance on subtest scores for the classification of aphasic patients. Like the *PICA,* the *WAB* provides a single overall score which is called the Aphasia Quotient (AQ); but unlike the *PICA,* the AQ reflects performance in only auditory and speech modalities, while the *PICA* overall score represents performance in all four major language modalities. The AQ has been used extensively by Andrew Kertesz and his colleagues in measuring recovery.

The basic battery for deriving the AQ consists of four sections: (A) Spontaneous speech, which includes questions to answer and a picture to describe, a line drawing from the *MTDDA;* (B) Auditory verbal comprehension, which includes tasks similar to the *BDAE* but with more yes/no questions and more instructions to follow; (C) Repetition, which includes single words, phrases, and sentences; and (D) Naming, which includes subtests of real-object naming, word fluency, sentence completion, and single-word answers to questions. The basic *WAB* can be administered in an hour to most aphasic patients. Kertesz (1979) described additional tests for reading, writing, and nonverbal functions from which he derived a Performance Quotient (PQ). The score derived from all subtests is the CQ, Cortical Quotient (Shewan and Kertesz, 1980).

The scoring and calculation needed to arrive at the Aphasia Quotient is what sets the *WAB* apart from the Boston Exam. A great deal of data in the literature on spontaneous recovery is reported in terms of the AQ. Forty percent of the AQ is derived from scoring the spontaneous speech sample, and two ten-point rating scales are used for this purpose (Kertesz, 1979). A rating of *fluency* has scale points defined with respect to length, grammatical completeness, use of jargon, word finding, and intonation. A rating of *information content* has scale points defined with respect to the communication value of the patient's

utterances, which is based largely on the number of correct responses to questions and completeness of picture description. A maximum AQ is one hundred points. Because the total of scores per subtest would be much greater than one hundred, some special calculations are used to derive the patient's AQ. Kertesz's 1979 description of this calculation differs from that reported in 1974 (also, see Shewan and Kertesz, 1980).

Norms were reported initially by Kertesz and Poole (1974; Kertesz, 1979) from samples consisting of 150 aphasics, 21 nonbrain-injured subjects, 17 with nondominant-hemisphere damage, and 21 with mixed-hemisphere damage. Mean scores and standard deviations for these groups and for eight aphasia syndromes were reported, along with graphic profiles for each type of aphasia. After 1974, 215 aphasics and 63 controls were added to the standardization sample (Kertesz, 1979). Criterion-related validity (called construct validity by Kertesz, 1979) was substantiated in a comparison of the *WAB* to the *NCCEA;* also, Kertesz found a significant relationship between the *WAB* and the *PICA.* Construct validity was examined by Kertesz and Phipps (1977), who used an elaborate clustering analysis of test scores to see if the mathematical procedure would generate groups of patients which correspond to the definitions of neoclassical syndromes. The computer-generated clusters corresponded closely to clinically defined syndromes. Also, two types of conduction aphasia, afferent and efferent, were derived from this analysis. Test-retest, interexaminer, and intraexaminer reliability coefficients were found to be high (Shewan and Kertesz, 1980).

Guidelines for interpretation with the *WAB* have been focused on differential diagnosis. Though it has been used to measure recovery, prediction in terms of the AQ has not been developed formally. The norms are suggestive for identifying different disorders. Kertesz (1979) established that an AQ below 93.8 is indicative of aphasia. A score at or above this level is most likely to be made by patients with diffuse or subcortical brain damage and by nonbrain-damaged persons. Normals in his two standardization samples had mean AQ's of 98.4 and 99.6. His two samples with nondominant (mostly right) hemisphere damage differed somewhat; the first group of seventeen averaged near normal at 97.1, but the second group of fifty-three averaged 92.9. Kertesz's norms also include average AQ's for the syndromes of aphasia.

The syndromes of aphasia are identified from patterns on the fluency rating, and scores on auditory comprehension, repetition, and naming. The guidelines are shown in Table 7–5, which was used to develop Figure 6–1 in the previous chapter. Conduction aphasia, for example, is recognized by scores which are low in repetition relative to a higher range of scores for fluency and comprehension. An unusual feature of the fluency rating is that a *5*, which places a patient into the fluent category, was defined in part as "Predominantly telegraphic, halting speech, but some grammatical organization . . . " (Kertesz, 1979, p. 41). A patient with moderate-to-mild Broca's aphasia could be described in this way.

SUMMARY AND REMARKS

Deciding on which test to use is not a simple matter. Many clinicians employ one battery faithfully because it is the test that has served them well for years. Learning a new test and getting used to its nuances are difficult processes of adjustment. A clinician working regularly with aphasic patients should have the *MTDDA, PICA,* and *BDAE* available, so that the clinician can be flexible as to purpose of assessment and can select from either the *MTDDA* or *BDAE* portions which might supplement assessment of individual cases. The clinician also should have at least one short test such as the *SAS* or the *ALPS* for a fairly complete screening given time and space constraints. Relatively new options, such as the *MAE* and *WAB,* should be explored. As research changes, enlarges, and refines theoretical understanding of aphasia, methods of diagnosis and assessment are forced to change. Test methodology may be more resistant to these forces than the conceptual basis from which results are interpreted. Therefore, the *MTDDA* still is a valuable procedure, but its results should be interpreted in light of ongoing research on primary deficits and syndromes.

Most of the tests reviewed in this chapter are summarized in Table 7–6.

TABLE 7–5. Criteria for classifying aphasias based on scores from the Western Aphasia Battery. *(Reprinted by permission from Kertesz, A., Aphasia and Associated Disorders: Taxonomy, Localization, and Recovery. New York: Grune & Stratton, (1979).*

	Fluency	Comprehension	Repetition	Naming
Global	0-4	0-3.9	0-4.9	0-6
Broca's	0-4	4-10	0-7.9	0-8
Isolation	0-4	0-3.9	5-10	0-6
Transcortical Motor	0-4	4-10	8-10	0-8
Wernicke's	5-10	0-6.9	0-7.9	0-9
Transcortical Sensory	5-10	0-6.9	8-10	0-9
Conduction	5-10	7-10	0-6.9	0-9
Anomic	5-10	7-10	7-10	0-9

TABLE 7-6. Most of the tests reviewed in this chapter are summarized. Characteristics include primary orientation of the test, such as for treatment (Tx) planning, and its administration time. Populations on which norms are available in the literature are cited; in some cases, certain data are not in the test manual. Sources for these norms have been cited in the text.

	Orientation	Administration Time	Comprehensiveness	Norms	Reliability	Research Use
MTDDA	Tx planning	2-6 hours	Strong	Aphasics Normals	Undetermined	Occasional
PICA	Measurement and Tx planning	1/2-2 hours	Good	Aphasics Normals RH and bilateral brain-injured	Strong	Frequent
BDAE	Classification and Tx planning	1-4 hours	Strong	Aphasics Normals	Undetermined	Frequent
SAS	Screening	15-60 minutes	Moderate	None	Undetermined	Rare
ALPS	Screening	20-30 minutes	Minimal	Aphasics Normals	Good	Rare
LMTA	Tx planning	1-3 hours	Good	None	Undetermined	By Wepman
NCCEA	Tx planning and measurement	1-3 hours	Good	Aphasics Normals Nonaphasic brain-injured	Undetermined	Occasional
WAB	Classification and measurement	1 hour	Good	Aphasics Normals Nondominant brain-injured	Strong	By Kertesz

These tests are similar in content, but their structure reflects different primary objectives. It is difficult to say that a test does one thing and not another, because the principal burden of diagnosis and assessment lies in the objectivity and interpretive capacities of the clinician. Most comprehensive tests can be used to serve all the major goals of diagnosis and assessment, when the clinician thinks carefully about the results and interprets them with respect to each test's unique characteristics and, especially, with respect to assessment strategies outlined in the previous chapter.

When there was a dearth of published aphasia tests in the 1940s and 50s, individual clinicians and clinical programs created their own tests. The speech-language pathology profession is no longer well served by continued use of individualized, unpublished, and unstandardized aphasia assessment and measurement devices. The continued development of commonly used tests enhances communication among clinical aphasiologists and among all professionals concerned with aphasia rehabilitation. In spite of the availability of many comprehensive tests, there will be a need for new tests or modification of current tests. If tests are to be helpful in identification of primary deficits (and, therefore, provide explanation for a variety of secondary symptoms), the test-makers will be responsive to valid and reliable findings from basic research on the hidden processes of normal language function, on the relationship between these processes and brain function, and on the bases for aphasic disturbances. That is, some of the information in Chapters 3 and 5 is suggestive of future developments in assessment and treatment.

8 Supplemental Tests and Measurements

Speech-language pathologists have confronted several clinical problems in an effort to enhance our ability to identify and measure particular aspects of the aphasic patient's disorder. We have had difficulty measuring communication outside the narrow clinical setting. Solving this problem is crucial for determining the true effectiveness of treatment. Another problem has been the detection and measurement of subtle language impairment. Also, thorough assessment of specific language functions, such as reading, has been done with methods borrowed from other professions rather than with methods designed for the adult aphasic population. Solutions to these problems enable the clinician to magnify certain components of aphasia in order to facilitate closer inspection of them.

TESTS OF FUNCTIONAL COMMUNICATION

The tests in this section are indicative of two perspectives on functional communication. We can focus on how well language is used in conversation and natural contexts outside the clinic. Also, we can attend to communication and look upon language as one mode of conveying messages. The previous tests measure how well language is used in structured tasks where natural context is minimized. Holland (1980a) remarked: "Clinicians who use aphasia tests are expected to generalize their findings not only to everyday life situations in which language is used, but to all communication, nonlinguistic and linguistic" (p. 2).

Functional Communication Profile (FCP)

The *FCP* was designed in 1956 by Martha Taylor Sarno to be part of a battery of tests used at the Institute of Rehabilitation Medicine, New York University Medical Center (Sarno, 1969). Later, she (Taylor, 1965) published a description of the test, and this article was reprinted in her book of readings on aphasia (Sarno, 1972). Complete administration and scoring instructions became available in 1969. The *FCP* is a test primarily of language as opposed to all modes of communication, and it focuses on the use of language in natural, everyday situations. The operational definition of functional performance, which is to be remembered by the examiner when scoring the patient's behavior, is that language is used "without assistance, cues, or artificial conditions" (Sarno, 1969, p. 15). In effect, the *FCP* is a measure of the aphasic person's independence as a language user.

The *FCP* is a rating scale of forty-five communicative behaviors, divided into five categories. These behaviors were considered to be "common functions of everyday urban life." The five categories are Movement (including gestures), Speaking, Understanding (auditory), Reading, and Other (including writing and calculation). The largest category is Understanding; its fifteen items comprise one-third of the measure. Also, the Speaking category contains ten items. The Understanding portion includes ratings of this function in certain contexts such as understanding conversation, television, and movies. Some attention is given to the linguistic adequacy of communicative behavior such as understanding object names and action verbs and, in the Speaking section, saying nouns, verbs, noun-verb combinations, and complete sentences. The examiner is instructed to use results of language tests in order to rate certain writing abilities, such as copying and writing to dictation.

Ratings are obtained partly from an informal interview with the patient which precedes formal testing. The test items should be memorized so that the clinician can be without test materials in a social situation designed for the clinician to get to know the patient. Scoring is done immediately after the interview. Each item is rated on a nine-point scale with reference to the patient's premorbid ability. The manual provides some general guidelines for rating a performance in terms of normal, good, fair, and poor. A single overall score can be obtained, and best performance is 100 percent. The patient's total score for each section is translated into a

weighted score, using a conversion chart, in order to arrive at an overall percentage of natural language ability that is retained.

Information on validity and reliability is provided in the manual of directions. Construct validity of the five categories is implied by the manner in which the current test organization was derived. Until 1964, the forty-five items were categorized as receptive or expressive. However, a factor analysis showed that the items clustered into five groups corresponding to movement, speaking, understanding, reading, and other. Also, the *FCP* was compared to subtests of the *MTDDA*, and rankings of performances were found to be similar between the two tests. Statistically significant correlations were found between the *FCP* and measures of auditory memory span. J.E. Sarno, et al. (1971) and M.T. Sarno and Levita (1979) compared the *FCP* to the *NCCEA* as to their sensitivity to recovery; they found that the *NCCEA* detected improvement of language which was not detected by the *FCP,* mostly during the first six months. Later, they found the opposite relationship, improvement on the *FCP,* during the six-to-twelve month period after onset. Holland (1980a) compared Sarno's test to the *Communicative Abilities in Daily Living* and found a correlation of 0.87. Interexaminer reliability of the *FCP* on twenty patients was 0.95 for the overall score and 0.87 to 0.95 for the section scores. Test-retest reliability was described as significant, but correlations were not reported (Sarno, 1969).

To aid interpretation, the manual provides two examples of performance profiles which are suggestive of differential diagnostic capability with this test. A profile of aphasia with apraxia of speech shows the typical severe depression of speaking relative to writing; and a profile of a patient with right-hemisphere damage and no aphasia shows mild reductions in all categories except Other, which was more severely impaired. The single overall score has facilitated use of this test to study recovery (see Chapter 9).

Communicative Abilities in Daily Living (CADL)

Audrey Holland (1977b) recommended that clinicians assess aphasic talking behavior, not only with an ear directed toward propositional or linguistic content, but also with an ear and eye toward whether an intended message was conveyed. In the *CADL,* communicative adequacy is the standard for measurement, a feature which is unique among commercially available measurements of aphasia. The test is unique also because real-life problems are presented to the patient; these problems include making an appointment with a doctor and shopping at a store. Holland (1980a) considered it to be a "practical" test of communicative ability; she wanted "to incorporate both more natural language activities and a more natural style in an effort to more closely approximate normal communication" (p. 47). The *CADL* is not intended to be a substitute or replacement for the measurement of language skills but, rather, is intended to provide another perspective on the problems of aphasic persons.

Description of the **CADL.** Several questions were posed in developing 68 items which would simulate daily-life activities. In what circumstances do normal people demonstrate comprehension and expression of different speech acts? In what circumstances does the average person read during the day? In what ways are numbers normally used? What are some adaptive strategies employed when miscommunication occurs? Settings from the home were rejected, because many activities within the home are sex-stereotyped and because typical home settings could produce additional difficulties for institutionalized patients.

The items are not organized according to language modalities, as they are in language-oriented aphasia batteries; instead, they are arranged according to settings being tested and, within these settings, according to the natural sequence in which specific behaviors would occur. The *CADL* begins with two items addressed to social greetings between the patient and clinician occurring away from the test site. It proceeds to a brief interview concerning name, address, age, and family. The only truly simulated situation, administered next, is a trip to the doctor. Twenty-one items proceed from arriving at the doctor's office to being interviewed by a "doctor." Subsequent situations are presented with drawings, photographs, and props representing problems in driving a car, shopping at a store, and using the telephone.

The communicative functions examined with the *CADL* differ from the modality-based conceptualization of language tests. Ten categories of behavior are assessed. More than one category may be tested by one item, while twenty-two of the sixty-eight items sample a single category. The categories of communicative behaviors are as follows (Holland, 1980a, pp. 29–30):

1. Reading, writing, using numbers to estimate, calculate, and judge time (twenty-one items). What can you buy for eighty-five cents?

2. Speech acts (twenty-one items). Certain test situations call for informing, explaining, negotiating (What is a good time for your doctor's appointment?), requesting, and warning.

3. Utilizing verbal and nonverbal context (seventeen items). What do you do when the gas gauge reads empty?

4. Role playing (ten items). A visit to the doctor's office requires the patient and examiner to pretend to assume certain roles. The clinician puts on a white coat and stethoscope and, probably, a change of personality.

5. Sequenced and relationship-dependent communicative behavior (nine items). These behaviors include dialing a phone number and recognizing the relationship between a speed limit sign and speedometer.

6. *Social conventions* (eight items). Near the end of the test, the clinician says, "I'm sorry this all took so long."

7. *Divergences* (seven items). Chapey's concept of divergent or multiple responses is referred to in the manual. Holland mentioned "more holistic communicative aspects," including some of the humor and metaphor items.

8. *Nonverbal symbolic communication* (seven items). Recognition of facial expression is one example.

9. *Deixis* (six items). This is defined as movement-related or movement-dependent communicative behavior such as demonstrating an idea through gesture; Gleason, et al. (1980) defined it as "verbal pointing" (see Chapter 5).

10. *Humor, absurdity, metaphor* (four items). "Look at these cartoons. Which one is funny?" These categories are thought to involve high-level cognitive-linguistic relationships; one is recognizing the contextually determined implication of an utterance such as "They shot the bull" (see Winner and Gardner, 1977).

These categories can be used to develop a functional profile for the patient in order to facilitate interpretation of test results.

Administration and Scoring. Test materials include vehicles for learning administration and scoring. An audiotape contains aphasic responses to each item, and the clinician can practice scoring these items. The manual contains two sample test forms for additional practice. A series of convenient steps for self-training had been sufficient to produce strong reliability.

The *CADL* takes thirty-five to forty minutes to administer. The test kit includes a set of pictures and a score booklet which contains item instructions and space for descriptive notes. Additional materials must be obtained by the examiner: the white jacket and stethoscope, a shoelace, soup packages, some coins, and other materials to enhance realism. A unique feature is the recommended testing style.

The examiner's manner should be relaxed and friendly, which is not especially unusual for any testing procedure. However, with regard to the use of props and role-playing, Holland (1980a) advised, "If you are able to do this with a flourish, or with humor, we believe this is both relaxing and helpful in terms of the informal mood we are trying to create, and we urge you to do so" (p. 49). When playing the role of doctor, the examiner, in effect, must become an actor in order to make the situation seem as real as possible.

The scoring system is a three-point scale applied to all items of the test. A score of 2 is assigned when the patient gets a message across. No matter how the message is conveyed, this score is given as long as the appropriate idea is understood by the examiner. This criterion differs from criteria in language batteries in which a specific level of linguistic performance is required for a maximum score. In the *CADL* a clearly inadequate response is scored 0. The 1 response is a broad category which, Holland explained, is between correctness and incorrectness, an "in the ballpark" response.

Standardization. Two studies were conducted in standardizing the *CADL*. In study I, Holland examined the validity and reliability of an early version of the test which contained seventy-three items. In study II, she had eliminated five items and obtained norms on 130 normal subjects and 130 aphasic persons with the current version of sixty-eight items. Additional studies, reported in the manual, involved giving the *CADL* to 30 trainable mentally retarded persons and to 30 experienced hearing-aid users.

In the test manual the two norming samples are described in detail, with special attention to distribution according to age, sex, and living environment. Different cutoff scores are provided, separating aphasic from normal performance for twelve groups defined in terms of these three variables. For example, the cutoff is 128/136 for noninstitutionalized males under age forty-six, while it is 111/136 for institutionalized females over age sixty-five and below eighty. Institutionalized aphasics, which included any group living environment, tended to have lower scores than noninstitutionalized aphasics. Patterns of performance according to the ten *CADL* categories are provided for five syndromes of aphasia (Global, mixed, Wernicke, Broca, and Anomic). Also, a distribution of types of performance by all aphasics on each test item is included.

Criterion-related validity was determined with respect to two types of measures. One measure was a direct observation of communicative behavior in the patients' living environment. Three proportions were obtained, involving total appropriate communicative behaviors to total communicative attempts. Correlations between the three proportions and the *CADL* score for eighty aphasics were 0.60, 0.62, and 0.62. Noninstitutionalized patients displayed generally higher correlations than institutionalized patients. All were significant at the 0.001 level of confidence. Regarding concurrent validity, the *CADL* correlated at 0.93 with the *PICA,* 0.87 with the *FCP,* and 0.84 with the *BDAE.* Interexaminer reliability with twenty patients was 0.99.

Interpretation. Determining how closely an aphasic patient's performance comes to normal is aided by the twelve cutoff scores mentioned previously. Furthermore, a patient's strengths and weaknesses as a communicator can be assessed with respect to the ten categories of performance. Only the global and mixed aphasics exhibited differentiations among the categories: with global aphasics, social conventions were distinctively stronger than the other categories; mixed aphasics were stronger in this area and, like the globals, were especially weak in reading and writing, speech acts, and sequenced behavior. Global aphasics had trouble role-playing, and mixed aphasics found nonverbal symbols more difficult than some other communicative categories.

An indication of the *CADL*'s value as a measure of recovery was reported by Holland (1980b). During data collection for Studies I and II, twenty-eight aphasic subjects were retested at intervals of between eight and fifteen months. The first test was at least four months postonset. The thirteen subjects who received treatment during this period improved from 70 percent to 77 percent on the *CADL.*

AUDITORY COMPREHENSION

Tests of the auditory language modality have had two orientations. First, they have dealt with the problem of assessing high level aphasics; comprehensive tests have been insufficiently difficult to measure the deficits of these patients. Morley, Lundgren, and Haxby (1979), for example, found that auditory subtests of the *PICA* and *BDAE* have a low ceiling for aphasics. Second, they have provided an opportunity to identify specific auditory deficits by the careful selection of stimuli and analysis of error patterns.

Token Test

Ennio DeRenzi and Luigi Vignolo at the University of Milano felt that it was difficult to identify mild aphasic auditory comprehension deficits during routine clinical examination with methods available in the 1950s. Mild comprehension deficits are most likely to be found in patients with Broca's and anomic aphasias. DeRenzi and Vignolo developed the Token Test to detect and measure these subtle deficits. A survey of this test is imposing, because there are several Token Tests.

The popularity of the Token Test is reflected in the frequency of its application to the investigation of comprehension deficits and to treatment. It has been used to study the effects on auditory comprehension of pauses (Liles and Brookshire, 1975), of stimulus repetition (LaPointe, Rothi, and Campanella, 1978), and of examiner experience (Salvatore, Strait, and Brookshire, 1978); it has provided a standard of auditory language comprehension to be compared with other measures of auditory processing (Swisher and Hirsh, 1972; Tallal and Newcombe, 1978); it has been used for comparing language capacities of the cerebral hemispheres (Zaidel, 1977, 1979); and it has been a model for treatment programs (West, 1973; Holland and Sonderman, 1974). Furthermore, a book of essays is devoted solely to this influential test (Boller and Dennis, 1979).

Original Version. The Token Test was introduced by DeRenzi and Vignolo (1962) as a task of following instructions. It was designed so that a correct response would be based on the processing of language without clues from the situational context, the test objects, and extraneous verbal context. The patient responds to a series of commands by manipulating tokens of different shape, color, and size. Five sections of the test reflect levels of increasing difficulty; Parts I through IV increase primarily in length of the command, while Part V contains commands of varying syntactic complexity. Parts I through IV contain ten items each. DeRenzi and Vignolo provided only a few examples of these commands. In their article, Part V contained twenty-one items for a total of sixty-one commands.

Boller and Vignolo (1966) presented the first complete list of commands. Although these commands contained some differences from the description in 1962, this version became the basis for most subsequent applications of the Token Test (Swisher and Sarno, 1969; Whitaker and Noll, 1972; Needham and Swisher, 1972; Brookshire, 1974; Gallaher, 1979). The following are examples from the 1966 version:

I. *Touch the yellow rectangle.*

II. *Touch the large blue circle.*

III. *Touch the red circle and the yellow rectangle.*

IV. *Touch the small yellow circle and the large green rectangle.*

V. (1) *Put the red circle on the green rectangle.*

(11) *Touch the white circle without using your right hand.*

(20) *After picking up the green rectangle, touch the white circle.*

The tokens are arranged in front of the patient in rows of five; ten tokens are used in Parts I, III, and V, and twenty in Parts II and IV. Complexity of Parts I through IV, analyzed by Whitaker and Whitaker (1979), increases in terms of the amount of attribution in a noun phrase and the compounding of noun phrases. Part V contains a variety of verbs and a varied sampling of syntactic structures. Boller and Vignolo (1966) added one item to Part V, example (11). Most subsequent versions of the complete Token Test contain twenty-two items in this section for a total of sixty-two items.

Differences between the 1966 and 1962 versions are of interest because the 1962 version was employed to some extent in a few studies (Poeck, Kerschensteiner, and Hartje, 1972; Poeck, Orgass, Kerschensteiner, et al., 1974). Morley, et al. (1979) referred only to the 1962 article, but their examples of instructions came from the 1966 revision. First, there is the difference in number of commands in Part V. Second, the first version had instructed patients to "pick up" the tokens in I and II and "take" the tokens in III and IV. The 1966 revision made the verb ("touch") in Parts I through IV consistent, and this change simplified the response.

Current Versions. Changes have been made to the content of Boller and Vignolo's (1966) original Token Test.

Variations from the 1962 version were inevitable because of the minimal detail provided concerning stimulus items, administration, scoring, and interpretation. A commercial version was not produced with interpretive guidelines based on sound normative data and validation, and so the test was vulnerable to modification of its content. As a result, the test has evolved in the hands of many investigators, and its history is cluttered with subtly different versions collectively referred to as the "family" of Token Tests by Berry (1973). Researchers are often careful to specify which version they are using and what tinkering they performed on the stimulus items. DeRenzi (1979) has incorporated many of the changes in his more recent short version of the test.

The most consistently employed modification was suggested first by Spreen and Benton (1969), who replaced *rectangle* with *square*. *Square* has more frequent usage in language; its occurrence is more comparable to *circle* (Whitaker and Whitaker, 1979). This change was maintained by Brookshire (1974, 1978), Lesser (1976), Noll and Randolph (1978), and DeRenzi, (1979). Poeck, et al. (1974) are among the few investigators who used the original *rectangle*.

DeRenzi (1979; DeRenzi and Faglioni, 1978) changed the color of one token from *blue* to *black*. The elimination of *blue* was due to difficulties by brain-damaged and normal adults in discriminating between blue and green. The *Revised Token Test* (McNeil and Prescott, 1978), which is presented later, includes blue and black (and green) while yellow was eliminated. This test might be called the "black-and-blue" version.

In giving the test to children, Whitaker and Noll (1972) changed the lexicon for size from *large* and *small* to *big* and *little*. This adjustment was not maintained by Brookshire or DeRenzi. McNeil and Prescott (1978), however, used *big* and *little*.

The most consistent version of the Token Test has been Boller and Vignolo's (1966) sixty-two items, with squares instead of rectangles. The version found in most studies consists of the following content:

Verb (I–IV).	*Touch the . . .*
Size.	*Large, small*
Color.	*Yellow, blue, green, white, red*
Shape.	*Circle, square*

Content will vary partly as to whether a certain short version is adopted. For example, Spreen and Benton's (1969) short version includes *show me* instead of *touch* as the verb element in their sections corresponding to Parts I through IV.

Berry (1978) proposed some supplemental tests which contain similar commands and common objects instead of tokens. Aphasic performance on these tasks has been reported (Tompkins, Rau, Marshall, et al., 1980). However, use of objects instead of tokens has been investigated more for the better understanding of aphasia than for the clinical assessment of patients (Lesser, 1979). In one study, aphasics were asked to point to houses and flowers of various sizes and colors in addition to circles and squares (Kreindler, Gheorghita, and Voinescu, 1971). The commands with shapes were more difficult to comprehend than the commands with objects. Martino, Pizzamiglio, and Razzano (1976) devised a "token test" with an envelope, cup, comb, brush, and pencil which were either black or white and large or small. Their subjects also did better with the objects than with the original Token Test. Of course, DeRenzi and Vignolo (1962) had wanted a more difficult test, one without clues from the nature of concrete objects; and these results are supportive of the original purpose. However, contradictory evidence has been reported. Lesser (1979) and

Lohman and Prescott (1978) found that concrete objects did not improve performance over shapes. So far, there is no object-version of the Token Test that has received wide acceptance as a clinical assessment device.

Another version of the Token Test was devised by Brookshire (1978c) as a means of isolating components of test performance and of distinguishing between aphasic patients and nonaphasic right-hemisphere-damaged (RH) patients. His Configurational version involved pointing to one of four arrangements of tokens drawn on a card as the mode of response for all five parts of the test. In effect, all items involved a single pointing response. Aphasic subjects found the configurational version to be easier than the standard version, while the RH subjects experienced equal success on these versions. A similar procedure, called the "Three-Figures-Test," has patients point to shapes on a card (Peuser and Schriefers, 1980).

Short Versions. Some of the modifications of content accompanied reductions in the number of items so that the test might provide the same information in a shorter time. The first shortened Token Test was developed by Spreen and Benton (1969) as the "Identification by Sentence" subtest of the *NCCEA*. Instead of sixty-two items there are thirty-nine items; and it contains six parts instead of five. Spreen and Benton broadened application of the test by adding an easier section involving identification by only shape or color ("Show me a square," "Show me a red one"). Spellacy and Spreen (1969) indicated that an even shorter version containing sixteen items is capable of being equally informative, at least, in the identification of auditory comprehension deficit.

DeRenzi (1978; DeRenzi and Faglioni, 1979) developed comprehensive norms for a thirty-six-item Token Test which incorporates most changes of content since the

original version of 1962. Like the Spreen and Benton short test, DeRenzi's version contains six parts, but it has three fewer syntactically complex commands in the last part.

Administration and Scoring. The Token Test is simple to administer. A complete list of commands is available in a few articles (Boller and Vignolo, 1966; Brookshire, 1974; Noll and Randolph, 1978). A set of plastic tokens has been available for years through purchase of the *NCCEA*. Now, plastic tokens come with the *Revised Token Test* (McNeil and Prescott, 1978), but two of the five colors are different from the original and *NCCEA* versions.

Different arrangements of the tokens have been recommended. DeRenzi and Vignolo (1962) recommended that when all twenty tokens are displayed the top two rows should be circles, large and then small, and the bottom two rows should be rectangles, large and then small. Brookshire (1974) used a squares-first arrangement. Spreen and Benton (1969), on the other hand, presented a large-small arrangement; large circles and squares formed the top two rows, and small circles and squares formed the bottom two rows. This arrangement was maintained by DeRenzi (1979).

Different scoring systems have been used. DeRenzi and Vignolo (1962) counted the number of errors made with respect to each element of each command. A total of 250 errors were possible considering size, shape, and color in sixty-one commands. Total errors was used in several studies of the Token Test (Orgass and Poeck, 1966; Spellacy and Spreen, 1969; Poeck, Kerschensteiner, and Hartje, 1972; Hartje, Kerschensteiner, Poeck, et al. 1973). Another scoring procedure, probably more common in the United States, involves assessing each item as either correct or incorrect and then counting the total correct. A total of sixty-two points is possible with the complete test (Boller and Vignolo, 1966; Swisher and Sarno, 1969; Gallaher, 1979).

Standardization. Normative data on the Token Test must be pieced together from several studies. With the sixty-two-point scoring method, seventy-eight normal adults have been given the Token Test in three studies (Boller and Vignolo, 1966; Swisher and Sarno, 1969; Noll and Randolph, 1978). Range of normal performance was 48 to 62; one mean score was 57 (Swisher and Sarno, 1969), and another was 59.7 (Noll and Randolf, 1978). A sample of mildly impaired aphasics ranged from 18 to 59 points, with an average of 43.5 (Noll and Randolph, 1978). An unselected sample of aphasics ranged from 0 to 58, with an average of 23 (Swisher and Sarno, 1969). Good comprehending aphasics performed well on Parts I through III and poorly on Parts IV and V (Boller and Vignolo, 1966); average errors by mild aphasics were 1.0 (I), 4.1 (II), 6.1 (III), 9.8 (IV), and 11.5 (V) in Noll and Randolph's (1978) study.

Norms have been presented for the short versions of the test. As part of the *NCCEA,* the thirty-nine item version comes with percentile equivalents for normal and aphasic persons. However, the normative samples were not described (Spreen and Benton, 1969). The thirty-six-item version is reported with scores from large samples of normal subjects, aphasics, and brain-damaged nonaphasics (DeRenzi, 1979; DeRenzi and Faglioni, 1978). DeRenzi established a cutoff score of twenty-nine for this version.

Validity of the Token Test as a measure of auditory language comprehension has been well established. Criterion-related validity was determined by significant correlations with the *FCP* (Swisher and Sarno, 1969), special syntactic and semantic tests of comprehension (Parisi and Pizzamiglio, 1970; Pizzamiglio and Appicciafuoco, 1971), a typical clinical assessment of comprehension (Needham and Swisher, 1972), and the auditory comprehension subtests of the *PICA* and Boston Exam (Morley, et al., 1979). Token Test performance was unrelated to a measure of nonverbal cognition (Boller and Vignolo, 1966), but there has been an indication that years of schooling is a factor (Orgass and Poeck, 1966; Boller and Vignolo, 1966; DeRenzi, 1979). The significant correlation between Token Test performance and scores on a picture-matching task draws attention to the subtle interaction between verbal and nonverbal cognition (Birchmeier, 1980).

Few studies have been focused on validity relative to the test's original purpose, namely, whether it identifies and measures subtle auditory language comprehension deficits which are not identified by standard clinical evaluation. To accomplish this, aphasic subjects should be defined as being at or near ceiling level performance on standard auditory assessment, and the Token Test should then show a deficit in these subjects that is not shown with nonaphasic brain-damaged and normal subjects. DeRenzi and Vignolo (1962) reported that thirteen motor aphasics and six recovered sensory aphasics, all with adequate comprehension on standard assessment, showed pronounced difficulty with Parts IV and V of the Token Test. This pattern was substantiated in thirty-four expressive aphasics by Boller and Vignolo (1966). These patients performed worse than right-hemisphere-damaged nonaphasics who were equal to a normal group. Noll and Randolph (1978) selected twenty-five aphasics with mild or no impairment registered with either the *MTDDA* or the *PICA.* The aphasics performed significantly worse than normals indicating that mild impairment can be identified with the Token Test. Morley, et al. (1979) found that the *PICA* auditory tests provide little information at high levels of aphasic performance, while Parts IV and V of the Token Test can measure a range of performance at high levels of ability. This range (eighteen through fifty-nine) was cited previously from Noll and Randolph's study, which is the only investigation in which mild aphasic subjects were selected based on current clinical batteries.

Other validation studies have consisted of a wider range of aphasics, which is indicative of an expanded application of the Token Test since 1962. The addition of an easier subtest in the shortened versions widened the test's sensitivity to more severely impaired patients. Several investigations determined that aphasia of any severity can be identified with this test in comparison with other brain-damaged groups. Therefore, the test measures a deficit which is characteristic of aphasia rather than of brain damage in general. Aphasics performed much worse than right-hemisphere-damaged nonaphasics (Swisher and Sarno, 1969; Hartje, et al., 1973; Lesser, 1976; Martino, et al., 1976; DeRenzi and Faglioni, 1978), and worse than left-hemisphere-damaged nonaphasics (Hartje, et al., 1973; DeRenzi and Faglioni, 1978). Aphasic subjects in these studies displayed impairments with all parts of the test. The deficient performance of the left-hemisphere nonaphasics in Boller and Vignolo's (1966) study led these authors to describe a "latent aphasia" found mainly with Part V of the Token Test (see Chapter 6).

Test-retest reliability was investigated by Gallaher (1979) who found high correlations between test administrations and no evidence of a learning effect due to repeated testing.

Interpretation. Although performance on the Token Test separates aphasics from other brain-damaged patients, clinical use of the Token Test does not include differential diagnosis. There has been some interest in whether performance differs between fluent and nonfluent aphasias, but average scores for these categories have not differed (Orgass and Poeck, 1966; Poeck, et al., 1972; DeRenzi, 1979). The problem with using fluent aphasia as a basis for grouping aphasics in research was discussed in Chapter 5. With their Revised Token Test, Mack and Boller (1979) found that fluent aphasics consisting of Wernicke's aphasia made more errors than nonfluent aphasics. When specific syndromes were compared with a standard version, there was a difference among groups (Poeck and Hartje, 1979).

The principal purpose of the Token Test has been the supplemental measurement of auditory language capacity, especially for mildly impaired patients. A single score from the number of items correct has been sufficient for this purpose. However, clinical investigators have pursued the possibility of identifying peculiar kinds of comprehension difficulty revealed by patterns of performance within and among items and parts of the Token Test.

Performance has been examined relative to the contributions of verbal short-term memory and of specific linguistic processes characterized as semantic and/or syntactic. Lesser (1976) noted that the commands increase in length from two units in Part I (*white square*) to six units in Parts IV and V (*small blue circle* and *large yellow square; Put* the *red circle* on the *green square*). A gradual increase of errors from Part I to Part V may indicate that reduced short-term memory capacity is the primary deficit. However, linguistic factors are embedded within these commands. A patient may have a semantic deficit reflected in errors concentrated on size, shape, or color. A significant increase of errors from Part IV to V may be indicative of normal memory capacity and problems with the varied syntactic operations of V.

Brookshire (1974) suggested that different patterns of Token Test performance are indicative of different kinds of auditory deficit. Test patterns were revealed with multidimensional scoring of each command and identification of the incorrect element within each command. A tendency to make errors on the first part of a command was indicative of "slow rise time," in which the auditory system needs more time than normal to reach an active state. A tendency to make errors on the final portion of a command was indicative of "noise buildup," in which the early part of a stimulus interferes with processing subsequent parts. This pattern could be interpreted differently, as Lesser (1979) suggested that deficient short-term memory would result in fewer errors on earlier elements. A third pattern described by Brookshire was increasing difficulty as length of the commands increased, but without a consistent pattern of error within each command. When pauses were inserted within the command, performance deteriorated. This suggested a "retention deficit" in which registration time of the input within memory is reduced. When the insertion of pauses resulted in improved performance, this was taken to indicate an "information capacity deficit." Each of these possibilities, associated with auditory processing or short-term memory, are related to position of errors or processing time. Such patterns are possible regardless of the semantic content or syntactic structure of a command. When these aspects of the Token Test are considered, the delineation of processing components for Token Test performance becomes much more complex.

Noll and Randolph (1978) concluded that any difficulty with Parts I through IV by mildly impaired aphasics is indicative of reduced short-term memory capacity. This deficit would have an impact on Part V performance, but difficulties in processing syntax are also revealed by errors on Part V. They found that aphasics with mild comprehension deficits made many more syntactic errors (wrong relationship between tokens, for example) than semantic errors (wrong shape or color) on Part V.

Lesser (1976, 1979) concluded, however, that there are several components of Token Test performance and that they are difficult to isolate in an analysis of test performance. She found that test scores were correlated to measures of auditory verbal short-term memory, visual short-term memory, and motor sequencing. Following a command on this test requires these processes as well as syntactic and semantic operations. Whitaker and Whitaker (1979) argued that it is very difficult to separate the semantic/syntactic requirements of the test from its short-term memory requirements. With respect to Parts I through IV, the different attributive phrase structures (*blue square, big green circle*) probably make different demands on memory than coordinate structures (*blue square and white circle*). Isolating specific kinds of syntactic problems, such as with certain prepositions, on Part V is impeded by the varied selection of structures in this section (Poeck, et al., 1974; Mack and Boller, 1979). Therefore, in order to determine possible specific syntactic problems, revisions of Part V have been constructed in which certain structures are tested repeatedly (Mack and Boller, 1979; McNeil and Prescott, 1978).

Revised Token Test (RTT)

A substantial revision of the Token Test was made commercially available by McNeil and Prescott (1978). Their purpose was to provide a standardized version that would replace the inconsistent applications within the family of Token Tests. A second purpose was to provide more information about a patient's auditory comprehension problem by reconstructing the presentation of certain syntactic structures from Part V and by developing a more elaborate scoring system.

The *Revised Token Test (RTT)* consists of ten sections with ten commands per section. Subtests I through IV are constructed on the same basis as Parts I through IV in the original Token Test. Semantic content is unique, however, in that the shapes are *circle* and *square,* the sizes are *big* and *little,* and the colors are *black, blue, green, red,* and *white.* The selection of this lexicon was based on the similarity of frequency of occurrence among all the items. The remaining six subtests were created as a means of focusing on a few of the original Part V items by using subtests that are homogeneous and that are an adequate sampling of each structure. Nine of the original twenty-two commands are represented in Subtests V through X of the *RTT.*

Subtests V and VI require the patient to place one token in a spatial relationship to another token. An example of V is *Put the black circle above the white square.* Subtest VI keeps the structure the same but increases the information load (*Put the big red square in front of the big white circle*). Several prepositions are tested, such as *before, on, behind, under, below,* and *beside.*

Subtests VII and VIII request the patient to put one token to the left or right of another token. As in VI, Subtest VIII represents an increased information load within the noun phrases.

Subtests IX and X present a variety of conditional clauses in each command, such as (IX) *Unless you have touched the white square, touch the green circle* and (X) *If there is a big white circle, touch the little blue square.*

Administration and scoring are fashioned after the *PICA.* A protocol booklet specifies each command and instructions for repeating and cueing. A multidimensional scoring system of fifteen scale points is applied to each linguistic element of each command. A command in Subtest III (*Touch the blue square and the black circle*), for example, has six units: a stated verb, an implied verb, two colors, and two shapes. Each of these elements is assigned a score, and the score for each command is the average of the element scores. The subtest score is the average of all element scores in

the subtest; Subtest III has sixty element scores. The number of scores derived from the *RTT* is awesome. The original Token Test, with its plus-minus scoring, yields a single score of number correct of a possible sixty-two and five average scores per Part. The *RTT,* on the other hand, yields one hundred mean command scores (fifty-eight mean scores per linguistic element), and ten subtest scores.

Norms are provided in the manual for normal adults (N = 90), RH-damaged nonaphasics (N = 30), and LH-damaged aphasics (N = 30). Percentile scores can be derived from raw scores for each of these groups. Concurrent criterion-related validity was determined in comparison with the *PICA.* Correlation with the average of *PICA* auditory comprehension subtests was 0.71. Reliability coefficients for test-retest and examiner consistency were high.

Percentile scores enable the examiner to determine the degree of deficit relative to the general disordered population. In addition, the numerous scores and profiles for summarizing these scores are intended to expose specific kinds of auditory deficits. The *RTT* manual provides several profiles representing these deficits. However, the existence of some of these deficits as discrete entities in individual patients has not been clearly demonstrated. As McNeil and Prescott (1978) stated, their profiles are "theoretical" possibilities which could be revealed by their test but have not been. Their examples "... do not necessarily represent actual cases, but rather general patterns of auditory processing deficit as they might be identified from *RTT* performance" (p. 49). These hypothetical deficits include a deficit associated with increasing stimulus length, fatigue/cumulative noise, short-term storage/tuning in/poor rise time, specific linguistic deficit, and intermittent auditory imperception. The value of such a test for treatment planning would be in its ability to identify specific deficits. If one of these deficits were to be demonstrated in a patient, then treatment could be planned with a more specific direction.

Auditory Comprehension Test for Sentences (ACTS)

The *ACTS*, developed by Shewan (1979), is designed to provide a quantitative assessment of degree of deficit in auditory comprehension of sentences; to determine contributions of length, vocabulary difficulty, and syntactic complexity to auditory comprehension deficits; to provide a qualitative analysis of the deficit; and to provide a guide to treatment planning through the identification of specific deficits. It first appeared as a research paradigm on the heels of psycholinguistic investigations of the 1960s, which focused on certain syntactic structures as a means of studying transformational grammar (Shewan and Canter, 1971). An error analysis was presented by Shewan (1976a) to provide the qualitative analysis. In this study aphasics were similar to normal subjects in their pattern of errors.

The test consists of twenty-five sentences, four practice items and twenty-one test items, which are read to the patient by the examiner. The patient responds to each sentence by pointing to the one of four pictures that represents the meaning of the sentence. The sentences are constructed according to three levels of length, vocabulary difficulty, and syntax. Three sentence lengths are defined by the number of critical units and number of syllables. The three vocabulary levels are defined by frequency of word usage. The three levels of syntax are defined by the number of optional transformations. The first syntactic level consists of a simple active declarative sentence (*The girl is reading a book*). The second level consists of one optional transformation, either a negative or a passive (*The dogs are not chasing cats*). The third level consists of two optional transformations (*The milk was not drunk by her*).

Each of the three incorrect picture choices is derived by a change of one semantic element in the test sentence.

The *ACTS* takes ten to fifteen minutes to administer. Each item is scored as correct or incorrect after the examiner has noted which picture was pointed to by the patient. The maximum score is twenty-one points. A five-point scale is suggested in the manual. A score sheet assists the clinician in scoring responses to facilitate error analysis.

Norms were obtained from 150 aphasics and 30 normal controls. Average scores and standard deviations are presented for 30 amnesic (anomic) aphasics, 30 Broca's aphasics, and 30 Wernicke's aphasics. Concurrent criterion-related validity was determined in comparison with an eight-point rating scale for comprehension which accompanies the Minnesota test. High reliability was found for internal consistency and test-retest consistency.

A cutoff score of eighteen is the objective basis for identifying a language-comprehension disorder. Education is a factor because of the vocabulary level of some items, and a score of seventeen is the cutoff for those with under eight years of schooling. The *ACTS*, however, is intended primarily to aid treatment planning by helping to identify particular difficulties relative to the three stimulus parameters and to type of error. Error type is defined relative to position in the sentence (first half or second half) and the form class of the error. Most error sampling is on nouns and verbs. Only a few response choices are directed to adjectives and pronouns.

Validity of the qualitative analysis poses problems which are similar to the validity of hypothetical profiles accompanying the Revised Token Test. Research reported by Shewan (1976a) and in the test manual showed that position of error was not a factor in differentiating among aphasias and that there was no difference between sentence positions. Therefore, the value of performing this analysis was not demonstrated. Also, a higher proportion of errors was made on nouns than on verbs, but all groups performed similarly relative to rank order of type of error. Shewan suggested that individual patients may produce informative patterns, but such cases were not presented in the manual. The normative data did reflect the common finding that more complex sentences are harder to understand than less complex sentences. Length, vocabulary usage, and syntax are common dimensions for organizing task hierarchies in treatment programs for auditory comprehension.

READING

Supplemental assessment of reading for aphasic patients is an area that has recently matured in clinical aphasiology. This maturation is indicated by a reduced need for dependence on other fields prompted by development of methodology designed for the aphasic person. Problems with using "borrowed" reading tests are that these tests were not constructed to deal with some of the special difficulties associated with aphasia, and that their norms, so valuable for interpretation, were derived from nonaphasic groups. The need for supplemental reading assessment is greatest for high-level aphasics, especially those to whom reading was an important activity and who request treatment especially focused on this skill. Reading in this section refers to silent reading for comprehension instead of reading aloud, which is as much dependent on speech processes as it is on reading processes.

Borrowed Tests

Brookshire (1978b) discussed four requirements of a reading test for aphasics. First, a test should measure reading efficiency as well as reading capacity. Efficiency is indicated by rate of successful reading, and capacity is indicated by accuracy of comprehension without time constraints. Second, a reading test should cover a range of reading levels. A low level is represented by single-word comprehension, which commonly is tested with picture-choice tasks. Reading versions of the *Peabody Picture Vocabulary Test* (Dunn, 1965) and the *Ammons Full-Range Picture Vocabulary Test* (Ammons and Ammons, 1948) have been used for aphasics; but performance on these tests is tied to individual differences in premorbid vocabulary size, and only the Ammons test has norms for adults. Third, responses required of the patient should be simple. Having been designed for persons without brain injury, borrowed tests may have answering formats which could be perceptually confusing and motorically demanding for the aphasic. Finally, the test should be as pure a measure of reading comprehension as possible, with minimal loading on recall, reasoning, and problem-solving. Test instructions and response modes may have to be modified in order to measure aphasia, and subtests may have to be selected to minimize the influence of individual differences in factors unrelated to aphasic disturbance.

Tests designed to measure reading skill of school-age children and adolescents have been borrowed for use with aphasics (Brookshire, 1978b; Porrazzo, 1978). Results are generally interpreted with reference to reading "grade levels" based on norms from elementary and secondary students. *Functional literacy* is the ability to understand commonly available adult reading materials; the level of most newspapers and magazines lies between the fifth and seventh grades (Porrazzo, 1978). Degree of aphasic impairment must be judged with respect to an estimated premorbid reading level which is based on the patient's years of schooling and occupation.

Tests reviewed by Brookshire and Porrazzo include the *Nelson Reading Test* (Nelson, 1962) and the *Gates-MacGinitie Reading Tests* (Gates and MacGinitie, 1965). The Nelson test examines a grade range of 2.0 to 10.5. Its word-comprehension (vocabulary) section consists of multiple-choice sentence-completion items, making it a sentence comprehension task for the aphasic. The second part of the Nelson test is paragraph comprehension measured by three multiple-choice questions with each paragraph. The Gates-MacGinitie test includes a series of tests (especially Primary A, B, and C) which tap into lower reading levels. It examines word comprehension with a format which is better designed for the aphasic. The examinee chooses from four words to match with a picture (see Brookshire, 1978b, p. 71). Sentence and paragraph comprehension is tested by matching the language stimulus to one of four pictures. Brookshire preferred this test for patients who would perform at the lowest grade levels.

Reading Comprehension Battery for Aphasia (RCBA)

The *RCBA* was designed by LaPointe and Horner (1979) to provide an assessment of the nature and degree of reading deficit in aphasic patients. Therefore, it minimizes potential obstructions to the viewing of reading disturbance by presenting clear and simple visual arrays, requiring simple pointing responses, and minimizing the involvement of other language modalities in performance of the tasks. Its character as a test for aphasics is derived also from its attempt to isolate primary deficits which have been postulated in investigations of aphasic reading.

One limitation is the absence of norms as well as of validation and reliability data within the test manual. Though LaPointe and Horner noted that such studies are under way, interpretation of patient performance is weakened without the frame of reference provided by samples of aphasic performance. Some norms, including validation and reliability studies, were reported by Van Demark, Lemmer, and Drake (1980) at the American Speech-Language-Hearing Association Convention. LaPointe and Horner provide some interpretation guidelines based on an analysis of errors and on some of the findings in the literature on reading disturbance. However, this literature has not yet clearly established the validity of dyslexia classification, especially when speech is not involved in the reading task.

The *RCBA* consists of ten subtests which progress from word to paragraph levels of difficulty. Patients often are slow and meticulous readers, and this test may take well over an hour to administer in some cases. In most tasks the patient makes a pointing response to one of three choices.

Subtests I through III involve single-word comprehension, and the three choices are printed words to match with a picture. The choices are similar visually (I), auditorily (II), and semantically (III), permitting the examiner to identify a surface dyslexia or a deep dyslexia. Subtest IV examines functional reading such as reading common signs, using a checkbook, and finding a number in a phone directory. Van Demark, et al. (1980) found that functional reading was among the most difficult of the subtests for twenty-six aphasics. This may occur because the patient must read a sentence-length instruction to carry out each functional task, thereby weakening the validity of this subtest. Subtest V has the patient match printed synonyms, and subtests VI and VII involve selecting a picture corresponding to a sentence and short paragraph, respectively. Each of these subtests (I through VII) contains ten items.

The ten items of subtests VIII and IX are based on the patient's comprehension of five paragraphs. Each paragraph is accompanied by four multiple-choice sentence completions pertaining to the paragraph. Two of the completions (ten items) involve factual information (VIII). Two of the completions (ten items) involve inferred information (IX). Van Demark found that inferential responses were more difficult than factual responses. These paragraphs also contain some instances of humor, and the examiner is asked to note the patient's reaction.

The last subtest (X) is designed to determine whether particular syntactic structures might contribute to a patient's reading difficulty. Five different structures are tested, with two items per structure. Some of these structures are fairly complex, involving relative clauses and indirect objects. This was the most difficult of the ten subtests in Van Demark's study but was equivalent statistically to functional reading (IV) and to two of the paragraph reading subtests (VII, IX).

VERBAL EXPRESSION

Special analytical and measurement techniques have been recommended which provide a qualitative analysis of spoken language or a measurement of degree of deficit especially in mildly impaired patients.

Word Fluency

While most tests of word retrieval require the patient to converge on one particular word in response (Chapey, et al., 1977), there has been some use of tasks in which the patient must produce multiple or divergent responses to a single stimulus. A word-fluency measure, investigated by Borkowski, Benton, and Spreen (1967), has been thought of as a measure of aphasia. Borkowski, et al. (1967) had used this procedure to study word retrieval impairment subsequent to brain damage. This procedure was incorporated into the *NCCEA* and the Boston Exam. The word-fluency measure is a controlled verbal-

association task in which the patient produces as many words as possible beginning with a specified letter or belonging to a semantic category. For example, Borkowski, et al. asked patients to say as many words as possible, as quickly as possible, which begin with the letter "B." Patients were given sixty seconds to produce associations to each letter. In the Boston Exam, patients must produce animal names within a similar time period.

Borkowski, et al. (1967) obtained norms on twenty-four letters from sixty-six normal adults. Six letters were determined to be difficult; *J*, for example, elicited an average of 4.83 associations. Seven letters were of moderate difficulty (*N* elicited 8.23 associations), and eleven letters were easy (*F* elicited 11.36 associations). The average number of verbal associations to letters discriminated between brain-damaged and normal subjects, with fewer words produced by the brain-damaged group. There was an indication that difficult letters differentiated between patients with right-hemisphere and left-hemisphere damage, with left-hemisphere damage resulting in fewer associations. Spreen and Benton (1969) used *F*, *A*, and *S*, three easy letters (11.36, 10.22, 11.50, respectively), as the word-fluency measure in the *NCCEA* battery. From Borkowski, et al.'s conclusions, the easy letters would not be expected to differentiate between left and right-hemisphere brain damage.

In obtaining norms for the Boston Exam, Borod, et al. (1980) found that 147 normal adults produced an average of 22.5 animal names with a standard deviation of 6.8 and a range of 9 through 41. Therefore, even within the normal population, word fluency to semantic categories appears to be highly variable.

The value of word-fluency measures for differential diagnosis is questionable. These measures do appear to be sensitive to brain injury, and they may differentiate between left and right-hemisphere damage. "A potential strength of the measure is its ability to assess mild aphasia" (Wertz, 1979, p. 245). Word fluency may provide a means for identifying these patients and for measuring their recovery. More research should be explored with this technique, especially with respect to qualitative aspects of word-retrieval performance. In the animal-naming task, aphasic patients sometimes appear to be facile in retrieving words from one subordinate category such as house pets or farm animals, but then they seem unable to shift to another subcategory in order to increase their association output.

The Reporter's Test

DeRenzi and Ferrari (1978) turned around the Token Test in order to create a measure of mild and moderate disorders of verbal expression. The patient becomes a "reporter" of performance carried out by the clinician with tokens of varying color, shape, and size. The Reporter's Test was intended to provide an objective measure of deficit in the production of connected speech. DeRenzi and Ferrari felt that verbal descriptions of the clinician's manipulations of tokens could be scored easily, because the words to be produced would be predetermined and would represent relatively unambiguous concepts. The test was introduced in a journal article, as was the Token Test in 1962, and it can be considered to be in a stage of development that is comparable to the status of the Token Test in the mid-1960s.

The test involves twenty tokens arranged according to a figure in the article (DeRenzi and Ferrari, 1978). Its five parts correspond to the five sections of the original Token Test. The Reporter's Test contains twenty-six items with four items in each of Parts One through Four and ten in the fifth part. Examples of the clinician's presentation and the expected verbal response for each part are as follows: (1) *Touch the green circle,* (2) *Touch the large yellow square,* (3) *Touch the red circle and the green square,* (4) *Touch the small black circle and the large yellow square,* and (5) *Put the red circle on the green square* and *Put all the circles into a box.* Among the ten items of Part Five are seven original Token Test instructions and three new items for the Reporter's Test.

DeRenzi and Ferrari always gave a shortened Token Test prior to administering the Reporter's Test. In an unusual twist of test administration, the clinician shields the tokens from view of an imaginary listener. The patient is instructed as follows: "... Imagine that a person is sitting beside you, but is prevented from seeing what I am doing by a curtain... Your task is to describe what I am doing as carefully as possible, so that this person would be able to repeat exactly my performance on another set of tokens..." (DeRenzi and Ferrari, 1978, p. 281). This is an attempt to create a more genuine communicative situation in which the patient's verbal expression is motivated by the goal of conveying new information to an uninformed listener.

Two methods of scoring responses were described. A pass-fail system allowed 1 point for correct responses, 0 for incorrect responses, and 0.5 for correct responses after a repeat of the stimulus. A maximum score was twenty-six. A weighted scoring system allowed one point for each adjective and noun retrieved in Parts One through Four of the test, and the maximum score was sixty.

The Reporter's Test was administered to seventy normals and sixty left-hemisphere-damaged aphasic patients who were described as having mild and moderate deficits. Based on the pass-fail scoring system, the normals averaged 23.09 and the aphasic subjects averaged 10.10, with a standard deviation of 6.14. The test separated aphasics from brain-injured subjects without aphasia. Twenty left-hemisphere-impaired nonaphasic subjects averaged 22.15, and twenty right-hemisphere-impaired subjects averaged 22.19. Only five of the sixty aphasic subjects scored above 18.35. The difficulty of the test for mildly impaired aphasic patients is indicative of the test's capability as a measure of recovery; however, this capability was not demonstrated in DeRenzi and Ferrari's article.

One limitation of the Reporter's Test is that its content is so specific that conclusions about results may not be generalized easily to language function as a whole. The authors stated, "A possible drawback of the test is that it involves a very limited number of words and does not tap, consequently, the wealth of vocabulary available to the patient" (DeRenzi and Ferrari, 1978, p. 281).

Further Attention to Connected Verbal Expression

With the Reporter's Test, we have begun to consider methods of assessment which have not been established as routine clinical procedures but rather have been used primarily as research procedures or as potential clinical options. The problem being investigated is a clinical problem: How can we describe and measure verbal discourse in a reliable and practical manner? Aphasia batteries have been criticized for being overly focused on eliciting convergent, single-word responses and for being insensitive to nuances of deficit in the extended verbal output of mild aphasia (Chapey, et al., 1977; DeRenzi and Ferrari, 1978; Yorkston and Beukelman, 1980).

Description. Descriptive methodology enables the clinician to identify pattern of expressive deficit in a way that facilitates comparisons among patients and that may lead to distinctive treatment objectives. Methods in clinical aphasiology have included rating scales of speech characteristics and linguistic description. Rating scales have arisen from the careful study of how aphasic patients differ from each other in their verbal expression. Linguistic description has been derived from methods used to characterize normal language. With both methods there has been an attempt to quantify the degree of deviation from normal. In its early stages this methodology can be cumbersome and relatively subjective; however, descriptive methodology is often a first step toward the development of convenient and reliable clinical measures of deficit and recovery.

The first requirement of any strategy for assessing spontaneous verbal expression is to obtain a sample of utterances from the patient. The more natural the circumstances, the more difficult it is to analyze the sample and to compare it with other samples. From a free-wheeling conversation about undetermined topics, it can be a challenge to resolve the ambiguities of aphasic speech so that semantic and syntactic units can be identified. Therefore, whenever conversation has been employed and a basis for comparison has been desired, certain common topics have been used such as "How did your speech problems start?" (Green, 1969a; Wagenaar, et al., 1975). A frequent procedure has been picture description, using, for example, the "Cookie Theft" picture from the Boston Exam (Goodglass and Kaplan, 1972). Pictures from the *Thematic Apperception Test* (Murray, 1943) were employed in several studies by Wepman and his colleagues (Fillenbaum, Jones, and Wepman, 1961; Fillenbaum and Jones, 1962; Spiegel, et al., 1965; Jones and Wepman, 1967). For linguistic description, more restrictive conditions have been used such as producing a sentence which contains a word given by the clinician (Schuell, Shaw, and Brewer, 1969).

The rating scale of the *BDAE* (see Figure 7–1) is based on six characteristics of verbal expression which Goodglass and Kaplan (1972) used to distinguish Broca's,

Wernicke's, anomic, conduction, and transcortical sensory aphasias. Other rating scales were built upon ten parameters of aphasic speech and were developed to investigate differences between nonfluent and fluent aphasias. Kerschensteiner, et al.'s (1972) scale consisted of three levels for each parameter: (1) word choice, (2) rate of speaking, (3) articulation, (4) phrase length, (5) effort, (6) pauses, (7) prosody, (8) verbal paraphasias, (9) phonemic paraphasias, and (10) perseveration. The frequency of pauses was not considered by Benson (1967). From ratings of forty-seven aphasic subjects, Kerschensteiner, et al. (1972) found that nonfluent and fluent aphasias were differentiated best by prosody, pauses, phrase length, and rate of speaking.

One of the first applications of linguistic methods to the analysis of aphasic spontaneous speech was by Fillenbaum, Jones, and Wepman (1961; Jones and Wepman, 1967). Their unit of description was the grammatical word class or form class. Jones, Goodman, and Wepman (1963) proposed a system of word classification that would be a manageable number of relatively unambiguous word classes. Spreen and Wachal (1973) used this system to code aphasic speech for computer analysis. Transformational grammar was also instituted so that relationships between words in a sentence would be captured in description of aphasic verbal expression. Schuell, et al. (1969) suggested that such description would be sensitive to small differences between impaired and normal language production. They compared the proportions of certain structures between two aphasic subjects and twelve normal controls. Myerson and Goodglass (1972) attempted a transformational analysis of three cases of agrammatism.

Crystal, Fletcher, and Garman (1976) developed "... a procedure for analyzing the syntactic character of language disorders, capable of being used routinely by anyone involved with the diagnosis, assessment and remediation of language disability" (p. 20). They called it *LARSP* (*Language Assessment, Remediation and Screening Procedure*). This profile of syntax usage in spontaneous speech was based on the development of syntactic structures in children. However, Crystal, et al. presented a case study of Broca's aphasia in order to demonstrate the applicability of *LARSP* to assessment of aphasia. Though they did not ascribe to the regression theory of aphasia (Chapter 4), they noted methodological similarities in dealing with child and adult language by citing Myerson and Goodglass (1972): "Taking samples from patients at various severity levels is analogous to examining speech samples from children at different ages" (p. 41). *LARSP* is a profile of the extent to which certain word classes and syntactic structures appear in spontaneous verbal expression.

Measurement.   Serious attempts have been made to quantify features of verbal expression so that patients can be compared (differential diagnosis) and so that recovery of more natural expressive performance can be measured (assessment). Comparison of spontaneous speech samples within and between patients is faced with the problem of unequal speech sample sizes, so that simple counting of units in the sample results in unfair comparisons. Therefore, much of the data has been stated as ratios to facilitate comparisons.

A common ratio for the characterization of spontaneous verbal expression has been the *type-token ratio* (TTR), a measure of diversity of vocabulary use. The TTR is the frequency of occurrence of different categories of items (types) relative to the frequency of the total number of items produced (tokens). When counting words, the TTR is a ratio of the number of different words relative to the total number of words, and appears as follows:

$$TTR = \frac{\text{\# different words (types)}}{\text{total \# words (tokens)}}$$

A more varied vocabulary is indicated by a larger TTR. Fillenbaum, et al. (1961) had computed type-token ratios separately for content words and function words in their aphasic spontaneous speech samples. However, they did not report the results because of sensitivity of the TTR to speech sample sizes; ". . . generally speaking the smaller the number of words spoken the larger the type-token ratio" (p. 96).

Other ratios have been defined relative to more specific linguistic categories. For example, Wepman and Jones (1966) used a noun-pronoun ratio. The semantically empty speech of anomic aphasia might be depicted with a much lower noun-pronoun ratio than the noun-laden utterances of agrammatic speech in Broca's aphasia. Wagenaar, et al. (1975) listed thirty variables of spontaneous speech which they used in a factor analysis of spontaneous speech. One reference point in their ratios (the denominator) was time: *number of utterances produced in six minutes.* Another reference point was the total number of content words produced: *number of verbal paraphasias expressed as a percentage of the number of content words.* Another reference point was total number of utterances: *function-word deletions as a percentage of number of utterances* and *word-order mistakes as a percentage of number of utterances.*

A *phrase-length ratio* (PLR) was used by Goodglass, et al. (1964) to distinguish between nonfluent and fluent aphasia. Their ratio was as follows:

$$PLR = \frac{\text{\# 5- or more-word groups}}{\text{\# 1- and 2-word groups}}$$

Long-phrase dominant patients scored 0.31 or more, while short-phrase dominant patients scored 0.15 or less. Of fifty-three aphasic subjects, none were between these PLR's, and fifty-one of these subjects were sorted accurately into nonfluent and fluent classifications with this method. The PLR has not been investigated as a measure of recovery reflecting possible treatment goals such as increasing phrase length in Broca's aphasia or decreasing phrase length in Wernicke's aphasia.

Speaking rate in words per minute (wpm) has been a powerful consideration in differential diagnosis among aphasias. According to Howes (1964), normal rate is 100 to 175 wpm, and Kerschensteiner, et al. (1972) confirmed this standard with twenty normal control subjects. Benson (1967) based his scale for speaking rate on the assumption that some aphasics speak faster than normal:

> below normal—fewer than 50 wpm
> normal—50 to 150 wpm
> above normal—more than 150 wpm

However, Kerschensteiner found no aphasics above the normal rate of 175 wpm, and so his rating scale was forged as follows:

> very slow—0 to 50 wpm
> slow—51 to 90 wpm
> normal—above 90 wpm

Of forty-seven aphasic subjects, seventeen were very slow, thirteen were slow, and seventeen were normal (Kerschensteiner, et al., 1972).

At a Clinical Aphasiology Conference, Yorkston and Beukelman (1977) introduced a method of measuring subtle expressive deficit in mild and moderate aphasia for the purpose of documenting change. This method focuses on the rate of verbal expression. In a later report of this method, they presented data from a larger number of aphasic subjects and presented norms from an older adult sample (mean age of seventy-three years) in addition to a younger adult sample (mean age of thirty-one years).

Yorkston and Beukelman (1980) investigated whether their measure is sensitive to expressive deficits in aphasic patients defined as mild (81 to 99 percentile from the *PICA*), high-moderate (66 to 80 percentile), and low-moderate (50 to 65 percentile). Spontaneous speech was elicited by description of the Boston Exam's Cookie Theft picture, and each sample was tape recorded. The clinician recorded the time of verbal description, the number of syllables produced, and the number of content units produced. A content unit was defined "as a grouping of information that was always expressed as a unit by normal speakers" (p. 30), and examples of these units were listed in an appendix to the article. Content units included "cookies," "from the jar," "mother," and "in the kitchen" (p. 36).

Three measures were employed: (1) *number of content units* as an indication of amount of information conveyed, (2) *syllables per minute* as a measure of speaking rate, and (3) *content units per minute* as a measure of efficiency in conveying ideas. Average scores and ranges were reported for the two normal adult groups and the three aphasic groups. Four of the five groups produced a similar amount of information, while the low-moderate aphasic group produced significantly fewer content units than the others.

Speaking rate (syllables/minute) and communicative efficiency (content units/ minute) were the most discriminating parameters. The two normal groups spoke at a faster rate than the three aphasic groups. The older adults produced 193 syllables per minute, while the mild aphasic patients produced 121 syllables per minute. The low-moderate patients were significantly slower than the less-impaired patients. Mild aphasia was also separated from normal performance with respect to communicative efficiency. Mild patients produced 18.7 content units/ minute, while normal older adults produced 33.7 content units/minute. This parameter may be sensitive to normal aging because the normal younger adults

produced significantly more content units than the older adults. Test-retest reliability was above 0.90 with each of the three measures. Golper (1980) used the two measures of rate to measure recovery of aphasic and nonaphasic subjects during the first month postonset.

Finally, Golper and her coworkers turned their attention to some different parameters of spontaneous verbal expression (Golper, Thorpe, Tompkins, et al., 1980), because they were confronted with two cases of mild aphasia in which speaking rate and communicative efficiency were equivalent to Yorkston and Beukelman's (1977) normal elderly adults. Golper's evidence for the existence of mild aphasia came from the Token Test and the patients' own reports of their language problems. She counted the occurrence of the following speaking deviations: (1) phrase and word interruptions or revisions, (2) phrase and word sequence interrupters, including noncontentive vocalizations such as "uhs", and (3) morphological, syntactic, and phonemic errors. These measures were examined by gathering speech samples in the same manner as the Yorkston and Beukelman (1977, 1980) study.

Like Yorkston's finding, Golper found that normal elderly adults, right-hemisphere-damaged controls, and mildly aphasic subjects did not differ as to amount of content produced. High-level aphasia in Golper's study was defined as the 79th to 95th overall percentile on the *PICA,* which was about the same range as Yorkston and Beukelman's (1980) mild group. Content rate, contrary to the two cases which stimulated this project, was lower for the aphasic group than for the nonaphasic groups. Golper's mild aphasics were slower in syllable rate (93.2) than Yorkston's mild group (120.8).

All three of Golper's parameters clearly separated mild aphasia from the nonaphasic groups. The occurrence of revisions, sequence interrupters, and grammatical errors was minimal in the nonaphasic subjects, while they occurred frequently in the mildly impaired aphasic patients. Therefore, these measures may be added to the parameters of syllable and content rate as indicators of mild aphasia and as measures of recovery.

A TEST
OF NONVERBAL COGNITION

Raven's (1962) *Coloured Progressive Matrices, Sets A, Ab, B (RCPM)* is used frequently by speech-language pathologists as an assessment of nonverbal visual perception and reasoning. The clinician's purpose is usually to obtain an indication of the aphasic patient's cognitive capability in areas other than the use of language. Of course, a more thorough and skilled assessment of other areas of brain function is provided by a neuropsychologist, who might administer the *Wechsler Adult Intelligence Scale (WAIS)* or the *Luria-Nebraska Neuropsychological Battery* (Golden, Hemmeke, and Purisch, 1980). However, a neuropsychologist is not always available, and Raven's test is convenient and easy to administer. It should be remembered that the *RCPM*'s content is limited in scope, and inferences about intelligence from the results should be made with caution. The manual was revised by Raven, Court, and Raven (1976, 1977). Strategies for problem-type and error-type analyses of *RCPM* results were reviewed by Horner and Nailling (1980).

The *RCPM* consists of a series of visual patterns from which a small segment is missing. With each item, the omitted segment is presented with five similar segments. The patient points to the one believed to be the missing segment. *Sets A, Ab, and B* consist of three sections of twelve items each, and each section increases in difficulty. The maximum score is thirty-six. The raw score is translated into a percentile for normal adult age groups from sixty-five to one hundred years. Normal adults vary widely in nonverbal in-

telligence, and so it is difficult to decide whether a patient's score represents a deficit. One guideline is to judge whether the score is consistent with the patient's educational and occupational background prior to onset of aphasia.

Aphasic performance on the *RCPM* is indicated in a study by Kertesz and McCabe (1975). Aphasic patients with severe auditory comprehension deficits were grossly deficient on this nonverbal test when compared with normal and brain-damaged nonaphasic control subjects. Global aphasics averaged 3.6/36; Wernicke's aphasics averaged 12.1/36. Groups of Broca's, conduction, and anomic aphasia had average scores of 16.6, 18.0, and 21.8, respectively. The normal controls of comparable age averaged 24.8, with a standard deviation of 6.6. Because people vary in nonverbal intelligence, scores were variable for normals and overlapped with scores by aphasic patients. However, all aphasic groups performed significantly worse than normal controls; Broca's, conduction, and anomic aphasias were equivalent to the non-dominant hemisphere damage group. Therefore, aphasia results in deficient performance on the *RCPM,* and the test appears to be sensitive to brain damage in general.

Although aphasic comprehension deficit was related to *RCPM* performance, Kertesz and McCabe concluded that cognitive processes underlying the test may be independent of auditory comprehension processes. A few patients with severe auditory deficits performed normally, and some brain-damaged controls with intact comprehension were unable to perform on the test.

SUMMARY AND REMARKS

A complete battery of tests for initial assessment might include one of the three major comprehensive language tests (see Chapter 7), a test of functional communi-

TABLE 8-1. Modality-focused tests and measures are summarized as to their most likely use as supplemental procedures with different types and degrees of aphasia.

Purpose	Test	Mild Aphasias		Mild Broca's	Moderate Broca's	Severe Broca's	Wernicke's
		Anomic	Conduction				
Auditory comprehension	Token Test	Yes	Yes	Yes	Perhaps	No	No
	ACTS	Yes	Yes	Yes	Yes	Yes	Yes
Reading	RCBA	Yes	Yes	Yes	Yes	Yes	Yes
Verbal expression	Word Fluency	Yes	Yes	Yes	Yes	Perhaps	No
	Reporter's Test	Yes	Yes	Yes	No	No	No
	Ratios	Yes	Yes	Yes	Yes	Yes	Yes
	Rate	Yes	Yes	Yes	Perhaps	Perhaps	No

cation such as the *FCP* or *CADL,* and a set of modality-specific tests and measurements. This is a potentially overwhelming undertaking of several hours, and so selectivity is exercised depending on the setting, time constraints, cost, and the deficits presented by the patient. Table 8–1 summarizes most of the modality-specific tests and measures according to their value for different degrees and types of aphasia. Because some of these tests were originally intended to detect and measure mild aphasia, the table reflects a tendency for most supplemental measures to be recommended for these patients. Time may not be a serious concern because high-level patients may take comprehensive tests very quickly. The most severely impaired patients, especially with global aphasia, may not be given high-level tasks; and more attention needs to be addressed to the development of special tests for these patients, simply for identification of their communicative assets.

9 Recovery, Prognosis, and the Influence of Treatment

Once the aphasic patient has received an initial speech and language assessment, the clinician is concerned with recovery of speech and language functions. The patient and his or her family usually want to know what to expect. They will ask: "Will he get better?" "How much better?" "How long will it take?" This chapter provides the available data concerning recovery from aphasia. An understanding of what is known and not known relative to recovery not only may assist the clinician in making predictions but also may contribute to decisions about a long-term plan of rehabilitation and about dismissal from treatment.

OBSERVING RECOVERY

Recovery can be observed readily in the natural circumstances of language use during the few days and weeks after onset of aphasia. A patient who has been speechless for a while will begin to utter a few words. Recurrent stereotypic speech may be replaced with differentiated utterances which are appropriate for the situation. Agrammatic spaces between words may occasionally become filled with functors, and utterances may lengthen from one word to two or three words. Streams of neologistic jargon may subside, with a few recognizable phrases starting to appear from time to time. However, after the first two months of aphasia, improvements come more slowly until they are difficult to observe from day to day or even week to week. After the first six months, aphasic patients come to believe they are getting better but cannot put a finger on exactly what it is that is getting better. At this time, improvements can be detected by clinical measurement using repeated administrations of sensitive and reliable tests.

Investigators have focused on measurement of changes in overall language function, in the four language modalities, and in performance on specific subtests of certain aphasia batteries. Recovery is also observed as the patient becomes successful with levels of increasing task difficulty during treatment. In effect, the patient is able to do something he or she could not do before. Most of our data on recovery from aphasia is addressed to changes in clinical performance or linguistic adequacy of performance. Clinical performance has been the most workable means of obtaining measurements on a regular and reliable basis.

However, clinical performance and functional performance are not comparable for many persons with aphasia; and the literature contains relatively little information on the recovery of functional language or communicative abilities in natural settings. Recovery of functional language has been measured with the *FCP* and, to a lesser extent, with the *CADL* (see Chapter 8). Sarno, Sarno, and Levita (1971) contended "that improvement which is not reflected in the patient's daily life is not improvement in fact" (p. 74). They attempted to determine whether standard measures of clinical performance would yield information about recovery comparable to measures of functional language. They compared auditory comprehension and naming subtests of the *NCCEA* with the understanding and speaking sections of the *FCP* relative to their detection of improvement in twenty-three severely impaired aphasic patients. Especially with the measures of comprehension, the *NCCEA* showed improvement which was not shown with the *FCP*. Although it is possible that the *FCP* is not as sensitive as the *NCCEA* in detecting improvement in language function, these investigators concluded " . . . that improvement as measured by higher test scores does not always reflect useful improvement, that is to say, the ability of the patient to function better in his day-to-day existence" (p. 77). The reverse may also apply; useful improvement may occur which does not show up in clinical reassessment.

PARAMETERS OF RECOVERY

Whether the clinician is interested in improvement of overall language function, a particular language modality, or a specific clinical function such as confrontation naming, there are several parameters of that improvement which can be addressed. The parameters are reflected in common questions posed to the clinician about recovery. Questions such as "Is he getting better?" or "How much is he improving?" are answerable from observations of the amount of positive change made by the patient. When these questions are formulated in the future tense, such as "How much will he improve?" the clinician is asked to predict amount of recovery; and the answer is based on clinical experience and published research. The question "What will she be like when you stop therapy?" can be dealt with from investigations of the outcome of recovery and the pattern of recovering specific language functions. The question "How long will it take to get there?" can be approached from research addressed to rate of recovery.

Amount

Amount of recovery is indicated by the difference between two assessments of a patient. In research where amount of recovery has been examined, the smallest time interval between assessments was two weeks (Culton, 1969). Amount is quantifiable with reliable assessments which yield a score, so that an earlier score can be subtracted from a later score resulting in a *difference score,* called a "change score" by Sarno and her colleagues. The total amount of recovery by a patient can be determined when the initial assessment is made at the point of maximum deficit (completed stroke, for example) soon after onset and when a later assessment is made after recovery has ceased.

Several aphasia batteries yield a single score for indicating amount of overall linguistic and communicative recovery. This parameter has not always been represented with the precision of a difference score, as early investigators had depicted amount in terms of subjective rating scales. For example, Butfield and Zangwill (1946) and Wepman (1951) rated recovery as much improved, moderately improved, or unchanged; Marks, Taylor, and Rusk (1959) classified amount of improvement as excellent, good, fair, or poor. Difference scores may be represented graphically, or actual difference scores are reported. Amount of recovery has been reported in a variety of ways, making studies difficult to integrate.

Recovery is sometimes investigated without a record of actual amount of improvement. Instead, the number of patients making a certain amount of recovery is reported (Basso, Capitani, and Vignolo, 1979), or the frequency of occurrence of recovery is reported (Kenin and Swisher, 1972).

In studies of patients who had suffered thromboembolic strokes, investigators often prefer to wait until the patient's medical status and, in some cases, pattern of language deficit stabilizes before presenting a formal test. In many of these studies, initial scores are obtained around one month after onset. This time of initial testing may coincide with maximum degree of deficit (completed stroke) in cases where stroke-in-evolution lasts a few weeks. However, Hanson and Cicciarelli (1978) and Bamber (1980) reported a few initial *PICA* scores obtained between four and nineteen days post onset. Sarno and Levita (1971) administered initial *FCP*s to twenty-eight patients at bedside within two days after onset, when some of these patients exhibited "... a total lack of responsiveness and, quite probably, total absence of consciousness" (p. 177). Whenever amount of recovery is reported, the time since onset of the initial assessment should be considered. If the measure is obtained later than one month after onset or after regaining consciousness, the difference score reflects only a portion of total recovery.

Outcome

The study of prediction in aphasiology has involved determining whether a level of language function can be predicted given certain information, such as another level of function determined at an earlier time after onset. More specifically, can a *PICA* score taken at one month postonset be used to predict a subsequent *PICA* score at six months or a year after onset, thereby predicting what in some cases may be the maximum level or outcome of recovery? Outcome is the endpoint of recovery and is often the point at which the patient is dismissed from speech-language treatment. Predicting this parameter is important for long-range treatment planning, and being able to determine this parameter when it occurs is important for decisions about concluding treatment.

When amount of recovery has been computed for research on recovery, the second assessment has not always been taken at the point of maximum recovery. This is because some investigations have dealt only with early phases of recovery within the first three or four months after onset (Lomas and Kertesz, 1978; Ludlow, 1977). Outcome of recovery was earmarked as a dependent variable in four studies of language recovery after CVA. Keenan and Brassell (1974) rated final level of language function at termination of treatment, based on an examination of clinical records. Kertesz and McCabe (1977) rated outcome after twelve months postonset for representatives of different syndromes. Deal and Deal (1978) computed difference scores based on the *final* administration of a test at or near termination of treatment. Hanson and Cicciarelli (1978) computed difference scores based on the *peak* test score, the highest score achieved during treatment. Final and peak scores may not represent the same assessment for any one patient, making it difficult to compare these two studies in this respect and raising a question as to what test score would be most representative of outcome.

Before outcome can be characterized with a single score, it should be determined that the patient has indeed reached the end of recovery. This is confirmed when measures of language no longer show an upward trend across time; and this plateau of language function is observed only with a series of assessments in order to be confident that recovery has stopped. Within a series of assessments comprising the plateau of recovery, there will be some variation of scores within which a peak score will be observed. A peak score usually appears in the context of previous and subsequent scores and, therefore, may be achieved prior to the final score. Sometimes patients remain in some form of treatment long past the occurrence of a peak score, for various reasons: (1) a peak score may not be recognized until the clinician has obtained several scores in order to be confident that a plateau has been reached; (2) some clinical programs include a period of modified treatment addressed to maintenance of an achieved outcome; and (3) the clinician may not be confident that the assessment of clinical language performance reflects maximal improvement, because other aspects of communicative behavior may continue to improve. An implication for the investigation of recovery is that, when we are interested in duration of recovery, the final score may not be the best indicant of completed recovery. The final score may be related to clinical decisions independent of the recovery process. Also, given that the peak score may be just the high point of fluctuation within the plateau of recovery, the best single indicant of outcome may be an average of the series of scores making up the plateau.

Rate

Rate refers broadly to the time, after onset of aphasia, that it takes the patient to reach the maximum level of recovery. The maximum level is usually reached sometime before the occurrence of a peak test score or final test score. Investigators who have reported amounts of recovery have also reported the time intervals from which difference scores were obtained, so that some information about rate is available.

However, some investigators examined only certain intervals within a complete recovery period; maximum level of recovery was not determined in some studies; and often the initial test score was obtained after some recovery had already occurred. Therefore, a picture of recovery rate from beginning to end has to be pieced together from several studies examining different intervals during the process.

Common time frames in the study of recovery are as follows: onset to three months postonset, three to six months postonset, six to twelve months, and twelve to eighteen months and beyond. For example, Kertesz and McCabe (1977) compared amounts of recovery for zero to three months, three to six months, and six to twelve months or more after onset of aphasia. Spontaneous recovery, which occurs without treatment, was examined by Sarno and Levita (1971) in the zero-to-three and three-to-six-month periods. The effect of language treatment on recovery was studied by Hagen (1973) in the six-to-twelve and twelve-to-eighteen-month periods after onset. Amounts of recovery reported by Sands, Sarno, and Shankweiler (1969) spanned four years after onset, and Broida (1977) presented amounts of recovery that occurred beginning at twelve months after onset. Of all the aphasic subjects used in studies of recovery, relatively few have been followed according to level of function at regular intervals from shortly after onset to a conclusive completion of recovery. One of the largest groups to be followed throughout the first year after onset was thirty-four of an initial sixty-seven subjects who were tested by Wertz, Collins, Weiss, et al. (1981) at approximately the intervals noted at the beginning of this paragraph.

Pattern

In addition to considering recovery in the unitary terms of overall language function, recovery can be assessed by comparing the four language modalities, subtests of an aphasia battery, or symptom patterns displayed in spontaneous speech. Pattern of recovery is reflected in the different amounts and rates of improvement which occur among the different language functions. With respect to spontaneous speech, Prins, Snow, and Wagenaar (1978) examined recovery of twenty-eight variables. Changes in the use of paraphasias, function words, perseverations and so on were recorded. Also, there has been speculation that some aphasias evolve from the symptom pattern of one syndrome to that of another syndrome (Kertesz, 1979, 1981).

One intriguing issue has been the pattern of recovery in multilingual (polyglot) patients with respect to differential improvement among languages learned by the patient. Over one hundred cases were reviewed by Paradis (1977) and Albert and Obler (1978). There have been three basic explanations regarding recovery patterns: (1) *The rule of Ribot,* which states that the first learned language should be less impaired and should recover first, (2) *The rule of Pitres,* which states that the most familiar or recently used language recovers first, and (3) *Affective factors* that may explain differential recovery when the other rules do not apply (Albert and Obler, 1978).

DESCRIPTION OF RECOVERY

In this section the description of spontaneous recovery is separated from the description of recovery made by patients receiving speech-language treatment, in spite of the fact that some of the characteristics of recovery are similar for untreated and treated aphasic persons. Studies of spontaneous recovery and of treated subjects have differed in a few basic ways, including classification of aphasic subjects and depiction of parameters. Also, amount of spontaneous recovery has been measured mostly with the *WAB*, while in treated subjects amount has been measured mostly with the *PICA, NCCEA,* and *FCP.*

Spontaneous Recovery

Some improvement of language functions is inevitable in most cases of aphasia irrespective of whether patients receive speech-language treatment. This recovery may stem from the functional substitution and reorganization described in Chapter 4. Spontaneous recovery of language was reported by Culton (1969), Sarno and Levita (1971), Lomas and Kertesz (1978), and Kertesz and McCabe (1977; Kertesz, 1979). Other data on spontaneous recovery can be obtained from untreated control groups in studies of treatment efficacy (Basso, et al., 1978; Deal and Deal, 1978; Hagen, 1973). Studies of spontaneous recovery are difficult to come by, because medical problems often prohibit thorough language testing during the first month after onset and because clinicians and physicians are reluctant to withhold treatment after the first month.

Amount: Overall Language. The proportion of untreated patients reported to have improved is not as high as clinical observation implies. Of twenty-seven untreated subjects in Vignolo's (1964) study, only 55 percent demonstrated improvement between language assessments. In the larger group studied by Basso, et al. (1979), 42 percent improved in auditory comprehension and 21 percent improved in oral expression. However, a patient was considered to be improved if there were at least two points of change on a five-point scale. This criterion probably excluded patients making small amounts of recovery. Another reason for these apparently small proportions is that they are based on amounts of recovery occurring at varying times after onset. Of those observed initially within two months postonset (Basso, et al., 1979), 50 percent improved in auditory comprehension and 33 percent improved in oral expression.

Percentage of improved patients does not indicate exactly how much improvement can be expected from untreated aphasic patients. Unfortunately, actual amounts of spontaneous recovery have seldom been reported, and the few available reports have been based on a small sample of the untreated aphasic population. The mean change in Aphasia Quotient (AQ) was 16.64 points by thirty-six mostly untreated aphasic subjects during the first three months after onset (Kertesz and McCabe, 1977; Kertesz, 1979). Variability of amount of recovery during this time is indicated by five subjects with global aphasia improving 5.16 points and four with Broca's aphasia improving 36.80 points. Deal and Deal (1978) reported spontaneous recovery of ten subjects examined initially with the *PICA* within one month postonset. The time of retesting was not specified. These cases improved an average of 1.30 points in terms of mean response level and an average of 12 percentile points. These cases varied from 0.34 to 2.72 points of improvement.

Rate: Overall Language. Rate of spontaneous recovery has been more clearly established, primarily with patients suffering CVA's. Sarno and Levita (1971) compared amounts of recovery with the *FCP* between the zero-to-three-month interval and the three-to-six-month interval in patients judged to be severely aphasic. Initial testing was done at 2 days postonset, and change scores were obtained for eighteen subjects during the first interval and for fourteen during the second. The three-month boundary was an average; it varied widely from 49 to 113 days after onset. Sarno found significantly more spontaneous recovery in the first three months. Kertesz and McCabe (1977) also found most recovery occurred during the first three months. Culton (1969) pinned down rate of recovery more specifically within the first three-month interval. Using his own language measure, he tested eleven

patients initially within one to four weeks postonset and compared amounts of improvement made during four subsequent two-week intervals. The only statistically significant change occurred during the first two-week interval. These results have been translated into a general recovery curve for aphasic stroke victims. This hypothetical curve is characterized by most spontaneous recovery occurring during the first month after onset, a substantial but smaller amount in the next two months, and a decelerated rate of change to a near plateau at six months postonset.

These findings indicate that almost no spontaneous recovery can be expected after six months, which is consistent with a long-established belief than spontaneous recovery lasts six months (Butfield and Zangwill, 1946; Sarno and Levita, 1971). However, as Sarno and Levita observed, there has been considerable disagreement as to how long it does last, with some aphasiologists suggesting that it could last for years. Culton examined another group of aphasic subjects after six months postonset and found no significant improvement. However, Kertesz and McCabe found some improvement by subjects after six months, and untreated subjects with Wernicke's aphasia made substantial gains between six and twelve months postonset. Hagen (1973) found some improvement of certain receptive functions in an untreated group after six months postonset. A definitive conclusion about spontaneous recovery after six months cannot be made from the available evidence. Some recovery is possible but the expected amount has not been established.

Outcome. Outcome of spontaneous recovery was examined by Kertesz and McCabe (1977; Kertesz, 1979), who followed forty-seven persons with aphasia due to CVA for one year or longer. The AQ values, taken at an average of 28.6 months postonset, were categorized as poor (zero to twenty-five points), fair (twenty-five to fifty), good (fifty to seventy-five), and excellent (seventy-five to one hundred). Almost all of the twelve global aphasias remained poor, and none progressed into the good or excellent categories. The twelve Broca's aphasics exhibited a range of outcomes, as five ended up fair, three good, and four excellent. The seven Wernicke's aphasics were just as varied, with three remaining poor and one improving to the excellent category. Most of the anomic, conduction, and transcortical aphasics achieved an excellent outcome. In fact, they comprised most of the 21 percent of all subjects who made "complete" recovery, defined as a minimum AQ of 93.8.

Pattern. One of the few studies of changes during the first month involved attention to the pattern of syndromes. Kohlmeyer (1976) concluded that type of aphasia changed during the first two to four weeks in only 13 percent of 303 cases of left hemisphere ischemias. This stability of deficit pattern was strong when the occlusion occurred in branches of the middle cerebral artery. More research needs to be done in order to determine the nature of deficits and of the rapid recovery which can occur during the acute stage.

Amounts of recovery within the first four months after onset were compared among eight tasks of the *WAB* (Lomas and Kertesz, 1978). There were two clinical tasks of auditory comprehension, one of repetition, and five expressive tasks primarily requiring single word retrieval. The investigators found that the yes/no question task for auditory comprehension improved significantly more than all other functions. The word-fluency task—retrieving animal names in one minute—was the only expressive task which did not show recovery significantly more than zero (see Figure 9-2, page 226). However, word fluency, when the patient is given a letter instead of the animal category, demonstrated significant recovery in a study of treated patients by Ludlow (1977).

Recovery of reading and writing was displayed by Kertesz (1979) for twenty aphasic patients. His graph shows that most improvement occurred in the first three months after onset. This pattern was consistent for each syndrome except global aphasia. Global aphasia was characterized as having some recovery of reading during the first three months but no recovery of writing throughout the first year after onset.

Kertesz and McCabe (1977) tabulated "the evolution of aphasic syndromes and the patterns of transformation from one clinically distinct group into another as defined by the subscores on subsequent examinations . . ." (p. 15). Of their ninety-three subjects, twenty-nine were noted to have ended up with a syndrome that was different from their initial symptom pattern. Kertesz and McCabe concluded that anomic aphasia is a common end stage of recovery, although only fifteen of sixty-eight initially nonanomic subjects had anomic aphasia at the completion of their recovery. Kertesz's (1979) conclusion from this data was a strong one: "Often global aphasia evolves to Broca's aphasia; Broca's, conduction and Wernicke's aphasics usually become anomic aphasics when recovery reaches a plateau" (p. 99). Yet only 33 percent of their subjects changed syndromes. It appears that symptom patterns remain stable during the first month after onset (Kohlmeyer, 1976) and that some changes occur afterward.

Because of the bimodal spontaneous recovery capability of Wernicke's aphasia in which some cases improve to a relatively large degree, the pattern of recovery from this initially severe disorder has received some special attention. Kertesz and McCabe found that four of thirteen Wernicke's aphasias ended up as anomic aphasia, thereby making a substantial amount of recovery. Authors have proposed stages through which a patient with Wernicke's aphasia may pass from the neologistic jargon found in the most severe form of this syndrome. These proposals, based on observation of a few cases, have been fairly consistent.

Though his terminology differed from the terms used in this book, Alajouanine (1956) described a progression from undifferentiated incessant jargon to neologistic jargon to semantic jargon. This sequence depicts recovery within the category of Wernicke's aphasia. Kertesz and Benson (1970) appeared to extend this progression by describing the following pattern: neologistic jargon to semantic jargon to circumlocutory anomic speech. The third stage could be misread to represent a transition to anomic aphasia, the syndrome; but Kertesz and Benson implied that it is a milder form of Wernicke's speech, because deficient auditory comprehension and repetition remain. Brown (1976) wrote that neologistic jargon may evolve to either semantic jargon or verbal expression containing literal paraphasias, as in conduction aphasia. Naeser and Hayward (1979) described a case which changed from Wernicke's aphasia two weeks after hospital admission to conduction aphasia three months later. If syndromes are indeed related to locus of lesion, one might wonder if the site of damage moved also. A repeated CT scan showed that, in effect, it did move as the hematoma from an intracerebral hemorrhage was absorbed by surrounding tissue.

Recovery by Patients Receiving Treatment

Considerably more data is available on recovery by patients who received speech-language treatment. While spontaneous recovery is of interest for determining the efficacy of speech-language treatment, the recovery of treated subjects is of interest for prediction. A prognosis is generally made for patients who are about to receive or who are receiving treatment.

Amount: Overall Language. Without standardized or sensitive techniques for measuring the amount of change, early investigators relied mostly on counting subjects who were making a certain amount of recovery, judging them with a rating scale. Actual amounts or rates of recovery were not reported until the 1970s. The early investigators did report that many but not all persons with aphasia do get better while receiving treatment. In studies mostly of traumatically injured veterans, 81 percent to 87 percent of the patients improved in language function to some degree (Butfield and Zangwill, 1946; Wepman, 1951). Of their 205 cases of CVA, Marks, Taylor, and Rusk (1957) found 50 percent made some improvement; Godfrey and Douglass (1959) found 37 percent of CVA cases could be rated as improved in language ability. The figures for CVA may be somewhat low, as Basso, et al. (1979) found 73 percent made obvious improvement in auditory comprehension and 46 percent made obvious improvement in oral expression. Cases of CVA making subtle but real change were not included in Basso's proportions.

Three studies show remarkable agreement in measured amounts of recovery, even though the sample size in each study was small. Hanson and Cicciarelli (1978) and Bamber (1980) each studied thirteen cases due to thromboembolic CVA. *PICA*'s were given first within eight to sixty-four days post onset in the former study and four to thirty-four days in the latter study. Difference scores were obtained relative to the peak score at an average of nine months after onset and thirteen months, respectively. Contrary to the amounts of spontaneous recovery reported earlier, Hanson's and Bamber's difference scores could be construed as representing the total amount of recovery in most cases. They found an average recovery of *3.24* and *3.25* points respectively on the mean response-level scale (35 percentile points). Deal and Deal (1978) reviewed seventeen cases tested initially within one month postonset. The final score upon termination of treatment was the second test. They found a similar average recovery of *3.38* overall points. Wertz, et al. (1981) reported a somewhat smaller average amount of recovery of 29 percentile points by eighteen subjects receiving direct treatment for one year. It would provide a secure feeling for speech-language pathologists if they could use these average figures to answer the question "How much will he improve?" In spite of the consistency of these averages from different samples of aphasia, these averages are not helpful for advising the individual.

The average amount of recovery of about 3.30 on the *PICA* scale loses its value because of the wide variability among aphasic persons already demonstrated with respect to spontaneous recovery. The range of difference scores reported by Hanson and Cicciarelli was 0.98 to 4.29, 0.10 to 6.18 by Bamber, and 0.51 to 7.16 by the Deals. Therefore, the range of difference scores for the forty-one subjects in these studies was *0.10* to *7.16.*

Rate: Overall Language. Rate of language recovery in treated patients is subject to the forces of spontaneous recovery. Most improvement by treated patients is made during the first three or four months after onset, which was demonstrated by Demeurisse, et al. (1980) and Wertz, et al. (1981). For patients in direct individual treatment until eleven months postonset, 65 percent of their recovery occurred between four and fifteen weeks (about four months) after onset (Wertz, et al., 1981). Sarno and Levita (1979; Sarno, 1981) followed thirty-four treated patients for one year with the *NCCEA* and the *FCP.* They observed little change on both measures between four to eight weeks postonset, but substantial recovery occurred between the third and sixth month. The final measure was taken six months later, and most patients continued to improve during this period. Rate is somewhat difficult to see on their graph of *FCP* change, because unequal time periods are spaced equally. From looking at the difference scores, it appears that the subjects improved at a constant rate throughout the year.

Information about rate of recovery is more likely to be obtained from treated than from untreated patients, because treated patients tend to be observed until they reach maximum recovery. Even if we could predict the amount of recovery, the data suggests that we would be hard pressed to predict how long it would take. A correlation between Hanson and Cicciarelli's (1978) amounts and times to peak performance shows no relationship, while Bamber (1980) found a correlation of 0.61 with her data. Inspection of data in both studies demonstrates the problem in predicting duration of recovery by patients receiving treatment. One patient took over seven months to improve 4.01 on the *PICA,* while another took about eight months to improve only 0.98 points. The duration of recovery can be very different between patients making similar amounts of recovery. Two patients who improved almost 3.00 points took about four and nineteen months to do so. Two who improved 4.84 and 5.22 points took 7.7 and 30.4 months, respectively. This data can be deceptive, however, because of the way outcome is defined, as was discussed earlier in this chapter. A peak score may occur long after the plateau of recovery has been reached. Therefore, durations to peak, especially the 30.4 months in Bamber's study, may be based on clinical decisions as well as on the process of recovery. The relationship between amount and time of overall language recovery remains unclear.

Outcome. The data from Hanson and Cicciarelli (1978), Deal and Deal (1978), and Bamber (1980) are suggestive of outcome for treated patients using the *PICA* overall score. Table 9–1 shows the initial

TABLE 9-1. Initial *PICA* overall scores and maximum level of recovery by aphasic patients in studies by (1) Hanson and Cicciarelli (1978), (2) Deal and Deal (1978), and (3) Bamber (1980).

	Initial Level		Maximum Level	
	Mean	*Range*	*Mean*	*Range*
(1)	9.48	6.63-13.16	12.72	10.64-14.88
(2)	9.13	4.00-12.47	12.36	8.69-13.90
(3)	8.40	5.85-13.56	11.65	8.72-14.00

and maximum levels of forty-one patients; most were tested first within thirty-two days after onset. Peak outcome score was taken by Hanson and Bamber, while the final score was taken by the Deals. The outcome of treated aphasics in these studies ranged from *8.69* to *14.88*. We can compare this range of outcome to the range of overall scores by 130 nonbrain-injured subjects, which was 13.40 to 14.99 (see Table 7–3). The proportion of aphasics in these studies ending up within this range was 32 percent, a figure which is larger than Kertesz's 21 percent who reached the AQ cutoff.

One way of depicting the outcome of recovery with reference to this range of *PICA* performance is to use Porch's (1971a) general descriptions of aphasic communication at different overall response levels. The lowest level reached by the subjects represented in Table 9–1 is the eight-to-ten range, which included 12 percent of the subjects in the three studies. Porch described these patients as possessing marked difficulty with most language skills. Continued reduction of auditory comprehension can be compensated for by context, but speech is still not functional. When above 10.00, the patient has reached a level of independent communicative function in a familiar environment. At the ten-to-twelve level, 26 percent of the subjects could be depicted as having good auditory comprehension with difficulty on complex instructions and as having verbal output which is at least appropriate and often accurate. Most subjects, 56 percent, achieved the twelve-to-fourteen range. These patients manage most communicative tasks; expression is still incomplete and includes delayed but accurate use of language. Only 7 percent reached the fourteen-to-fifteen range, where there is minimal communication difficulty. Verbal expression contains some hesitancy, slowness, and self-correction, but at this level patients show more concern about recalling what they read. Therefore, 89 percent of treated patients ought to reach at least independent communicative function in familiar settings.

Schuell presented the outcome of recovery by her five groups of aphasics in terms of the proportions that returned to school, entered vocational training, or obtained gainful employment (Schuell, et al., 1964). With simple aphasia, the youngest and least-impaired group, 14 percent entered school or vocational training and 19 percent resumed gainful employment. Success was greater with Group 3 (as with Broca's aphasia), as 33 percent entered vocational training and 27 percent returned to gainful employment. Schuell noted that the former group had trouble accepting employment with lower language requirements than their previous employment, while the latter group was the most determined of all the groups to improve and adjust. Within the most impaired groups, none entered vocational training or employment. Many of these were older patients and, therefore, had retired before onset of aphasia.

The individual language functions

which achieve the highest levels upon completion of recovery are the receptive and imitative functions. The mean peak score on the *PICA* gestural subtests by Hanson and Cicciarelli's thirteen subjects was 14.00. The nonverbal visual matching tasks averaged 15.00 at the peak of recovery, but these were relatively unimpaired at the beginning. The two auditory comprehension tasks, Subtests VI and X, ended up at 14.78 and 14.68 respectively. The two reading tasks, V and VII, peaked at 13.70 and 14.03. Copying, another nonverbal function, reached 14.37; while word repetition peaked at 14.43. These maximum levels were products of different amounts and somewhat different rates of recovery, which are considered here relative to the pattern of recovery.

Pattern. A basic pattern of recovery across varieties of aphasia was indicated in the study of spontaneous recovery, in that auditory language comprehension improved a greater amount than did verbal expression. As Ludlow (1977) pointed out, such comparisons among modalities are possible when each modality is tested in a similar fashion with equivalent scoring systems. The auditory-versus-verbal pattern has held up in a variety of circumstances. Basso, et al. (1979) found a higher percentage of patients improving in auditory language than in speech. Prins, Snow, and Wagenaar (1978), in a study of patients for one year beginning at least three months after onset, found auditory function improved while several parameters of spontaneous speech remained unchanged. Kenin and Swisher (1972) observed that receptive function at the word level, along with imitative functions, showed more improvement than pure expressive functions in a group of treated nonfluent aphasics. Some subtle aspects of this pattern need to be examined more carefully, especially because the spontaneous recovery research (Lomas and Kertesz, 1978) and studies by Kenin and

Swisher and Ludlow were done within four months postonset.

Search for a more subtle relationship between auditory and oral language recovery seems necessary when we see that Ludlow's (1977) ten treated subjects improved more on the *NCCEA* in sentence construction than in sentence comprehension within three months after onset. Hanson and Cicciarelli's (1978) tabulation of difference scores relative to duration of recovery for each *PICA* subtest are suggestive of a more refined description of recovery pattern. Having followed recovery to its peak instead of to three or four months postonset, they found that verbal functions improved a larger amount than auditory functions. Object naming (IV) and description of object function (I) improved 5.29 and 6.36, respectively, while pointing to objects by name (X) and by function (VI) improved 2.56 to 3.30. One reason for this difference is that auditory function is less impaired to begin with and therefore has less room to show measured improvement. Furthermore, these auditory functions reached their peak sooner, at 5.7 and 5.4 months postonset, than the expressive functions at 7.8 and 8.6 months. Therefore, auditory function may show more improvement within three or four months after onset, because this function improves faster; while improvement of verbal function is slower but relentless, continuing beyond six months after onset. Verbal subtests together improved 4.69 in 7.4 months, yet gestural subtests together improved 2.22 in 4.7 months. Receptive peaks were reached sooner than verbal peaks. Sarno and Levita (1979) found a similar pattern with the *NCCEA*.

The comparison between auditory and oral language functions in recovery can be summarized as follows: Auditory function reaches a higher outcome than expression and reaches its peak sooner. Verbal expression is likely to continue improving after auditory function has reached its peak and to show a greater amount of recovery in terms of standard measurement. Variations from this pattern depend partly on the method of measuring changes in modalities and on the investigator's statistical analysis. Lomas and Kertesz (1978), finding auditory function improving more than oral, used an analysis of covariance which, in effect, made the starting points of these functions more equivalent than they actually were. Still, their comparison was made within four months after onset. Also, pattern of recovery will vary somewhat depending on the initial pattern of aphasic symptoms.

Whether the patient changes from one syndrome to another was reviewed earlier in this chapter relative to spontaneous recovery. Kertesz and McCabe (1977) indicated that some aphasics recover in this fashion. With the *WAB,* Kertesz (1979) compared sixty-four acute aphasics, 2 to 6 weeks after onset, with eighty-three chronic aphasics more than 330 days after onset. The results of a cluster analysis of each group showed a large group of Wernicke's aphasics in the acute stage and very few in the chronic stage. The chronic group had a larger cluster of anomic aphasics and of patients surpassing the 93.8 AQ cutoff. There were clusters of Broca's aphasia in both groups, indicative of the saying, "Once a Broca's, always a Broca's." On the other hand, Clark, Crockett, and Klonoff's (1979) factor analysis of *PICA* results showed the same groupings after five months of treatment which indicated that patterns of aphasia do not change.

Nevertheless, when a Wernicke's aphasic improves from severe to moderate auditory deficit and his jargon disappears, replaced by a carefully monitored limited production, the pattern of deficit becomes more like an expressive disorder. In terms of a test score pattern, as with the *WAB,* this patient may appear to have become a Broca's aphasic. It might be more accurate to say that the patient, still with a posterior lesion, has a different version of Wernicke's aphasia, a product of recovery and of response to training.

Wertz, Kitselman, and Deal (1981) pointed out how data on changing syndromes can be an artifact of the method for labeling symptom patterns. They reviewed the data from their longitudinal study (Wertz, et al., 1981) and classified their subjects at different times during recovery according to the *WAB* criteria (see Chapter 7). Patients did change in symptom pattern, and some nonfluent aphasias became fluent which is contrary to the "Once a Broca's . . ." observation. On the *WAB* fluency scale, five to ten is the range of scores for the fluent aphasias; but the description of a five corresponds to nonfluent expression (see Chapter 7). Therefore, a Broca's aphasic could become a "Wernicke's" or "anomic" aphasic by progressing up this fluency scale to a five.

Regarding recovery of languages in multilingual patients, a variety of patterns do occur. Obler and Albert (1977) observed that the rule of Pitres accounts for pattern of recovery more often than the rule of Ribot. The rule of Pitres stated that the *most recently used* language recovers more rapidly than other learned languages. Patients over age sixty were less likely to follow the rule of Pitres than younger patients. This rule is more likely to be followed in multilinguals than in bilinguals (Albert and Obler, 1978).

PROGNOSIS

To a certain extent, prognosis has been a guessing game for the clinician, partly because of the wide variability among patients in amount and rate of recovery. Porch and his colleagues defined three approaches to prognosis (Porch, Collins, Wertz, et al., 1980). The prognostic variable approach has been the most common; the behavioral profile approach has been used minimally; and the statistical prediction approach has only recently begun to be developed.

Prognostic Variable Approach

The clinician "compares a patient's biographical, medical, and behavioral characteristics against how these variables are believed to influence change in aphasia" (Porch, et al., 1980, p. 312). A judgment is made as to whether the cumulative impact of these variables is favorable or unfavorable. Authors have been fairly consistent in their listing of numerous patient variables thought to determine the course of recovery. Occasionally these variables are noted simply as contributing to better or poorer prognosis without an indication of their degree of influence on the different parameters of recovery. Also, some of these variables are mentioned based on common sense or clinical experience rather than on an experimentally controlled demonstration of correlation.

The variables can be classified generally as either endogenous or exogenous factors. *Endogenous factors* arise from within the patient and are usually present at the time of onset and of initial language evaluation. They tend to be beyond the control of a clinician. Rubens (1977b) classified these factors as lesion variables, such as type, location, and size of lesion; and as patient variables, such as age and degree of language lateralization to one cerebral hemisphere. Patient variables are characteristics of the individual existing prior to onset, while lesion variables arise, of course, at the time of onset. Also, lesion variables contribute to attributes of the patient's aphasia such as initial severity and type of aphasia, the behavioral counterparts to the lesion variables. *Exogenous factors,* on the other hand, arise outside of the patient and tend to be subject to manipulation by the clinician. These include the ad-

ministration of language treatment and other environmental influences. The time since onset of initiating treatment has been a prominent factor which may or may not be manipulable by a clinician.

One problem with this method is that patient characteristics often do not all line up on the side of either a good or poor prognosis. When a patient possesses a mixture of favorable and unfavorable prognostic indicators, the clinician can be only guarded about a prediction. Also, as indicated by Porch, et al. (1980), the prediction is an adjective such as *good* or *poor* or *guarded,* and so is vague as to amount, rate, pattern, and outcome. Such specifics are not yet available with respect to many of the relevant factors. The influence of factors such as type and site of lesion has been demonstrated largely according to percentages of patients attaining a certain general level within a certain time, without the measurement of amount or observation of the complete recovery process. Much of the evidence indicates that certain factors are influential, but the measurement of that influence has been lacking.

Behavioral Profile Approach

This approach "involves evaluating the aphasic patient with a variety of listening, reading, speaking, and writing tasks; constructing a profile of his performance; and comparing this profile with the change made by previous patients with a similar profile" (Porch, et al., 1980, p. 313). This is Schuell's approach, described in Chapter 7. Though this is a data-based approach, its value is limited in the degree to which a variety of aphasics can be matched to a behavioral profile. Schuell's profiles do not differentiate among types of aphasia. Even if the Boston classifications were used, only 50 percent of the clinical caseload could be easily related to a syndrome category.

Statistical Prediction

Development of statistical prediction has accompanied increasing use of the *PICA*. Broida (1979) advised families that this test can be used to predict language level at six months with a test administered at one month postonset for patients with ischemic CVA's. The HOAP methods and Peak-Mean Difference method were described here in Chapter 7. These methods are reasonable guidelines based primarily on theoretical considerations. Debate surrounding the validity of these methods was cited in Chapter 7.

Studies have been undertaken to determine whether recovery *can be* predicted based on test scores and age. Porch (1974) had shown that the overall score from the *PICA* could be used in some instances to predict recovery of a group of aphasic patients with mixed etiologies. The overall score at one month postonset predicted the overall at three months postonset at a correlation of 0.90 accuracy for sixty-three patients. The overall at three months postonset predicted the overall at six months postonset with 0.93 accuracy for thirty patients.

In a more recent study, Porch and his colleagues (1980) examined whether modality summary scores—gestural, verbal, and graphic—would be adequate predictors of recovery by 144 patients with thromboembolic CVA's. With a stepwise multiple regression analysis, they wondered what would be the best combination of these scores obtained at one, three, or six months postonset for predicting later overall scores at three, six, and twelve months postonset. The three modality scores and age had different degrees of effectiveness in prediction, depending on the time interval between initial test and subsequent test. The most consistent predictor was the gestural mean, and the least successful predictor was age. The main conclusion was that statistical prediction with the *PICA* is possible. Another study applied Porch's formula to prediction for 90 aphasics and was supportive of the possibilities for the statistical method (Deal, Deal, Wertz, et al., 1979b).

Porch, et al. (1980) warned that clinical application of a formula based on test scores and age is premature until (1) ample replication of the original study is done, (2) the predictive power of other variables is determined, (3) the method is developed for treated and untreated groups, and (4) a more systematic schedule of reassessing patients is followed on a larger scale.

ENDOGENOUS PROGNOSTIC FACTORS

The prognostic variable approach to prediction is elaborated in this section, with a survey of its data base. The endogenous factors are partly responsible for the variability among patients in parameters of recovery. Therefore, initial predictions are based on a careful analysis of the patient's status as regards each of these factors.

Etiology

In Chapter 2, it was indicated that the different causes of aphasia have different effects on brain structure and operate differently over time. Most of the research on recovery of language function in aphasia, especially since World War II, has dealt with recovery from stroke. Ischemic strokes are usually distinguished from hemorrhagic CVAs in recovery research. The typical recovery curve of gradual improvement discussed previously is attributable primarily to ischemic CVA. After hemorrhage, absorption of the hematoma may not begin for weeks or even months after onset of aphasic symptoms (Rubens, 1977b). There may be alternating periods of plateaus and improvement with a hemorrhage. Recovery from traumatic injury depends on the extent of damage which can be reflected in the length of unconsciousness or coma subsequent to injury. Luria (1970b) demonstrated that penetrating (open) wounds resulted in more severe aphasias than nonpenetrating (closed) wounds. Tumors develop out of supportive brain tissue, and malignant forms produce progressively increasing amounts of brain damage. Aphasic symptoms may occur subsequent to surgery, and recovery depends in part on success of removing malignant tissue.

Kertesz and McCabe (1977) compared spontaneous recovery subsequent to thromboembolic CVAs, hemorrhages, and trauma. Of their ninety-three aphasic subjects, only seven were traumatic in origin; but the authors concluded that traumatic injury is responded to with a greater amount and faster rate of recovery than is found generally after CVA. Their graph of recovery in these cases illustrates dramatic change, with two cases improving fifty AQ points within three months after onset. The average for thirty-six cases with CVA was almost seventeen points. The cases of hemorrhage showed wide variation in recovery with some as large and rapid as traumatic patients and others showing little or no recovery. Twelve subjects were identified in the text of Kertesz and McCabe's article as having subarachnoid hemorrhages, but the graphic display of this variation in recovery referred to twelve with subarachnoid and intracerebral hemorrhages. Therefore, the type of hemorrhage represented by this data is somewhat unclear.

In spontaneous recovery from head injury, Luria (1970b) found differences between penetrating (open) and nonpenetrating (closed) wounds. Most cases of penetrating injury to primary language areas, 93 percent of seventy-three cases, continued to be clinically aphasic after two months postonset; however, 63 percent of sixteen cases of nonpenetrating injuries to primary zones remained aphasic after two months. Though the sample of nonpenetrating wounds was relatively small, data on damage to marginal language areas also indicated that more patients with nonpenetrating wounds made total recovery. In studies of closed head trauma, Groher (1977) and Levin, Grossman, Sarwar, et al., (1981) observed patients who recovered language to a functional level for conversation by four months postonset and to normal levels on the *NCCEA* by six months, respectively. Persistent deficit was associated with persisting left-hemisphere hematomas. After reviewing studies of recovery from closed head injury (CHI), Levin (1981) summarized: " . . . the studies of long-term recovery of language after CHI show an overall trend of improvement that may eventuate in restoration of language or specific defects ('subclinical' language disorder) in naming or word finding in about two-thirds of the patients who are acutely aphasic" (p. 441).

Direct comparisons among etiologies have been difficult to achieve because clinical caseloads have been dominated by one type of lesion or another. Early studies illustrate this point in that Butfield and Zangwill (1946) and Wepman (1951) examined mostly traumatic cases, while Marks, Taylor, and Rusk (1957) and Godfrey and Douglass (1959) primarily studied cases of CVA. A comparison among these studies suggests that more patients with traumatic lesions improve in language function than those with CVAs. However, if age is a factor, this comparison should be considered in light of the large age difference between the traumatic and cerebrovascular cases in these studies.

Site of Lesion/
Type of Aphasia

Site of lesion has a pronounced influence depending on whether damage is within the primary language zone of the left hemisphere, the borderline or marginal areas around the language zone, or structures deep to the cerebral cortex (Luria, 1970b; Rubens, 1977b). Type of aphasia, the behavioral consequence of site of lesion, is studied more frequently because it has been more readily observable. Primary-zone damage produces Broca's, Wernicke's, conduction, anomic, or global aphasias. Marginal-zone damage produces the transcortical aphasias, motor or sensory.

Several patients with traumatic damage to marginal zones were found by Luria (1970b) to make rapid and complete recovery. Of 130 cases with penetrating injuries to marginal areas, 83 percent were aphasic initially and 52 percent remained aphasic after two months. Of the 73 cases of penetrating injury to primary zones, 97 percent were aphasic initially and 93 percent remained aphasic after two months. The rapid and total or near-total recovery of a few transcortical aphasias has been observed by Rubens (1977b) and Kertesz and McCabe (1977). Kertesz (1979) found few transcortical aphasias in the 84 chronic aphasics of his cluster analysis.

Damage to other areas of the brain results in aphasic symptoms or related disorders which are relatively temporary. Kohlmeyer (1976) reviewed fourteen cases with slight anomia and alexia due to CVAs in the posterior cerebral artery which supplies blood to the posterior region of the cortex. All of these cases recovered completely within five to ten days. He concluded that if language disorders due to infarction are going to recover completely within a few days after onset, the most likely location of the occlusion would be in the posterior cerebral artery and the internal carotid artery. Kohlmeyer found about 30 percent of the latter cases to make such recovery. In addition to damaged marginal and posterior areas of the cortex, hemorrhages in the thalamus resulting in aphasic symptoms have been followed by complete disappearance of these symp-

toms by the end of the second month (Rubens, 1977b).

A CVA in the middle cerebral artery or trauma to the primary language zone generally produce permanent aphasias (Kohlmeyer, 1976; Luria, 1970b). Kertesz and McCabe (1977) compared amounts and rates of spontaneous recovery among global, Broca's, Wernicke's, conduction, and anomic aphasias. Data on subjects within each group represented varying time intervals after onset, and some subjects were followed much longer than others. Amounts of recovery were reported for thirty-six of ninety-three subjects. Broca's aphasia had the greatest average amount of recovery, and conduction aphasia showed almost as large amounts and reached nearly maximum AQs in some cases. These two types also had the fastest rates of recovery. The smallest amounts of recovery were found in global and anomic aphasias. Global aphasia results from too large a lesion to have a chance for much recovery, while patients with anomic aphasia have high initial AQs (an average of 85.5) leaving little room for much improvement on the *WAB*. Global and anomic aphasia also had the slowest rates of recovery. Thirteen patients with Wernicke's aphasia showed a bimodal distribution of recovery, as some improved little and others improved by at least twenty AQ points. Some of the latter cases, however, took six months to a few years to make this recovery without treatment. Wernicke's patients with higher initial test scores and less jargon did better than the other Wernicke's patients.

Lomas and Kertesz (1978) made a careful study of spontaneous recovery with thirty-one aphasic subjects divided into four groups based on initial levels of comprehension and fluency. These subjects were tested initially with the *WAB* within one month postonset and were retested 2¹/₂ to 4 months later. The relative amounts of recovery, weighted for a statistical analysis of co-variance, are shown in Figure 9-1. The low-fluency/high-comprehension group made the most recovery, corresponding to findings with Broca's aphasia. As in the findings with global aphasia, the low-fluency/low-comprehension group made the least amount of recovery. Making moderate amounts of recovery were the two high-fluency groups. Of these, the low comprehenders correspond to Wernicke's aphasia, and the high comprehenders could include anomic and conduction aphasia (see Figure 6-1).

When the aphasias are classified more broadly as nonfluent and fluent, the results from different studies are mixed. Prins, et al. (1978) found no difference between these groups, but they added that 80 percent of their subjects were mixed aphasias without clear specific classification. The nonfluents and fluents in Sarno and Levita's (1979) study had the same outcomes on the *FCP* at twelve weeks and one year postonset. Their fluents were more severely impaired at four weeks and caught up with the nonfluents at eight weeks. Wertz, Kitselman, and Deal (1981) found a significant difference favoring the nonfluents. These were primarily studies of treated subjects.

The bulk of evidence suggests that amount and, perhaps, rate of language recovery are related to site of lesion and, therefore, type of aphasia. The only evidence to the contrary was reported by Basso, et al. (1979), who did not find an effect of type of aphasia for untreated and treated groups. However, their dependent variable was the number of subjects making a certain minimal and demonstrative amount of recovery. This research strategy may have been insensitive to small changes falling below their criterion. Also, subjects in this study were assessed at varying intervals after onset, including a few months afterward. The studies which demonstrated an effect of syndrome involved data gathered when most spontaneous recovery occurs.

Most of the earlier research involved the classical divisions of expressive and receptive aphasia. Marks, et al. (1957) is difficult to interpret because 115 of 159 cases were labeled as having expressive aphasia. Only 30 were expressive-receptive, and only 6 were receptive. Their conclusion, however, was in agreement with those of Butfield and Zangwill (1946) and Godfrey

Figure 9-1. The overall amount of spontaneous language recovery differs among groups defined according to level of comprehension and fluency. These amounts are from the first four months after onset. *(Adapted by permission from Lomas, J., and Kertesz, A., Patterns of spontaneous recovery in aphasic groups: A study of adult stroke patients.* Brain and Language, 5, 388–401, 1978)

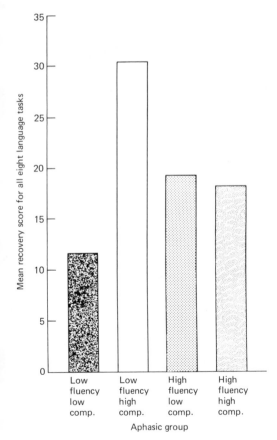

Mean recovery score for all eight language tasks

| Low fluency low comp. | Low fluency high comp. | High fluency low comp. | High fluency high comp. |

Aphasic group

and Douglass (1959), all of whom stated that patients with expressive aphasia make the most recovery. Broca's aphasia, which is a predominantly expressive deficit, was found by Kertesz to make the most spontaneous recovery. The conclusion that Broca's or expressive aphasia makes the largest amount of overall recovery is a consistent one.

Ludlow's (1977) comparison of Broca's and fluent aphasias indicated that the pattern of recovery among *NCCEA* subtests is different between types of aphasia during the first three months. In Lomas and Kertesz's (1978) study of spontaneous recovery, a significant interaction between tasks and subject groups also indicated that patterns differ (Figure 9–2). The most

severely impaired group showed substantial improvement in answering yes/no questions; auditory comprehension and repetition were the only language functions to recover significantly. The high fluency/low comprehension group (as with Wernicke's aphasia) had a similar pattern, except that answering questions with single nouns (responsive naming) also improved significantly. The two high-comprehension groups were similar to each other in that all tasks except word fluency exhibited significant recovery. Therefore, aphasic subjects with low comprehension improved primarily in receptive functions, while aphasic subjects with high comprehension improved receptively and expressively.

Figure 9-2. Pattern of spontaneous recovery among eight language tasks differs somewhat among groups defined according to level of comprehension and fluency. This pattern is from the first four months after onset. Other research suggests that amount of recovery in verbal expression would be relatively higher when measured six months or later. *(Reprinted by permission from Lomas, J., and Kertesz, A., Patterns of spontaneous recovery in aphasic groups: A study of adult stroke patients. Brain and Language, 5, 388–401, 1978)*

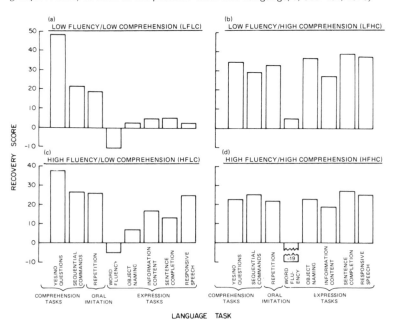

Severity of Aphasia

Initial severity of deficit is related to size of the brain lesion. Kertesz, Harlock, and Coates (1979) correlated lesion size with *WAB* difference scores. Though they concluded that the negative correlation between AQ and lesion size indicated that larger lesions are related to less recovery, their correlation was not statistically significant.

Sands, et al. (1969) stated, "It is generally agreed that there is a negative correlation between severity of aphasia in the early recovery period and the amount of improvement which occurs during the recovery process whether or not speech therapy is given" (p. 204). Because syndromes differ in overall severity, one might expect that initial severity would be related to recovery. When considering amount of recovery, however, this relationship would not be a simple correlation between overall severity and amount of change. The most severely impaired patients, global aphasia, have small amounts of recovery; but the least impaired, anomic aphasia, also have small amounts of recovery relative to the scoring ceilings built into tests.

Initial severity has sometimes been measured within a few days after onset. Sarno and Levita (1971) tested patients at two days postonset, when some were unconscious. In a hospital record survey, Gloning, Trappl, Heiss, et al. (1976) attended to initial measures taken within seven days after onset. In both studies there was no relationship between severity and recovery. Severity measured this soon may not be a good predictor of recovery because of the generalized acute effects of brain damage and unstable medical conditions. The actual severity of disorder may not appear until three weeks to a month after onset.

Statistically significant correlations between early severity and amount of recovery were found by Hanson and Cicciarelli (1978) and Bamber (1980) when etiology was thromboembolic CVA. Aphasic patients with lower initial scores, or greater severity, tended to make the most change. This finding suggests that initial or early severity is a positive prognostic sign relative to *amount* of recovery, contrary to the conclusion of Sands. Considering the well-established observation that global aphasia involves minimal amounts of recovery, this correlation may not be representative of the entire range of initial severity in aphasia. Hanson's subjects started between overalls of 6.63 and 13.16, and Bamber's started between 5.85 and 13.56. Only one subject below the fifteenth percentile was included in these correlations. These results might have been different if a more complete range of initial severity had been represented in these studies.

Kertesz and McCabe (1977) concluded that initial severity within Wernicke's aphasia was related to the amount of recovery made by these patients. Considering all of their subjects, initial overall severity related more linearly to the final outcome of spontaneous recovery.

Having found that high-comprehending subjects made much more recovery than low-comprehending subjects, Lomas and Kertesz (1978) concluded that initial level of auditory comprehension might be related to the amount of improvement in expressive language. This supports an earlier observation by Schuell about the prognostic value of auditory comprehension (Osgood and Miron, 1963).

Persons with global aphasia still make some measurable improvement, even after three months postonset. Sarno and Levita (1981) tested seven of these patients at several intervals until one year postonset. These subjects received three to five sessions of treatment per week. Tests included the *FCP* and certain subtests of the *NCCEA*. Significant improvement was noted primarily in auditory comprehension and use of gestures, and most of it occurred between six to twelve months postonset. During early spontaneous recovery, low-comprehending patients did improve in comprehension but not verbal expression (Lomas and Kertesz, 1978). Wapner and Gardner (1979) observed unimpressive "recovery" of auditory comprehension in global aphasia; but they did not state when the measures were taken postonset, and change was observed only during a one-to-two-week interval. Recovery by global aphasics may be restricted to certain functions and may not appear until after a period of training. Attention to the nonverbal mode of communication suggests that recovery of communicative skills, and not just language, brings a more encouraging outlook to prognosis.

Severity of aphasia has frequently been identified with respect to initial test in studies of treated subjects. Darley's (1972) list of factors in recovery included "severity of aphasia at the beginning of therapy" (p. 18). The "intake score" was used by Sands, et al. (1969) in their study of thirty patients. The five patients making the greatest improvement had an average intake score on the *FCP* that was over twice the intake score of the five with the least improvement. Almost half of their subjects started treatment after three months postonset, so that their results are indicative of intake scores whenever they are obtained, not of severity "in the early recovery period." Butfield and Zangwill (1946), who had found a higher incidence of recovery in moderately and mildly impaired patients, used some subjects who started treatment more than six months postonset and others who started at unspecified times within six months postonset. Basso, et al. (1979) found that severity on initial examination was significantly related to the incidence of recovery across treated and untreated groups. For the purpose of making predic-

tions, the speech-language pathologist can always obtain the severity of deficit at intake but does not always have access to initial severity. This is why test scores at various times after onset have been studied for their predictive value (Porch, et al., 1980).

Age at Onset

Age at onset is the most frequently investigated endogenous factor. It appears to be associated with etiology, type of aphasia, and severity of aphasia (Davis and Holland, 1981). Proposing age as a factor suggests that with the same type, location, and size of lesion, a seventy-year-old aphasic should make a different amount or rate of recovery from that of a forty-year-old patient. When we consider the possibility of functional substitution or reorganization involving the right hemisphere, aging may become a factor because of the apparent stability of left-hemisphere efficiency and decline of right-hemisphere efficiency with age (Johnson, Cole, Bowers, et al., 1979; Kocel, 1980).

However, chronological age by itself is not very meaningful, as indicated by Kimmel (1974) who wrote that "when we find age changes or age differences, it is important to keep in mind that these findings only point to changes that occur with age but do not indicate the possible causes of these changes" (p. 33). Growing older is accompanied by changes in biological structure and function, in susceptibility to complicating medical problems, in social milieu and living environment, and in certain cognitive functions (Birren and Sloane, 1980). Each of these factors may have implications for recovery. Although these changes occur in predictable stages, chronological age may not be the best predictor for when they occur. Because these changes do occur, it makes sense that age would be considered in recovery either reflecting the state of the individual at the moment of onset of aphasia or the ability of the central nervous system to respond to injury. For example, the bilateral reduction of blood flow subsequent to a focal infarct has been shown to be more prolonged for patients older than age sixty than for patients younger than age sixty (Meyer, Kanda, Fukuuchi, et al., 1971).

Little experimental evidence has been found to show that age is related to any parameter of recovery. Culton (1969) had not looked at age as a factor with only eleven subjects; however, upon reexamination of his data, he found his older subjects had improved more than the younger ones (Culton, 1971). Correlations between age and amount of spontaneous recovery were not significant in two studies (Kertesz and McCabe, 1977; Sarno and Levita, 1971), and it has not been a factor in studies of treated patients (Basso, et al., 1979; Keenan and Brassell, 1974; Messerli, et al., 1976; Rose, et al., 1976; Sarno, et al., 1971; Sarno, 1981). Vignolo (1964) did not have a large enough sample size in his youngest group to make a valid comparison. Investigators impressed by age as a determinant of recovery were Sands, et al. (1969) who called it "the most potent variable influencing recovery" (p. 205). The five patients making the most change averaged forty-seven years, and the five making the least change averaged sixty-one years. Age cannot be ruled out as a predictor of recovery because of the many conditions which are associated with it.

Extent of Language Lateralization

A few people appear to possess bilateral or more diffusely represented language function (see Chapter 3). Broader language representation implies that focal lesions are more likely to leave unscathed some cortical areas controlling language. Therefore, there is a small portion of the population which may have less severe aphasias and a better likelihood that un-

damaged regions of the brain can support recovery of impaired language functions.

Chapter 3 included some clues indicative as to who would have more diffuse or bilateral representation of language function in the cerebral cortex. The relationship between language lateralization and recovery has been studied primarily with respect to handedness. Luria (1970b) was interested especially in recovery by overt left-handers (4.8 percent of his patients) and those with subtle left-handedness and/or a familial history of left-handedness. Most pure right handers (75 percent of sixty-four) remained severely aphasic after two months. On the other hand, most right handers with slight left-handedness or left-handedness in the family (63 percent of seventy-three) recovered quickly. It should be remembered that these subjects were young and traumatic in origin, so that results from a CVA may be characterized by much lower incidence of complete recovery. However, they are a strong indication that not only left-handedness but also this tendency in right-handers are positive prognostic signs. Sex differences in recovery were not found by Sarno and Levita (1971), Gloning, et al. (1976), and Kertesz and McCabe (1977).

EXOGENOUS FACTORS: LANGUAGE TREATMENT

The effect of language treatment on recovery is as difficult to determine as the effect of any other single factor. The issue, outlined in an important paper by Darley (1972), is whether treatment enhances recovery beyond that which is already attained in spontaneous recovery. Answering this question involves a comparison of some kind between the presence and absence of treatment. Further questions delve into the somewhat varied strategies of treatment proposed since World War II. Types and variations of treatment can be compared. Also, the optimal amount of treatment needs to be examined in order to determine the most gain for the least cost. Amount can be defined in terms of length of time in treatment and its intensity (such as hours per week). The intensity of treatment reported in studies of treatment efficacy has varied from three to five hours per week to eighteen hours per week. The generalizability of findings depends partly on whether the treatment being studied is typical of most clinical settings.

A Survey of Opinions

" . . . most neurologists are skeptical of applying these methods to patients and, in general, believe the extent of long term recovery from a lesion is a function of the individual's capacity to realize repair and has little to do with external therapy" (Gazzaniga, 1974, p. 204).

"A long-standing hindrance to the acceptance of aphasia rehabilitation by neurologists has been a deeply entrenched and widely taught adage that therapy for aphasia is ineffective . . . that the improvements gained through formal therapy merely represent the anticipated spontaneous recovery" (Benson, 1979b, p. 187).

"There is a considerable literature on aphasia rehabilitation (e.g., by means of speech therapy) but it is probably fair to say that this is dominated by statements of opinion and belief rather than by empirically validated evidence" (Miller, 1980, p. 531). The neuropsychologist continued: "As yet there is no attempt known to this writer aimed at proving that psychological manipulations are powerful enough to make a real difference to the handicapped person's everyday life . . . " (p. 533).

These opinions, held in much of the medical profession, continue to be faced by the speech-language pathologist. This bleak view of treatment is understandable considering our current understanding of the mechanics of aphasia, namely, the permanence of destroyed brain tissue; and considering the difficulty of measuring recovery, which can be attributed to intervention. Some of the concern is aimed more at the evidence for treatment effectiveness than at treatment itself. Many physicians in the hospital during a patient's acute phase of recovery never observe improvements by the patient after he or she leaves the hospital. Many physicians are simply not aware of the goals and methods of language rehabilitation. Other professionals are not very aware of the evidence that is available concerning the efficacy of language treatment.

The view of neurologists is changing, however. Rubens (1977b) stated that " . . . the brain is not a totally static and hard-wired organ, and there are many factors which tend to reduce the severity of initial deficits and which interact positively with specific rehabilitation programs" (p. 31). After reviewing some research on the effect of treatment, Benson (1979b) wrote in the *Archives of Neurology* that " . . . language therapy has a demonstrated effectiveness in the treatment of aphasia and, as such, occupies a place in the therapeutic armamentarium of the neurologist" (p. 189). A review of several studies enabled Darley (1979) to state "aphasia therapy works." Two approaches have been used to identify recovery due to treatment as opposed to recovery attained spontaneously. These are the no-treatment group comparison and the post-spontaneous recovery comparison.

No-Treatment
Group Comparisons

In order to identify the effect of treatment during the first six months after onset of aphasia, recovery during treatment should be compared with recovery when treatment is withheld. If treatment enhances recovery, this comparison would enable us to determine the extent of this influence beyond spontaneous recovery. Unfortunately, the first publication of a comparison with an untreated group was of *severely impaired* patients at averages of twenty-seven to forty-one months postonset (Sarno, Silverman, and Sands, 1970). Treatment made no difference at these times after onset. Only one well-controlled no-treatment group comparison during the spontaneous recovery period has been reported in the literature. The major obstacles to conducting such studies are the difficulty in obtaining two groups which match in terms of the endogenous factors and the ethical problems of deliberately withholding treatment from a patient.

In a study begun by Vignolo (1964), Basso, Capitani, and Vignolo (1979) minimized these obstacles by accumulating data on large enough samples so that both groups would be equally representative of the aphasic population and by not deliberately withholding treatment. It took thirteen years to complete the study. They compared 162 treated patients with 119 untreated patients who "were prevented from attending therapy for extraneous factors, such as family or transportation problems . . ." (p. 191). Benson (1979b) noted that the comparability between groups in this study was weakened be-

cause the selection process was not random. The basis for group assignment may have made these groups different in ways affecting recovery, as in the possibility that the untreated group may have been less motivated to receive treatment than the treated group. However, Basso, et al. argued that selection was based on "objective difficulties" unrelated to the aphasia per se and that information about the untreated patients did not indicate a lack of motivation. Indeed, Benson was impressed with the similarity between groups in terms of educational and socioeconomic levels, distribution of types of aphasia, etiology, and sex.

In the data analysis, each group was divided further according to the time of initial testing after onset, coinciding with the time treatment started for the experimental group. Table 9–2 shows the comparison between groups for auditory comprehension and oral expression in terms of the percentage of subjects within each group that made at least a two-point improvement relative to a five-point scale. Focusing on the groups assessed during the period of maximum spontaneous recovery, the under two-month and two-to-six-month groups, one can see that substantially more treated subjects improved than did untreated subjects. This data indicates that treated subjects are

TABLE 9–2. Percentage of subjects within each of six groups, showing at least a two-point (of a five-point scale) improvement in test performance (derived from Basso et al., 1979). Groups are defined as treated or untreated, with the first test administered either within two months, between two and six months, or after six months postonset.

	Time postonset		
	<2 months	2–6 months	>6 months
Auditory Comprehension			
Treated (N = 107)	88	65	50
Not treated (N = 86)	50	48	16
Oral Expression			
Treated (N = 162)	59	39	29
Not treated (N = 119)	33	9	4

more likely to have substantial recovery soon after onset; however, it does not provide data in terms of actual amount and rate of recovery relative to spontaneous recovery alone.

Deal and Deal (1978) found differences in amount of recovery favoring treated groups during the spontaneous recovery period, but they readily acknowledged "...weaknesses and limitations of this report" (p. 73) such as small groups which were not matched for site of lesion or type of aphasia.

A comparison between two treatment strategies can provide an indication of a singular effect of one kind of treatment on the recovery process. For example, Seron, Deloche, Bastard, et al. (1979) compared two word-retrieval treatment strategies, one involving drill with many words and the other with only a few words (see Chapter 4). Two groups (N = 4) received twenty sessions in two months. Independent measures of finding words which were not included in therapy were given before and after the treatment period. The few-word strategy was associated with more improvement, but the period after onset of this treatment was not stated. On a larger scale, Wertz, Collins, Weiss, et al. (1981) compared an intensive individual treatment program with a group treatment program beginning at one month post-onset. Both strategies were administered eight hours per week until about one year after onset. In order to obtain matched groups, this study commanded the co-operation of several Veterans Administration Medical Centers. Twenty-nine patients per group received eleven weeks of treatment; and, due to attrition, a total of thirty-four were treated for forty-four weeks. There were significant differences favoring individual treatment.

Single case research designs have some potential for finely controlled comparison between the presence and absence of treatment during the early recovery period (Davis, 1978a; LaPointe, 1977, 1978b).

The subject serves as his own control in these paradigms. The *alternating phase or A-B-A-B design* permits comparison by alternating the presence and absence of treatment. Regular measurement of a criterion behavior should be taken during each phase. A specific variable within a treatment program could be assessed in this way by alternating the presence and absence of that variable; with this strategy, treatment need not be withheld. The *multiple baseline design* permits comparison between behaviors or functions, one which is treated and another which is not treated for a period of time. Texts on these strategies are available (Hersen and Barlow, 1976; Kratochwill, 1978; McReynolds and Kearns, In Press).

A few single subject experiments with adult aphasics have been published. Rosenbek, Green, Flynn, et al. (1977) alternated periods of treatment and no-treatment with a patient beginning six months after onset. The patient's largest improvements came during periods of treatment. Measures were taken at the boundaries of the alternating periods rather than continuously during these periods. Multiple baseline designs require independence between compared functions, which cannot be assumed when two language functions are compared. Bisset and Davis (1978) compared "distant" functions of verbal repetition and reading comprehension. Treatment of reading was delayed, while repetition was exercised. Repetition improved, while reading remained at a low and variable level. When treatment of reading began, this function showed a steady improvement above previous levels. Rosenbek, Becher, Shaughnessy, et al. (1979) reported similar effects when treatment was introduced sequentially for different phonemes in a case of apraxia of speech.

In a study of two bilingual aphasics, Watamori and Sasanuma (1978) treated one language but did not treat the other. Both languages were impaired equally when treatment began at two and three months postonset. Treatment continued for several months. Most improvement occurred decidedly in the language that was treated. As in the other single subject experiments, treatment was shown to have an impact on recovery.

Postspontaneous Recovery Comparison

Several investigators have examined recovery of treated subjects whose treatment began or continued after the period of maximum spontaneous recovery, so that the subjects' recovery was compared, in effect, with an *assumed* minimal recovery if there had been no treatment. Speech-language pathologists frequently use this principle of comparison to note the value of their treatment administered after six months postonset.

Wepman (1951) found that sixty-eight aphasic patients, whose treatment had begun at least six months after onset, improved from an initial grade level of 3.8 to a final level of 9.1 and from 1.8 to 3.9 on a rating of speech performance.

Fourteen cases reported by Broida (1977), where treatment was started at least twelve months postonset, improved an average of ten overall percentile points on the *PICA*. Three of these subjects improved as much as twenty-two and nineteen points.

Hagen (1973) compared groups of treated and untreated patients relative to several language functions, a study which " . . . commenced when all subjects were discharged from the physical rehabilitation program six months post-onset" (p. 456). Relative to the language functions where there was a difference between groups, the untreated group showed no change while the treated group showed substantial improvement. The untreated group did show continued improvement in certain receptive functions.

Wertz, et al. (1981) and Sarno and Levita (1981) reported on treated aphasics who continued to improve substantially after six months.

Other investigators have used the postspontaneous recovery comparison either in comparing groups that differ according to when treatment was initiated or in studying new treatment procedures started after the spontaneous recovery period. An early example of the former is Butfield and Zangwill's (1946) study, which included thirteen aphasic patients whose treatment was begun no sooner than six months after onset. Ten of these subjects improved in spoken language according to a rating scale. Basso, et al. (1979) examined a similar subgroup of treated subjects in which 50 percent improved in auditory comprehension and 29 percent improved in speech (Table 9–2). This was in contrast to untreated controls measured after six months postonset, where only 16 percent and 4 percent, respectively, improved in these modalities. Deal and Deal (1978) found a significant improvement in *PICA* overall scores with a group of nine patients whose treatment was not started until four to seven months postonset.

In the study of particular treatment procedures, Sparks, et al. (1974) found improved language test scores when Melodic Intonation Therapy was initiated after no change had occurred six months previously; five of Skelly, et al.'s (1974) patients learned Amerind after at least six months of prior treatment; and some of Holland and Sonderman's (1974) subjects improved in auditory comprehension with a treatment program begun at least four months postonset and on an average of 5.6 years postonset. Helm-Estabrooks, Fitzpatrick, and Barresi (1981) administered their Syntax Stimulation Program to a patient who had been severely agrammatic for three years. The patient made substantial improvements in expressive function after treatment was initiated. All of these studies indicate that aphasic patients can improve in impaired language functions or learn new communicative strategies at a time after onset when little or no recovery would be expected without treatment.

Does Starting Time Make a Difference?

Because treatment methods have been shown repeatedly to make a measurable difference in recovery, one remaining question is when treatment should begin relative to onset. There is an apparent disagreement in the literature as to whether it is best to start very soon after onset or to wait a few weeks. This debate is elaborated in Chapter 10, but the pertinent research is presented here. The disagreement may be more apparent than real because of differences in the way treatment is defined in this argument and because of vague criteria as to the effect of starting time on recovery.

The time of initial test or the start of treatment after onset of aphasia has been a frequently mentioned factor in recovery. This variable makes a difference in the prediction of amount of recovery from the time a patient is first seen in a speech-language clinic, and it may make a difference relative to the patient's overall recovery. The former implication of this variable has been determined more adequately than the latter. This is because when times since onset have been compared, there has been no measure of the recovery made prior to the initial test. Using time of initial test simply as a predictor does not attribute any effect on the recovery process to this factor.

A relationship between time since onset of initial test and amount of recovery would follow from the nature of the recovery curve. Recovery is represented by steadily increasing test scores through the three-to-six month period after onset, reaching a plateau sometime after six months postonset. Considering the pattern of recovery, auditory function may level off sooner, and verbal expression may level off later. The later an initial test score is obtained, the less recovery should be subsequently expected. This relationship would be reflected in a negative correlation between the number of days or months after onset of the initial test and the difference score for amount of recovery occurring afterward.

For a perspective on this factor, we should consider a hypothetical comparison between *one month* postonset and *four months* postonset as times for beginning direct treatment of language functions. Treatment which is started within one month postonset, in effect, latches onto the processes of spontaneous recovery and rides them as far as it can. The possible effects of early treatment include (1) acceleration of spontaneous recovery where a certain amount of recovery occurs sooner than it would without treatment, (2) a higher peak level of recovery than would occur without treatment, or (3) both, namely, acceleration to a higher level. Treatment beginning at four months postonset or sometime thereafter follows on the heels of maximum spontaneous recovery and may cause additional recovery to occur, as found in postspontaneous recovery comparisons.

The central problem in comparing effects of different treatment starting times lies in finding a common basis for comparison. Comparing amounts of recovery *during equal lengths of treatment* poses the problem that with a four-month starting time most spontaneous recovery has already occurred; on the other hand, maximum spontaneous recovery is included in the amount recorded with a one-month start. Therefore, subjects compared on this basis are not comparable with respect to the interval postonset which is measured. Although five months of treatment for a four-month group may be associated with a smaller difference score than the same amount of treatment for a one month group, both groups could be at the same level nine months after onset. With respect to a time after onset common to both groups, treatment starting time still may or may not make any difference. Therefore, the selection of a parameter common to both groups is essential in making such a comparison. We would want to know, for example, whether early treatment results in higher functioning at termination of treatment than does later treatment or whether early treatment produces the same end result but produces it sooner.

The first study which has been used to support the early start of treatment was Butfield and Zangwill's (1946) comparison between fifty-two subjects starting earlier than six months postonset and fourteen subjects starting later than six months. Fifty percent of those starting earlier were much improved, while 33 percent of those starting later were much improved. Even if the validity of this comparison were strengthened with a comparable number of subjects in each group, one still cannot say whether the late starters were worse off, because their previous spontaneous recovery was not included in the measure of their extent of recovery.

The same reservations could apply to Basso, et al.'s (1979) data in Table 9–2. Though the proportion of treated subjects making substantial improvement decreased with later initiation of treatment, initial testing coincided with the start of treatment and, therefore, not at the same point relative to onset for each group. The changes made by the two late starting groups do not include the previous recovery made by these groups. What these data do indicate is that the same amount of treatment does not result in the same amount of recovery *during the period of treatment* as a function of when treatment begins. Such data does not indicate

whether starting time has anything to do with the total amount of recovery from time of onset or with the outcome of recovery.

Hanson and Cicciarelli (1978) provided at least one common parameter for comparison, namely, peak overall performance measured with the *PICA*. They reported the number of days between onset and initial overall score for each of thirteen patients, and this interval ranged from eight to sixty-four days. They also reported the amount of recovery during treatment. However, because Hanson and Cicciarelli were interested in other questions, they did not report correlations between treatment starting time and either amount or peak of recovery. The present author did these correlations and found them not to be significant. Bamber (1980) had the same results in a similar study. The different starting times in these studies were within a narrow range of time, namely, within the first two months after onset; so this variable may be more influential across a much broader expanse of time. Hanson and Cicciarelli's strategy for data collection could be expanded with a wider range of treatment starting times and a larger number of subjects in order to determine the effect of starting time.

We can be fairly certain that starting time does not matter within the first two months with respect to the outcome of recovery. However, regarding the question of the effect of starting treatment after this period, there has been no data to provide an answer with respect to total amount of recovery, rate, or outcome. As discussed earlier, time postonset does serve as a predictor of *subsequent* amount of recovery.

Other Factors

Several other characteristics of aphasic patients have appeared in lists of prognostic factors, but these have generally not been subjected to formal investigation. Potential factors existing prior to onset include educational experience, intelligence, style and level of language use, social status, and general health. Complicating factors include level of awareness of deficit, emotional state and motivation, and coexisting sensory and motor speech problems. Some of these factors are manipulable by the clinician, physicians, hospital staff, and the patient's family. Holland (1980a) found that institutionalized aphasics performed less well on the *CADL* than did aphasics living at home. Though these groups were matched for age, the institutionalized group could have been placed in that setting because of more severe aphasia than those living at home. Nevertheless, the potential influence of social milieu and living environment on recovery has led to counseling programs for families (Chapter 12) and environmental manipulation in nursing homes (Chapter 10).

Several factors may relate more to the ability of the patient to perform maximally in treatment than to the recovery process per se. *Motivation,* for example, should enhance the likelihood of a successful treatment outcome (Eisenson, 1949, 1973; Shill, 1979, Wepman, 1953). Eisenson (1949) suggested that *personality* makes a difference in that an outgoing and easygoing patient adapts better to treatment than the introvert. Horner (1979) identified a new consideration for anticipating the patient's responsiveness to treatment. She attempted to measure the patient's *learning potential* in terms of speed of learning, response stability, carryover, and other factors. Finally, Wepman (1958) addressed a specific aspect of severity which may be indicative of the patient's ability to achieve independence as a communicator. He listed several levels of *self-correction ability,* in which recognition of errors and readiness to modify responses would be indicative of a more favorable outcome in treatment.

SUMMARY AND SUGGESTIONS

Statements about recovery from aphasia, whether they appear in clinical reports or at the conclusion of a publication, can be much more explicit than "the patient is getting better" or "the patient improved a great deal." Different types and levels of behavior are observed to change over time, and the clinician or researcher should attend to exactly what is getting better or has improved. Furthermore, this improvement can be depicted with respect to different parameters such as the amount, outcome, rate, and pattern. Some aphasics improve a large amount but not to as high a level as other patients, whose amount of improvement is relatively small. Combining these two considerations leads to more precise statements such as "The patient improved *x* amount in retrieving words on a confrontation naming task."

In making a prognosis for a patient, the clinician considers all factors.

Etiology: A traumatic injury, especially closed head injury, may result in a greater and more rapid recovery than an ischemic CVA. Ischemic CVA exhibits a gradual rate of recovery, most of it occurring in the first three months. The only data on hemorrhage indicates that either large or small amounts of recovery can be expected; clinical observation has shown that recovery may begin a few weeks or months after onset. Type of lesion appears to be unrelated to pattern of recovery.

Site of lesion: Damage to marginal areas produces more complete and a more rapid rate of recovery than damage to primary language areas. Comparisons of amounts and patterns of recovery have been done with respect to syndromes which are indicative of site of lesion within the primary zone.

Type of aphasia: Broca's and conduction aphasias demonstrate the largest amount of recovery. Anomic aphasia results in the best outcome. Wernicke's aphasia has demonstrated a mixture of poor and good recovery which may occur at a slower rate. Global aphasia has a poor prognosis for improvement of verbal expression, but auditory comprehension does improve with treatment as late as six to twelve months postonset.

Initial severity: Overall severity of deficit at about one month postonset has not been studied adequately. There appears to be a nonlinear relationship to amount, with the most severe and mild forms resulting in less recovery than moderate aphasias. There is a more direct relationship between initial severity and outcome, which is the basis for statistical prediction with the *PICA*. Severity of auditory comprehension deficit may be predictive of overall recovery. The clinician probably relies most on initial severity of deficit, especially in comprehension and in motor speech overlay, to predict extent of recovery.

Age at onset: Though most of the evidence indicates that age is not a factor, most studies have had inadequate controls to examine age. Chronological age may still make a difference because of the medical, psychological, and social complications which can accompany aging.

Lateralization: Luria's research showed a more rapid rate of recovery in left-handed patients and patients with a tendency toward left-handedness.

Time since onset: Because of the general rate of recovery, a later observation after onset means that less recovery can be expected subsequently.

Treatment: It has a favorable impact on recovery no matter when it occurs after onset of aphasia. Its value is judged with respect to linguistic and more general communicative goals.

Statements about prognosis should be framed with respect to *what* is likely to improve. If speech is the only consideration, positive prognosis will be less frequent than when communication is a consideration. Patients with severe expressive deficits or global aphasia may have a relatively positive outlook with respect to auditory comprehension and nonverbal modes of communication—not the breadth of improvement we would like, but improvement nonetheless.

10 Treatment Principles

Treatment of aphasia is a long-term process which is usually measured with respect to weeks or months. It involves a special relationship between the speech-language pathologist and the patient. Similar procedures have been derived from different viewpoints, which have been based on understanding of the neurological and cognitive bases of aphasia, on theories about recovery, on principles of behavioral management, and on experience with what works with aphasic patients. Brookshire discovered that direct treatment of language functions possesses a certain invariant interaction structure (Brookshire, Nicholas, Krueger, et al., 1978). There are other methodologies. Yet many apparent variations found in professional literature and commercial programs can be characterized by a common set of goals, principles, and procedures.

OBJECTIVES OF TREATMENT

The overriding objective of treatment for aphasia is *to improve the patient's use of language in comprehension and expression.* Furthermore, as the definition of aphasia in Chapter 1 was expanded to include language within a broader category of symbols, the main objective of treatment can be expanded to include improvement in the use of all symbols. Because aphasia is a central and, therefore, multimodality disorder, there are more specific goals subsumed within the main one, namely, *to improve auditory language comprehension, to improve reading comprehension, to improve spoken language, to improve written language,* and *to improve representational gesturing.* As we consider more specific goals such as these, they assume different degrees of importance depending on the unique backgrounds, abilities, and needs of each patient. Until we understand recovery better and are able to predict specific levels of recovery, our goals remain couched in terms of "improvement" more than in terms that state what the patient will be like at a certain time in the future. There is one inescapable fact, however, which modulates the long-range objective: necrotic cortical tissue does not regenerate. Our objectives should be realistic in that no patient with aphasia can return to functioning as before onset of the language disorder.

Goals of treatment are refined with respect to the purposes for which language is used. The purpose of language which appears to have the greatest and most general importance to patients and their families is the use of language for direct interpersonal communication. Other uses of language include the comprehension of electronic media (radio and television), comprehension of the printed word (product labels, newspapers), and writing for oneself (lists, diaries) and for others (memos, letters, checks, forms, and so on). All of these can be said to be communication in that they involve receiving ideas from another source and conveying ideas to someone else or self. Language is used for thinking and imagining, for remembering and planning ahead. However, direct interpersonal communication has been the primary need of patients and the main interest of clinicians in designing treatment paradigms. A main goal of treatment, therefore, is *to improve the patient's ability to communicate his or her thoughts and feelings.*

The emphasis on improving communication has at least four implications. These are derived from recognition that the goal of participants in a conversational dyad is to convey messages. At any given moment in a conversation, a sender and receiver of a message share responsibility in seeing that the sender's message is received.

1. Language is but one mode by which messages are conveyed, albeit an extremely important one. Improving facility with language goes a long way toward improving communicative ability. However, expanding other modes of communication is helpful also.

2. The relative importance of improving or changing certain symptoms is evaluated with respect to the symptom's impact on communication. Mild agrammatism, for example, may have a minimal impact on message conveyance; the adaptive strategies described in Chapter 5 convey the same ideas conveyed by omitted grammatical markers.

3. Communication is maximized by modification of the nonaphasic participant as well as by changes made by the aphasic participant. Shared responsibility implies that the non-

aphasic speaker may use communicative strategies which assist the aphasic listener in comprehension. Therefore, treatment is directed to the potential communicators with the patient as well as to the patient per se.

4. Treatment is directed toward improving the patient's use of language *where* the patient uses it most of the time. Treatment is directed toward developing the patient's communicative skills independent from the clinician; the patient should become better able to use language when the clinician is not around to help. The content and format of treatment should reflect the patient's use of language in his or her living environment.

Another objective involves the maintenance of achievements attained in a regular and sustained treatment schedule. "Maintenance therapy" is less frequent and regular than a standard treatment schedule and is usually done once maximum recovery has been reached. It is directed toward minimizing a return to or development of bad communicative habits and to ensuring that learned communicative strategies continue.

One other objective is to facilitate the patient's psychological or emotional adjustment to the communicative deficit. Part of the adjustment involves developing realistic expectations about recovery and the outcome of language treatment. Many patients strive toward and believe they can reach their premorbid language capability. This unrealistic expectation results in frustration and discouragement over time. Another part of the adjustment involves dealing with a new self-image created by changes in speaking and in physical appearance. A reasonably positive view of self must somehow be borne out of the potentially shattering sound of an awkward, seemingly childlike, and sometimes strange new form of utterance.

It is helpful if the patient, family, and other professionals share the range of objectives cited here. The traditional label "speech pathologist" has led other professionals to assess the efforts of speech-language pathologists with respect to spoken expression only. Even the additional term "language" connotes expression to many people without consideration of comprehension. Directing everyone's attention to the goal of improved communication can enhance their sensitivity to the accomplishments of a patient in treatment. Recovered comprehension skill goes a long way toward improving communicative ability even if verbal expression does not change much. Newly learned strategies for conveying messages—either adding a gesture system to the patient's repertoire or modifying the speaking patterns of others to the patient—are accomplishments of clinical training and advice.

WHEN TO BEGIN

The patient should be seen by a speech-language pathologist in the hospital as soon as the patient is medically ready to visit with people. Especially when the first visit is at bedside soon after onset, the clinician need only assure the patient that someone is available to help with the communication problem. If, after brief introductions, the clinician wishes to take five minutes to assess the language deficit, an assessment can be done within a carefully structured conversation, including a couple of simple questions requiring a yes/no or pointing response to see if the patient comprehends. Most patients will try to talk. This is a delicate time. Attempts to stimulate the patient to talk may lead to unnecessary frustration and discouragement because of the temporary deficits existing during the first two or three weeks after onset (see Chapter 4).

The literature contains apparent disagreement as to when treatment should begin. Rubens (1977b), a neurologist, wrote, "I like to see aphasic patients enter therapy as early as possible, and I believe

that the therapy should be as intensive as the general medical situation will allow" (p. 1). Eisenson (1973) insisted that treatment begin "as soon as the patient is able to take notice of what is going on about him" (p. 144). The research showing that earlier treatment is accompanied by more recovery encouraged the sooner-the-better view. On the other hand, R. J. Duffy (1972) argued that there is little empirical support for this view; as shown in Chapter 9, treatment starting times have not been compared adequately in order to answer the question of whether this variable has an impact on the recovery process. Duffy (1972) and Wepman (1972) suggested that the intensive drill of direct treatment be delayed a few weeks after onset. However, there is also little empirical support for delaying treatment this long. These opinions can be analyzed best relative to the reasoning behind them; and the disagreement may be more apparent than real.

The difference in views might be understood better with reference to Wepman's (1972) position. He recommended delaying intensive direct treatment of language functions, not putting off the involvement of a speech-language clinician altogether. During the acute phase, the clinician should provide "a supportive psychological role." Although it appears that he recommended delaying direct treatment for at least three months, he did not dwell on a specific time period. Instead, Wepman presented certain considerations which are variable among patients: (1) the patient is emotionally unstable during the few days after onset and (2) the spontaneous recovery period, which lasts three to six months, presents an unstable picture of the residual deficit as the vascular system restabilizes and edema subsides. Because of the first consideration, direct treatment may produce a negative reaction to treatment and may be psychologically harmful. Because of the second consideration, the clinician may be treating problems that will disappear anyway.

Wepman's views were based on some assumptions which now are either erroneous or without empirical support. First, spontaneous recovery, which indeed may last three to six months, appeared to be equated with diaschisis, which usually lasts only two or three weeks. This distinction was explained in Chapter 4. The temporary deficits which cloud the permanent residual deficit usually clear away in this short period of time. The clinician can be confident that within one month the permanent deficit becomes evident in most cases. Wepman (1972) wrote; ''To be ultimately successful, it is argued, aphasia therapy should begin with the residual, permanent problem and not with the temporary one'' (p. 206). If he meant that the residual problem appears upon the fading of diaschisis, his recommendation is appropriate. However, if he meant that the residual problem appears after completion of spontaneous recovery, his recommendation is inappropriate, because spontaneous recovery is a natural amelioration of the residual problem. Second, the psychological devastation which Wepman said is likely to occur from treatment has not been substantiated. The patient does have psychological problems to deal with subsequent to onset, but these problems may be attributed more to a natural reaction to having aphasia than to a reaction to treatment.

Delaying the establishment of specific language goals and the judicious application of treatment activities may be much more harmful psychologically. It can be argued with equal plausibility that patients may develop a lasting depression and poor communicative habits if direct treatment is delayed three to six months. The initial shock of stroke may fester for too long without the experience of accomplishment which can be achieved by treatment drills administered in a sensitive

manner. Eisenson (1973) suggested that early treatment discourages development of counterproductive communicative strategies, such as an unwarranted shift to alternative modes, and of inhibitory reactions which keep communicative skills buried deep within a traumatized psyche. The patient may give up quickly or try not talking at all. Carefully applied treatment drills may sometimes merely unlock closed doors in addition to facilitating change in deficient functions.

Most clinicians agree that direct treatment should begin when the patient is medically and psychologically ready to establish goals and pursue regular drills. When care-givers provide encouragement tempered by an empathic understanding of natural reactions to sudden onset of aphasia, many patients become eager to work on their deficits within a few days. Their desire to talk better is too great for treatment to be deferred.

APPROACHES TO TREATMENT

The most basic and inclusive distinction between styles of treating language function is Wepman's (1972) distinction between direct and indirect approaches. **Direct approaches** focus the clinician-patient interaction on the exercising of specific language processes. They are referred to as stimulus-response training, in which the clinician elicits specific language responses from the patient. They are structured around tasks which are designed so that the patient is using discrete functions such as auditory language comprehension or word retrieval. **Indirect approaches,** on the other hand, are generally unstructured; and they often take the shape of informal conversation. Certain group methods such as ''coffee-hours'' for socialization belong in this category.

The standard direct approach to aphasia treatment was founded primarily on Hildred Schuell's principles of controlled auditory stimulation (Schuell, Carroll, and Street, 1955; Schuell, et al., 1964; Jenkins, Jimenez-Pabon, Shaw, et al., 1975). The clinician presents a stimulus designed to elicit a particular response from the patient. Schuell emphasized the use of auditory stimulation to elicit verbal responses. The term *stimulation* refers to what the clinician does in standard direct treatment; the frequently used term *facilitation* refers to the effect of stimulation upon the patient. The clinician stimulates the patient *in order to* facilitate the patient's comprehension and expression.

The literature is filled with many apparently different approaches to treatment. However, they generally do not represent mutually exclusive categories of procedures but, rather, represent slight variants of a fewer number of approaches. Psycholinguistic and cybernetic are terms which have been associated with treatments; these terms refer to assumptions about the processes being treated. The procedures associated with these categories continue to be consistent with the stimulation-facilitation approach. Treatment methods have also been identified as being programmed or operant, which characterize certain refinements and extensions of stimulation-facilitation instead of representing a truly different form of methodology. The point is that the aphasia literature presents an unnecessarily large number of terms for treatment, just as it presents numerous redundant schemes for the classification of syndromes.

Chapter 10 will present general principles and styles which characterize most specific treatment strategies found in the literature. The reader is encouraged to study primary sources for more complete details of clinicians' preferences. Direct and indirect treatment strategies will be related to the basic goals of improving language functions. Variants of these strategies will be shown to originate from the broader aim of improving communication. Specific procedures will be linked to selected symptoms in the next chapter.

DIRECT TREATMENT OF LANGUAGE FUNCTIONS

Direct treatment consists of tasks designed for the exercise of specific language functions. The task is defined in terms of the stimulus presented by the clinician and the response expected from the patient. Once the patient's primary deficits have been identified, each task is planned carefully so that it indeed will exercise a specific impaired process.

The Session

Depending on the setting, size of caseload, and needs of certain patients, the aphasic may be seen in three to five sessions per week, with each session lasting from thirty to sixty minutes. One of Brookshire's (1978b) principles of treatment is "Begin each treatment session with familiar tasks, in which the patient is generally successful" (p. 143). He called this a "warm-up" time which should always precede introduction of new materials and procedures. Also, the session should end with an easy task so that the patient may leave on an encouraging note.

Tompkins, Marshall, and Phillips (1980) presented data indicating that aphasics' linguistic performance is better in the morning than in the afternoon. This would be anticipated in a rehabilitation setting where the patient receives other more physically taxing therapies during the day. To suggest that all language treatment should be given in the morning is unrealistic, but the factor of fatigue should be recognized in the evaluation of performance during a session. Tompkins and her colleagues suggested that time of day should be held constant for an individual for reassessment and clinical research.

Planning the Task

In Chapter 6, it was said that treatment plans are developed from identification of the patient's primary deficit or deficits and from identification of the patient's specific communicative strengths and weaknesses. Primary deficits are the source of specific treatment objectives. If a primary deficit is the comprehension of complex syntactic relationships, then one objective is to improve comprehension of these relationships. If a primary deficit is word retrieval, then an objective is to improve word retrieval. Communicative strengths lead to specific strategies of treatment in which the strengths are expanded and are used to raise the level of weaker functions. In terms of neural structure and function, treatment takes advantage of the intact regions remote from damage and their connections with defective but structurally intact regions close to the destroyed area.

Two approaches to treatment planning are possible, and each depends upon the way the patient's deficits have been identified. One approach was referred to in Chapter 6 as "pure task blindness," which is a weak approach. The other approach involves inferring primary deficits from performances on several tasks used in assessment, which was illustrated in Tables 6–3 and 6–4.

Pure task blindness limits the range of procedures which might be considered for treatment. Basically, it involves the identification of a slightly deficient task performance and then the repeated use of that task in treatment. The progression of treatment becomes a movement up the hierarchy of tasks contained in a test battery. Once efficiency with one task is achieved, the patient is presented with a task which is more difficult. The crucial mistake is that the primary deficit is not identified; and, in effect, a true diagnosis is not made. The planning of treatment becomes merely a mimicry of diagnostic procedures. Procedures are limited to the small sampling of possible language behaviors depicted on the test.

The strong approach involves designing *procedures which reflect the broad range of possible language variables implied by the identified primary deficit.* The *PICA*, for example, samples receptive syntactic processing primarily with a prepositional phrase structure in the visual modality (reading). A problem with identifying the spatial relationships in prepositions may reflect a more general and central deficit described by Luria (1966) as a problem comprehending "logical-grammatical relations." Therefore, treatment would be directed toward a variety of syntactic relationships presented auditorily and visually. When the deficit is identified as a common thread underlying several tasks (see Table 6–4), it follows that the deficit can be treated with a variety of exercises. Brookshire's (1978b) eighth principle of treatment—"Direct treatment toward general abilities, rather than specific responses, whenever possible" (p. 146)—reinforces the recommendation of the strong approach to planning. As he put it, "the objective of the clinician should be directed toward the process represented by the stimulus-response pair, rather than to the stimulus-response pair itself" (p. 146).

The major advantage of the strong approach is that it opens up the clinician's thinking to a range of tasks involving the impaired process. When the several variables affecting a process are considered, a single task can be adjusted in several ways to create several versions. A very structured and artificial set of procedures can be made to reflect a wide variety of processing demands which might be encountered outside of the clinic. In this way, direct treatment of primary deficits generalizes to the possible circumstances of language use. Thinking of a deficit as one of "word retrieval" implies a variety of circumstances in which this process is employed (see Chapter 5). On the other hand, thinking of it as a "naming deficit" is a concept restricted to a particular activity in which word retrieval is employed. Determining the possible circumstances in which a language process can be exercised involves being aware of the influential variables found in research with normal and aphasic adults.

Determining the patient's linguistic and communicative strengths contributes to planning a task in the manner indicated by Brookshire's (1978b) first principle: "Structure treatment programs so that most of the patient's experiences are with tasks at levels of difficulty such that performance is slightly deficient, but not completely erroneous" (p. 138). *Most responses on a task should be correct, with deficiency reflected in efficiency of the accurate performance.* As one guideline, Brookshire suggested that treatment tasks be carried out by the patient at the level of ten-to-thirteen performance with respect to the *PICA* scoring system. Responses would be delayed, incomplete, or self-corrected. Porch (1981a) recommended a range of nine to fifteen. This requires the clinician's stimulus to be adequate in eliciting an accurate performance (Schuell, et al., 1964).

Brookshire (1972, 1976) has shown that the production of errors seems to reduce subsequent performance and that errors in treatment tend to cluster (Brookshire and Nicholas, 1978). Errors enhance frustration, which reduces attention to treatment objectives and presses upon the processes being exercised. Brookshire (1978b) suggested that *no more than 20 percent of responses on a task be errors.*

An important reason for creating a task at a level of moderate success is that accurate responding ensures that a targeted normal process is being exercised. When many errors are produced, the patient is engaged in unproductive processing of a kind that cannot be identified.

Planning a task which exercises a deficient process at a level of success requires consideration of several variables of task structure and content. The first considera-

tion is the *modality* to be exercised. If a receptive function is to be exercised, such as auditory comprehension or reading, then the task usually entails a linguistic input and a nonlinguistic response. When a verbal response is contemplated for an exercise of comprehension, the response is within the patient's capability so that it is not a factor in success on the task. If an expressive function is exercised, such as verbal expression or writing, there may be a nonverbal input (referent) or a verbal input and a linguistic response. When language is used to stimulate verbal expression, the stimulus is within the patient's capacity so that the exercise clearly focuses on expressive processing.

The second consideration involves identifying the *cognitive process* within the modality which needs practice. For example, when the intent is to exercise comprehension, the task should require the patient to make a decision about the meaning of a linguistic stimulus. Finding a printed word which matches a spoken word, for example, need not involve semantic decisions and, therefore, is not a comprehension task. If the printed word to be matched is a synonym, then a semantic decision is involved.

Creating a task to stretch short-term memory capacity or to exercise comprehension provides another example of relating the activity to the targeted process. If the intention is to exercise comprehension, a stimulus level would be selected which is performed at 80 percent success in relating a concept to the stimulus. The stimulus might be a word, a phrase, or a sentence. When the clinician wishes to expand capacity of working memory for comprehension, a linguistic level is selected which is comprehended at 100 percent accuracy and efficiency so that the internal mechanisms of comprehension are minimized as a factor. The stimulus might be sequences of words or phrases in which each unit is well within comprehension ability, but the length of sequence taxes the patient's processing at 80 percent accuracy. In this way, the patient stretches processing capacity within his or her ability to comprehend or exercises comprehension within capacity of working memory.

As shown in Chapter 11, expressive tasks may be oriented toward stimulation of word retrieval or stimulation of syntax formulation. Both processes interact when discourse is stimulated, but tasks can differ in their emphasis on these processes. When stimulating production of single words or a series of words, emphasis is on word retrieval. With cases exhibiting agrammatism, single-word retrieval is a prerequisite skill for tasks which encourage sentence production. The patient is asked to produce structured multiword utterances, in which each word is within single-word retrieval ability.

Tasks are defined further as to the *semantic content* of language and referents. This content is usually based on its familiarity, everyday usefulness to the individual, and its naturalness in terms of the patient's dialect and preferences. These considerations are also elaborated in the next chapter (pages 283–285).

Any structured task in direct treatment is a means to an end, and not an end in itself. The clinician's overriding objective is improvement of natural language function. We are interested in the patient's improvement of pointing, naming, and repeating only to the extent that these improvements push natural language function forward.

The Clinician-Patient Interaction

In carrying out the direct treatment of specific language processes, the clinician and patient engage in a fairly standard form of interaction. This interaction comprises the trials of each task. It was described by Brookshire, et al. (1978) as consisting of the *clinician's stimulus,* the *patient's response,* and the *clinician's feedback* to

the patient's response. A task is defined in terms of the clinician's stimulus and the clinician's *expected response* from the patient. The clinician's feedback varies depending on whether the patient's response is consistent with the expected response (an acceptable response) or does not measure up to the clinician's expectations (an unacceptable response). The key to exercising a productive language process lies in the clinician's use of stimulation which facilitates acceptable responding on at least 80 percent of the trials and the clinician's judicious use of feedback when unacceptable responses occasionally occur (see Chapter 11, pages 278–281).

Progression

So far, discussion of direct treatment has been focused on the planning and structure of clinician-patient interaction at any one point in time during the months of rehabilitation. Yet, in addition to the present, planning also entails looking ahead to what will be done next. Treatment over time for an individual has usually been conceived as a hierarchy or continuum of tasks, involving modifications of tasks in the direction of increasing their complexity. Precision in defining the progression of treatment has been enhanced by the principles of programmed instruction.

Programmed instruction was introduced to clinical aphasiology in the 1960s. The first application of programming principles to aphasia was by Rosenberg (1965) and Edwards (1965; Rosenberg and Edwards, 1965) who trained visual perception with teaching machines. Automated training has been tried by a few other clinicians (Doehring, 1968; Brookshire, 1968, 1969; Sarno, Silverman, and Sands, 1970; Lozano and Gaeth, 1977; Culton and Ferguson, 1979). Wepman (1968) had a strong reaction to automated presentation of stimuli; he referred to the teaching machine as "a devil's box" which interferes with the clinician-patient relationship, and accused clinicians who use them of fearing contact with people. Programmed instruction, however, does not necessarily entail automation. In explaining her application of programming principles to treatment, Holland (1970) noted that machines were used infrequently because of their inflexibility and cost. These principles have been applied primarily to assist the clinician in defining clinician-patient interaction in behavioral terms and in planning the progression of this interaction (Brookshire, 1967; Holland, 1969, 1970; Bollinger and Stout, 1976; Keenan, 1977; LaPointe, 1977; Goldfarb, 1981; Seron, Van Der Linden, and Van Der Kaa-Delvenne, 1978).

Costello (1977) explained the application of programmed instruction for speech-language treatment in general. Her components with respect to interaction structure, namely, the stimulus, the response, and the consequences of the response were mentioned earlier. Her principles of progression will be discussed in this section.

Initial and Terminal Responses. Treatment begins with what the patient can do communicatively when first seen by the clinician, and the endpoint of treatment is always at a level of language function which lies between the patient's starting point and normal language function. We exercise the patient's strengths, exhibited either as a level within a deficient function or as a relatively spared ability, such as gesturing, in order to augment or substitute for a deficient function. In addition to finding an initial response level in formal test performance, the clinician may find responses to build from in the patient's spontaneous utterances. Helm and Barresi (1980) developed programs for patients with severe expressive deficits by starting treatment with the patient's only spontaneous utterances, such as verbal stereotypes. Their programs involved

movement toward voluntary control over involuntarily produced utterances.

The terminal response represents either a long-term goal of treatment or a short-term goal from which springs a series of terminal responses as each short-term goal is achieved. As Costello (1977) instructed, the terminal response is a short-term goal which is stated in behavioral terms and serves as the last step of a treatment program. The terminal response might be the description of a picture with a sentence containing the agent, action, and object; the initial response might involve the patient's ability to say only the name of the agent (see Holland and Levy, 1971).

Terminal responses defined with respect to structured tasks, such as picture naming or description, are always intermediate steps of treatment in the long term. The final goal of treatment is expressed with respect to the patient's use of language in his or her daily living environment. The final step of Taylor and Marks' (1959) naming program is the use of their core vocabulary in the patient's "... everyday life without the help of a picture, a word card, or a therapist" (p. 16). Florance, Rabidoux, and Mc-Causlin (1980) reported on directing their treatment of apraxia of speech toward the transfer of trained skills to the patient's normal communicative contexts. Terminal responses were defined with respect to the "environmental impact" of treatment.

Small-Step Progression. Once the initial response is identified and the terminal response is defined, a treatment program entails moving the patient from the initial response to the terminal response. Treatment progresses by *successive approximations* from a response related to the terminal response toward the terminal response itself. The successive approximations are a series of small, carefully graduated steps. Dimensions along which these steps proceed may be characterized in several ways: (1) from maximum dependence on the clinician for success to independence from the clinician for equivalent success, (2) from clinically structured demands on the patient which foster success to the kinds of demands which the patient finds in everyday life, or (3) from the involuntary control of utterances to the voluntary control of utterances.

The small steps are created by the clinician's control of stimuli to the patient and by a realistic expectation of responses from the patient. A procedure of *fading* cues from maximal stimulus support to minimal stimulus support is often applied to adjustments of stimuli. A procedure of *shaping* is sometimes applied to verbal responses, whereby the clinician reinforces imperfect utterances which come closer and closer to the terminal response.

The next step in treating a deficit comes after the patient has been proficient with the previous step; so if the next step is similar to the previous step, the abilities used in the previous step can be applied readily to the subsequent step. The basic principle behind making small changes in a task is the same principle used in making experimental comparisons to analyze the effect of a variable, namely, *change one variable of a task at a time.* In a comprehension task, for example, the next step might entail an increase in stimulus length, an increase in the number of response choices, an increase of stimulus rate, *or* an increase in time between the stimulus and response. In an expressive task, the next step might entail a request for an increased length of response, a decrease in the familiarity of content, *or* a request for a quicker production. In this regard, the progression of treatment becomes variable from patient to patient. Some patients tolerate a change of one variable more readily than another variable. Some tolerate only a one-variable change, while other patients maintain a high success rate when more

than one variable is changed from one step to the next. The direction and distance between steps depends on the abilities of each patient and therefore is not the same for all patients.

Several examples of small-step progression have appeared in the literature. One approach has been to create steps in terms of different functions. Taylor and Marks (1959) and Keenan (1966) proposed such programs. In the former, the steps began with matching a printed word to a picture (reading), then pointing to a picture upon hearing a word, then copying a word, and then writing the word from memory, and so on. Keenan (1975) asked patients to recognize, then repeat, and then recall each word. The approach was a series of steps per word in which the steps changed according to language function.

Progression has been developed within individual language functions. This has been especially evident in the treatment of auditory language comprehension. Holland and Sonderman (1974) fashioned steps for a program based on the changes of length and phrase complexity in the Token Test. Culton and Ferguson's (1979) steps developed out of increases in stimulus length. Flowers and Danforth (1979) reported on a program administered by a patient's family members in which small steps were defined according to length of command. Different phases of Martinoff, et al.'s (1980) comprehension training include answering yes/no questions, following commands, and auditory sequencing; and, within each of these sections, steps are defined according to increasing length. One example of a progression toward sentence production was Holland and Levy's (1971) training of constituents of a sentence in steps toward the terminal response of a complete sentence.

Some attention has been given to small differences of syntactic structure in defining small steps of treatment. A complete program of syntax training for aphasia has not appeared in the literature. One reason for this is that such programs, if they are developed empirically, will be difficult to apply generally because of the individual differences among patients as to the relative difficulty of sentence types. One patient's hierarchy of difficulty, especially with respect to subtle differences of syntax, will probably not be another patient's hierarchy. Treatment programs which show a minimal influence from linguistics represent differences in difficulty according to the number of words or phrases in a stimulus or expected response and according to categories of simple sentences, complex sentences, and paragraph-length material. Ross and Spencer's (1980) task hierarchies are not strongly influenced by syntactic precision; Martinoff, et al.'s (1980) program for auditory comprehension reflects a little more attention to certain syntactic details. Clinical research has not demonstrated that a linguistically impoverished approach to planning task continua produces results that are different from a linguistically precise approach.

One of the best examples of combining principles of programmed instruction to create a progression of treatment is found in Melodic Intonation Therapy (Sparks and Holland, 1976; Sparks, 1981). MIT employs melodic intoning as a means of facilitating verbal production. The program contains four levels or phases, with the first level designed to orient the patient toward producing melodic patterns. The initial response requires the capacity to repeat an utterance as intoned by the clinician. Early facilitators or cues in the program include the clinician's intoning the utterance, repetition in unison, and an accompanying rhythmical hand-tapping with the clinician. Terminal responses for each level include repetition after the clinician, answering a question with part of the original utterance, and answering varied questions related to information in the utterance. Steps proceed from involuntary

to voluntary production. The aforementioned cues are faded from one step to the next within each level. Responses are shaped from the initial unnatural intoned pattern to a more natural pattern without intoning. Furthermore, the patient must be successful with one step before going on to the next one.

Response Criterion. In programmed instruction, learning is possible because each step is tuned to the learner's abilities. Furthermore, the next step is so similar to the current step that mastery of the current step should facilitate reasonable success on the subsequent step. These principles are applied to the stimulation of aphasic patients so that they are exercising language processes and continually are challenged to improve the operation of these processes. Mastery at one step is the criterion for moving to the next step.

There are at least three types of criterion used in making decisions about treatment. One is the task-selection guideline of 80 percent accuracy. At this level of success, the patient still may be somewhat incomplete or delayed in response. Repeated exercise at a given step is designed to improve this level of success to 100 percent accuracy with a more complete and quicker response.

This mastery, another criterion, is the basis for moving on to the next step of treatment. The criterion for moving to the next step, like other criteria, varies from patient to patient. A level of 90 to 95 percent accuracy may be as far as the patient can go given the continuing presence of a damaged brain, but the patient may still be proficient enough to apply present abilities to the next step of a treatment plan.

The third criterion which is often recommended in programs is related to the terminal response or objective of each phase in a program. Keenan (1977) and Martinoff, et al. (1980) offered guidelines as to terminal objectives whereby the steps of treatment lead to 80 to 90 percent accuracy at some advanced level of function. When this type of criterion is reached, a new phase of treatment is entered by the selection of a different type of task to exercise the same basic function or selection of a different function to be exercised. While performing at 80 percent or more in a treatment task, such as phrase repetition, the patient may be at a much lower level with respect to a task which reflects the terminal objective, such as picture description. Still, picture description might be measured regularly as a probe in order to monitor the patient's recovery.

VERSIONS OF DIRECT STIMULATION/FACILITATION

The emphasis in the previous sections was on the exercise of single modalities and processes within these modalities. Tasks were considered to be focused on either auditory comprehension or reading and on either spoken word retrieval, sentence formulation, or writing. However, clinicians have approached direct stimulation in other ways.

Multimodal Stimulation and Response

Instead of concentrating a task on a process within a single modality, many clinicians have involved multiple modalities as the patient deals with each word, phrase, or sentence. Several strategies of treatment can be represented as multimodal in that input modalities may be presented simultaneously or input and output modes may be used sequentially. In sequential stimulation and response, less-impaired modalities may precede more severely impaired modalities or vice versa. Each variation may be viable for a single patient.

Multiple Functions per Word. Early multimodal approaches to stimulation and response were borne out of general or vague conceptions of language function and aphasia. Schuell, et al. (1964), for example, presented procedures under the heading "Techniques for the Stimulation of Language" (p. 352). She did not address procedures to each language modality as independent treatment goals. Also, she did not aim her procedures at specific symptoms such as paraphasias or agrammatism. Treatment was viewed as "stimulation of language" and was directed primarily at improvement of verbal expression.

An example of multiple function stimulation is outlined in Table 10–1. With each word, the patient is asked to recognize it by pointing to a picture and then by pointing to a printed word. After doing this, the patient is either *expected* to repeat or read aloud under these circumstances or is *asked* to repeat. While repeating, the patient may be copying. Then, the patient is to say the word as if naming the picture. While saying the word without cues, the patient may be writing it also.

After all of this stimulation, picture naming is a matter of recalling the word as it had been given by the clinician and repeated by the patient. Under these circumstances, picture naming need not be a genuine retrieval of the word from long-term memory. Having the patient practice multiple functions with each word makes sense for one basic reason, namely, that aphasia is a central disorder and multiple functions should stimulate and reinforce each other. One limitation of this strategy is that it confounds interpretation of recovery of single-language functions if the clinician chooses to measure performance on the treatment task itself. However, this need not be a problem if probes independent of the treatment are used to measure improvement during treatment.

Pairing and Fading Stimuli. A slightly different form of multimodal stimulation is the *simultaneous presentation of auditory and*

TABLE 10-1. The sequence of stimulus-response trials in *multiple functions per word* is contrasted with modality-focused treatment, which has been emphasized in previous sections.

Modality-Focused Treatment	Clinician Stimulus	Expected Response
Comprehension task	Says "key"	Points to picture
	Says "fork"	Points to picture
	Says "apple"	Points to picture
Expression task	Says "key"	Repeats "key"
	Says "fork"	Repeats "fork"
	Says "apple"	Repeats "apple"

Multiple Functions per Word	Clinician Stimulus	Expected Response
First word *key*	Says "key"	Points to picture
		Repeats "key"
	Says "key"	Points to printed word
		Reads aloud
	"Write key"	Copies word
	Points to picture	
	"What is this?"	Says "key"
		Writes "key"
Second word *fork*	Same as above	Same as above

visual language stimuli. Saying and showing a word at the same time is considered to be a means of increasing the power of a stimulus to elicit an appropriate response, especially if one modality is stronger than the other. It may be directed at improving either auditory comprehension or reading.

The direction of fading one modality reflects which of these goals is being pursued, when one modality is stronger than the other (see Table 10–2). If the goal is to improve reading, then pairing auditory and visual language inputs is followed by fading the auditory input so that reading

TABLE 10-2. Similar to modality-focused drills, the *pairing and fading of inputs* involves two stimulus-response trials per word. The faded input is considered to be the stronger of the two inputs in each task.

Pairing and Fading Stimuli	Clinician Stimulus	Expected Response
Auditory comprehension	Says "key" and shows word	Points to picture
	Says "key"	Points to picture
	Says "fork" and shows word	Points to picture
	Says "fork"	Points to picture
Reading	Says "key" and shows word	Points to picture
	Shows word	Points to picture
	Says "fork" and shows word	Points to picture
	Shows word	Points to picture

can be exercised without auditory support. If the goal is to improve auditory comprehension, then this pairing is followed by fading the visual input so that auditory comprehension can be exercised without visual support. In both of these strategies, *the faded input is the stronger modality* which was used to facilitate processing of the weaker modality. The strategy of pairing and fading could be thought of as a form of "deblocking" but, as will be seen in the next section, the originator of this term referred to a subtly different procedure.

Deblocking. The patient's practice of multiple functions per word—comprehension, repetition, and recall or retrieval with all modalities—was described as a general procedure based on the idea that stimulating the central processes of language by any means would facilitate any one function, especially verbal expression. Also, the temporal proximity of comprehension and imitation, speech and writing, and so on would permit one function to facilitate or reinforce performance of another function. The concept of deblocking may also be invoked to explain the effect of this strategy on the patient. Deblocking is an idea developed by Weigl and his colleagues as a means of determining the linguistic competence retained by patients but masked by severe deficits in particular modalities or functions (Weigl and Bierwisch, 1970).

Weigl observed what he called a deblocking phenomenon in aphasic patients *when an impaired function was preceded by a relatively unimpaired function involving the same semantic content.* For example, a patient with impaired word reading was able to read a word after hearing the word. The reading impairment was considered to represent a blocking of semantic analysis through that modality which could be deblocked by a prior semantic analysis through the relatively unblocked modality. Sentence copying was used to deblock writing to dictation which generalized to

syntactically similar sentences. This phenomenon was evidence for the retention of semantic and syntactic competence in spite of the particular disrupted performance capability. Subsequently, clinical aphasiologists have adopted this concept as the basis for certain treatment procedures (Ulatowska and Richardson, 1974; LaPointe, 1978a; Rao and Horner, 1978).

Deblocking, as described by Greimas, et al. (1970) in their review of Weigl's research, is not necessarily a simple sequential pairing of input or response modes for the same semantic content. The prior stimulation with an intact mode was called a *prestimulation* phase of the task trial which the patient should perform without conscious awareness of its link to the subsequent presentation of an impaired mode. For example, a goal might be to deblock the impaired auditory channel. Prestimulation might include a printed word or picture representing the content to be deblocked. Moreover, the targeted content would be included in a series of words or pictures in the prestimulation phase (see Table 10–3). The patient merely views the series of stimuli *without response.* Then, the targeted item is presented in the auditory mode. Prestimulation is thought to "activate" the linguistic content, thereby making it easier to process in the more impaired modality. Prestimulation can be of three types: (1) direct, in which the key word appears in the prestimulation phase, (2) indirect, in which a related word, synonym or antonym, appears in the prestimulation phase, or (3) direct and indirect prestimulation. Therefore, deblocking is not an association between two inputs by pairing them, but rather it is an attempt to prepare or activate central semantic structures through an unblocked route of access. This is a normal cognitive process called "priming" by Collins and Loftus (1975).

Podraza and Darley (1977) compared the effects of direct and indirect pre-

TABLE 10-3. Weigl's *deblocking,* especially as described by Greimas, et al. (1970), involves a prestimulation phase for each stimulus-response trial. Prestimulation involves a relatively intact modality. (1) Auditory mode to deblock reading; (2) Reading mode to deblock naming; (3) Indirect deblocking, semantically related word to deblock naming.

Weigl's Deblocking Clinician Prestimulation	Clinician Primary Stimulus	Expected Response
(1) Says "apple, key, fork . . ."	Shows "key"	Points to picture
(2) Shows "apple, key, fork . . ."	Presents picture "What is this?"	Says "key"
(3) Says "This is a fruit."	Presents picture "What is this?"	Says "apple"

stimulation on picture naming by five aphasic subjects. Direct prestimulation was three words such as *line, bee, goat.* Then a picture of a bee was presented. Indirect prestimulation consisted of *sting, honey, hive* prior to presenting the picture of a bee. Direct prestimulation facilitated picture naming when compared to naming without cues. However, indirect prestimulation actually resulted in decreased naming by three of the subjects.

A prestimulation phase was used by Waller and Darley (1978) to study the influence of context on paragraph comprehension. Paragraph-reading tasks were preceded by a relevant picture, a verbal description, or both. This prestimulation contained information which was related to the paragraph. The antecedents containing verbal description improved paragraph-reading performance by the aphasic subjects.

Other references to deblocking have been more general. Ulatowska and Richardson (1974) associated deblocking with intersystemic reorganization. These two concepts indeed may overlap to the point that they are two ways of conceptualizing the same treatment strategy, namely, using an intact functional system to facilitate improved performance of a more impaired different functional system. However, these concepts are different. Intersystemic reorganization implies a change in the way a goal is achieved, while deblocking strives for im-

proved status of a function as it has always been performed. LaPointe (1978a) defined deblocking as " . . . maximizing residual skills by stimulating the channel that is most functional for the patient" (pp. 138–139). Deblocking is a concept which may explain a variety of multimodal stimulation/facilitation techniques, and Weigl's prestimulation procedure may merely be one way that deblocking is achieved.

Intersystemic Reorganization

Luria (1970b) wrote that the majority of compensatory mechanisms which develop following focal brain damage stem from either intrasystemic or intersystemic reorganization (see Chapter 4). "We can summarize both types by the general statement that recovery is brought about by the incorporation of some new type of *afferation* into the disturbed functional system" (p. 386). New sources of input to an impaired system might come from established connections with other regions of the brain. In *Traumatic Aphasia,* Luria was explicit about intersystemic reorganization as a means of treating the language deficits in aphasia. *An intact function, which is not normally involved in the impaired function, is introduced into the operation of the impaired function.* Usually this intrusion is designed to bring to conscious awareness the means by which a function is carried out mentally, a function which is normally performed without conscious awareness. This treatment strategy sometimes changes the clinician-client interaction from simple stimulus-response to a more complex interaction involving instruction and the use of special cues which encourage the patient to be more analytical in comprehending or formulating an utterance.

For patients who can comprehend words individually but have difficulty when they are in grammatical relationships, intersystemic reorganization was clearly applied. With Broca's aphasia, Luria (1970b) introduced repetition into the act of comprehending an utterance. Also, diagrams which "differ little from those used in common grammar texts" (p. 441) were used to make the relationships between words more explicit to the patient, thereby facilitating a conscious effort to integrate words into a whole idea. Constructions like "Point with the pencil at the comb" and "Mother's daughter" were broken down into component parts so that the patient could "consciously analyze the rule" (p. 442) underlying the construction. With instrumental constructions, the patient was asked to focus on "What is used to point." With genitive relationships, pictures were presented which separated the meanings of each word. A demonstrative pronoun was added—"*this* mother's daughter"—as a cue to which of the two nouns is the modifier. Abstract diagrams were used to cue the patient to the relationships represented by certain prepositions. In general, these methods were designed "to externalize the meaningful relationships implied by the constructions and compensate for the inner schemata which the patient lacks" (p. 443).

The idea of *substituting external aids for missing inner dynamic structures* was applied to facilitate sentence production, particularly with Broca's aphasia (Luria, 1970b; Luria and Tsvetkova, 1968). Luria presented cues as simple as three pieces of paper to represent the three components of

an agent-action-object relationship. In describing a pictured event the patient would point to each cue focusing on each component separately but in sequence. The complete sentence was produced slowly and with conscious awareness of each part. This was the basis for a sentence construction board developed by Davis (1973). Once a patient could produce an utterance fluently while pointing to these cues, the pointing and the visual cues were faded. These visual representations of grammatical relationships are a clear use of a new function, not normally involved in sentence formulation, being introduced to facilitate sentence formulation.

The "new type of afferation" implicated in the aforementioned examples of intersystemic reorganization is from the visual system in the left hemisphere, right hemisphere, or both. Another example of introducing a new source of input to an impaired system is the infusion of nonverbal auditory input to the process of formulating utterances in Melodic Intonation Therapy (Berlin, 1976; Sparks, 1981).

INDIRECT APPROACHES

Indirect approaches, like the direct approach, are intended to improve specific deficient language functions. The term "indirect" has been associated with a variety of clinical activities, with the common features of being less formally structured than specific tasks and of being less directed toward a single language process. These activities have included conversation, social groups, role-playing, and field trips. The term has also been associated with the use of direct treatment exercises of one language function which, for some patients, facilitates the exercise of another function. For example, some patients retrieve words readily only during a task designed to exercise auditory comprehension; and so this task is used to stimulate word retrieval "indirectly."

Content-Centered Discussion Therapy

Wepman took "a new look" at aphasia treatment and advocated a "nonlanguage, content-centered discussion therapy" for some patients. The procedure is conversation of a special kind. In Wepman's (1972, 1976) three examples, the clinician and patient discussed topics from the patient's vocational interests. The clinician's role was to keep the patient on the topic, focused on ideas rather than on words. The patient was directed away from "struggle for accuracy in word-finding" and toward thought processes underlying the use of words. Wepman asked a lawyer to discuss specific cases with visual aids, charts, and tables. The lawyer's associates were enlisted to exchange ideas about a particular litigation familiar to the patient. A psychoanalyst was asked to talk about old therapeutic cases and his own dreams. These patients were not asked to think about their use of language; the clinician never tried to elicit any particular verbal expression.

The goal was still to improve verbal expression, but by not focusing directly on it. Two of the examples were described as having had direct language stimulation treatment for some time without positive results. The lawyer " . . . never improved beyond the word-by-word struggle through over three years of effort" (Wepman, 1976, p. 134). The psychoanalyst, characterized as having a global expressive deficit, spoke almost entirely with " . . . automatic repetition of over-learned socially acceptable phrases despite over a year of direct linguistically oriented therapy" (p. 135). Wepman observed remarkable positive changes in verbal expression after his discussion therapy was initiated. This indirect approach primarily represents a shift in thinking about treatment, partly due to a festering dissatisfac-

tion with the outcome of direct stimulation for certain patients.

Wepman considered these cases to be evidence for a theoretical position that limitation in thought processes is the basis for certain aphasic language deficits. Content-centered discussion was effective, according to Wepman, because it dealt with the true problem of the patient, which was an impoverishment of ideas rather than of words. He viewed the thought deficit to be most pronounced in the jargon (Wernicke's) aphasic, although only the case of 1972 was described as having this symptom when indirect treatment began. Martin (1981a) elaborated on the theoretical bases of Wepman's treatment approach. Martin associated thought-centered discussion therapy with a communication-centered frame of reference for clinician-patient interaction. DiSimoni (1981) thought that Wepman's approach encompasses group psychotherapy and family counseling; however, this was not indicated in Wepman's two articles on the procedure.

Divergence

Content-centered discussion therapy places the patient in a position to exercise divergent language behavior where emphasis is on "variety, quantity, and relevance of output" and where the patient must " . . . provide ideas in situations where a proliferation of ideas on some topic is required" (Chapey, 1981b, p. 155). Chapey's investigation of aphasic impairment of divergent language and her analysis of diagnostic procedure were discussed previously in this book. She turned her attention to divergent language tasks as a means of broadening the patient's practice of word retrieval. Content-centered discussion and divergent verbal tasks are examples of treating the primary deficit of word retrieval rather than a task-specific deficit called "naming." Treating word retrieval with convergent and divergent procedures expands treatment to include a greater variety of real-life implications of the deficit than is done by using only convergent tasks.

Aphasic performance on single administrations of a few divergent tasks had been reported in comparison with normal adults (Chapey, Rigrodsky, and Morrison, 1976). For example, in a task of listing objects in a class, such as objects that roll, aphasic subjects ranged from 2 to 32 different words (average, 13.6) while normals ranged from 21 to 61 different words (average, 41). These tasks are difficult for many aphasic patients; patients with mild aphasia were impaired only in divergent word-retrieval tasks, while patients with severe aphasia were impaired in both divergent and convergent tasks. If treatment is to be instituted at a level of success with only slight impairment, divergent tasks may be best suited for mild aphasia. Severely impaired aphasic patients experience much frustration in attempting such tasks. Chapey (1981b) referred to ''some severely impaired patients who fail to produce any divergent verbal responses after two months of this type of intervention on a biweekly basis...'' (p. 159); and she suggested nonverbal divergent tasks for these patients.

The divergent model of treatment includes two stages (Chapey, 1981b). The first involves the patient's observing a group of normal adults, perhaps recorded on videotape, responding to a divergent task. The purpose is to orient the patient to the task and to provide a model for the patient to emulate later. In the second stage the patient carries out divergent tasks, and '' ... intervention should focus upon strengthening the ability to retrieve numerous and varied semantic responses through continuous reinforcement of relevant responses'' (p. 160). Convergent techniques, such as cues to specific words, can be used to facilitate retrieval of words which had not been produced on a divergent basis. Chapey's several examples of divergent tasks included instructions to

(1) say words that begin with or include a particular sound, (2) list problems inherent to a common situation, (3) list uses of an object, and (4) put a word in different sentences. Patients can be asked to name as many items as they can think of in a familiar category such as countries, states, familiar streets, or favorite foods.

A COMMUNICATION FRAMEWORK

The relationship between language and communication and the impact of aphasia on communication have been frequent concerns in this text. Considering the relationships between language and contexts and the functional uses of language in the planning of treatment has been referred to as the *pragmatic approach*. Early in this chapter, a primary goal of treatment was said to be improvement of the patient's ability to communicate. As stated then, this goal has four implications for how the language deficit might be treated and for how additional behaviors might be considered in broadening the scope of treatment. These implications are elaborated in the following sections.

Different Means but Same End

For Silverman (1980) in his *Communication for the Speechless,* having a communication orientation in speech-language treatment implies that the clinician should promote the patient's use of any mode of conveying messages, especially when speech has been severely reduced or eliminated as a means of communication. He defined nonspeech modes as ''procedures for encoding and transmitting messages without their being directly encoded into phonemes by the vocal tract'' (p. 3). Direct encoding into speech sounds was contrasted with indirect encoding into speech, which includes the operation of machines that talk. Silverman wrote that there are more than one hundred nonspeech communication modes. His elaborate review encompassed three general categories: (1) *gestural modes,* which involve only muscle movement, instrumentation not being required; (2) *gestural-assisted modes,* which contain "a readout device (or display) that is activated directly or indirectly by muscle gestures, or movements" (p. 58); and (3) *neuro-assisted modes,* which consist of "a readout device or display that is activated by *bioelectrical* signals" (p. 60). These modes have been developed primarily for children and adults who have motor deficits which have devastated their capabilities in speech and/or writing and for which prognosis is poor for treatment of the speech mode. These deficits include cerebral palsy, dysarthrias, severe apraxia of speech, and glossectomy (surgical excision of all or part of the tongue).

Usually patients with global aphasia or with aphasia and severe verbal apraxia have received formal training in a non-speech mode. The treatment goal is either the substitution of a new system to compensate for loss of the speech mode or the augmentation of communicative ability by supplementing the speech mode with additional modes. Silverman wrote that non-speech modes can be used on a temporary or a permanent basis by aphasic patients. For example, a communication board might be used during the first months postonset until more natural modes improve to a functional level. Often non-speech modes are invoked upon failure of treatment to facilitate functional improvement in the speech and writing modalities. Sometimes writing provides more clues to a message than speech, and so writing is encouraged (and it may serve to deblock the speech modality). Silverman has found that instituting any means of communication soon after onset can push motivation for improving speech on to greater intensity.

Of the many nonspeech modes reviewed by Silverman (1980) and DiSimoni (1981), only a few have actually been demonstrated with genuinely aphasic subjects. In the gestural category, these include natural gestures (Davis and Wilcox, 1981), pantomime (Schlanger and Schlanger, 1970), and manual sign language (Chen, 1968, 1971; Eagleson, Vaughn, and Knudson, 1970; Skelly, 1979; and Simmons and Zorthian, 1979). Kirshner and Webb (1981) reported teaching American Indian Signs and American Sign Language for the deaf to an unusual patient with bilateral focal brain damage and symptoms of aphasia. The patient learned to sign printed sentences. "Her spontaneous expressions by signs, however, have remained limited to one- and two-word phrases and to very concrete subject matter" (p. 167). Peterson and Kirshner (1981) provided a comprehensive review of gesture in aphasia, finding evidence for symbolic impairment and reason to continue investigating this line of treatment (also see R. J. Duffy and J. R. Duffy, 1981).

Gestural-assisted modes included the manual selection or manipulation of nonverbal symbols (Gardner, Zurif, Berry, et al., 1976; Glass, Gazzaniga, and Premack, 1973) and mechanical speaking devices, such as the Handi Voice (Rabidoux, Florance, and McCauslin, 1980). Klor (1980) demonstrated the presentation of commands with nonverbal visual symbols to aphasic subjects. Colby, Christinaz, Parkison, et al. (1981) have begun to explore the possible use of a portable computer to assist patients with anomia in retrieving words. The program capitalizes on patients' ability to retrieve partial information about an intended word (see Chapter 5 on the TOT state). Their brief case example was a patient with a thalamic lesion and mild symptoms of aphasia. Communication boards, which involve pointing to a specially organized set of printed words and/or pictures, may be employed with aphasic patients (Cohen, 1977).

Neuroassisted modes involve biofeedback via muscle action potentials and brain waves (Silverman, 1980), and their use by aphasic patients has not been demonstrated.

The possible pitfalls in training aphasic patients to use some nonspeech modes pertain to the central impairment of symbol function in aphasia and to the symbolic characteristics of a few nonspeech modes. Duffy, Duffy, and Pearson (1975) were skeptical of teaching patients new symbol systems when their deficit lies in the use of previously learned and highly automatic symbol systems. This problem does not necessarily exist with glossectomy, dysarthria, or cerebral palsy. The promotion of symbolic nonspeech modes for aphasia can be based on two faulty assumptions. One is that because cerebral palsy, mental retardation, and aphasia are neurological disorders, then all can benefit from the same treatment strategy. However, Bliss symbols may become functional for a cerebral-palsied child because of certain differences from aphasia, such as the maintenance of a cognitive system supportive of linguistic function. Ross (1979) reported successful training of the Bliss system to a nineteen-year-old with a traumatic brain injury, but this case was described as having no receptive language deficit and severely dysarthric speech. The second faulty assumption is that all nonspeech modes are considered equally. For example, DiSimoni (1981) used the aphasic person's maintenance of natural nonverbal modes as an argument for the use of any nonverbal mode. However, nonverbal modes vary widely from natural gestures to fairly complex semantic and syntactic systems.

As DiSimoni (1981) wrote, " . . . most of these methodologies have not been adequately tested with aphasic groups" (p. 333). Chen's (1971) subjects, for example, were described only as "26 patients with speech disturbance due to various causes" (p. 381). Then, Chen wrote that "patients with a sensory aphasia were unable to learn the manual alphabet" (p. 383). The best example of investigating these methods is Skelly's (1979) report on American Indian Gestural Code. Twelve of twenty aphasic patients achieved "propositional use" of the code. Two patients used all of the 200 signs presented, while nine patients achieved functional use of 14 to 80 signs. From field reports on the teaching of AMERIND code to sixty-seven other aphasic patients, "there was almost universal dissatisfaction expressed concerning transfer from the cued retrieval/replicative stage to self-initiated use" (p. 40).

The Patient's Capabilities with Language

Much of aphasic symptomatology possesses communicative value. This value sometimes is not recognized in the testing situation, which is designed to minimize the natural participation of the listener in a communicative interaction. Often the clinician simply counts the presence or absence of certain behaviors and compares linguistic behaviors against a standard of complete and accurate performance. However, in natural conversation the listener is formulating hypotheses about the patient's message by using the patient's limited or vague verbalizations as cues and by filling in gaps or disambiguating utterances with knowledge of the topic, patient, and situation. Recognition of the communicative value of aphasic behaviors can have an impact on what existing behaviors the clinician chooses to reinforce and on what new behaviors the clinician chooses to train the patient to use.

Holland (1977b, 1978) suggested that the criterion for reinforcing aphasic responses should involve a compromise on linguistic accuracy in favor of the communicative value of the utterance. That is, a clinician should shift from a tendency to frown upon circumlocutions or mildly agrammatic utterances toward a tendency to reinforce these productions and encourage their continued use. Though they are inefficient, circumlocutions often contain enough semantic information to convey the intended message. Adaptive strategies in Broca's aphasia (see Chapter 5) can be encouraged; these include a stressed opening word, adverbs to express time, and concatenation of phrases. Spending a great deal of time on training the inclusion of articles and verb tense markers may have less communicative value for the patient than training more efficient operation of an existing word-retrieval mechanism. Holland (1978) remarked that it is okay for the patient to be "in the ball park, rather than pitching a verbal no-hitter." This orientation to treatment leads to maximizing the patient's independence as a communicator.

What can your patient already do verbally which can facilitate communication? Many patients are able to comprehend better by learning to ask a speaker to "repeat please," "wait," or "slow down"; and these strategies can be taught in an hour (Holland, 1978). Also, patients possess self-cueing and self-correction strategies which enhance their communicative effectiveness. Luria (1970b) has described recovery as the response of intact brain to damage of one of its parts. This response was described by Mysak and Guarino (1981) as "the organism's intrinsic self-adjusting processes" (p. 215). Self-cueing and self-correction are behavioral manifestations of these hidden processes. Self-generated strategies for facilitating comprehension of *Revised Token Test* commands include (1) vocal or subvocal rehearsal of the stimulus, (2) delay of response, (3) immediacy or an unusually fast performance of the first part of a two-part command, (4) request for a repeat of the command, and (5) request for a second repetition (McNeil and Kozminsky, 1980). Vocal or subvocal rehearsal and immediacy were the most successful strat-

egies at 61 percent and 59 percent effectiveness, but they were not necessarily the most frequently used strategies. Therefore, some encouragement of these strategies might be warranted.

Self-generated cues to further verbal expression (Berman and Peelle, 1967) and self-correction strategies (Farmer, 1977; Farmer, O'Connell, and O'Connell, 1978; Marshall, Tompkins, Rau, et al. 1980) have been examined to some extent. Marshall, et al. investigated the frequency and success of self-correction behaviors in structured short-answer and single-word tasks "where behaviors can be easily defined and recorded" (p. 39). They identified three types of successful verbal self-correction behavior: (1) immediate, (2) effortful or non-immediate, and (3) cued, in which a self-generated related response leads to the correct response. The frequency of self-correction increased as the task became more difficult from verbal repetition to picture naming. Yet the proportion of successful self-corrections was the same for all tasks. Comparative use of the three types of successful self-correction was not reported in this article. The results do not suggest a clear path to a treatment strategy for improving the success of self-correction behavior. Easy tasks provide little opportunity to exercise these strategies; more difficult tasks may not be at a success rate which would be useful for a treatment exercise. Marshall indicated that these behaviors require additional study.

Environment and Significant Others

Silverman (1980) suggested that there are three reasons for an aphasic person to have limited motivation to communicate: (1) depression, (2) little or no need to communicate because needs are anticipated by others and there are limited opportunities to communicate, and (3) lack of positive reinforcement for communicating. The patient's environmental context can contribute to the presence of each of these factors. The effectiveness of communication with an aphasic patient can be improved not only by changing the patient but also by changing the patient's environment, which includes communicative settings and communicative partners. Lubinski (1981a) called this orientation *environmental language intervention.*

When the aphasic patient is living at home, this setting is often supportive. Familiar surroundings and the family contribute to the patient's adjustment and recovery by minimizing depression and providing opportunities to communicate and encouragement. However, when the patient is living in an institution such as a nursing home, the factors which reduce motivation can be present. Lubinski (1981) described the "communication-impaired environment," and the following are some of its characteristics:

1. It has rules that govern where, when, to whom, and what kind of communication might occur. There are few reasons to talk.

2. There are few places within the setting to have a private conversation.

3. The administration and staff do not value or reinforce communication among the residents or between residents and staff.

4. The problems of the residents themselves, many with dementia or aphasia, contribute to the limited communication opportunities.

5. Seating arrangements, poor lighting, and poor acoustics reduce communicative opportunities and efficiency (pp. 352–353).

Lubinski pointed out the wide variation among nursing homes as to whether they possess these characteristics, and she added that "successful communication . . . occurs in a climate that encourages interchange, that values and socially reinforces communication attempts and that minimizes the rules prohibiting communication" (p. 352).

The clinician's primary role in alle-

viating these communicative inhibitors is to evaluate the setting by looking for the presence of these conditions and then to assist the staff in making the necessary changes. Lubinski (1981a) provided a detailed checklist for assessing the communication environment. A responsibility commonly assumed by clinicians is conducting in-service programs for educating institutional staff about aphasia and communication with an aphasic resident. Frequent individualized follow-up with staff members is usually necessary in order to help them identify communicative strategies and more comfortable circumstances. Towey and Pettit's (1980) treatment of global aphasia included staff training in a small hospital. The clinician can work cooperatively with administrative staff to effect environmental changes in the most economical manner. Lubinski has made several specific suggestions for improving communication environments in general (Lubinski, 1981a) and nursing homes in particular (Lubinski, 1981b).

Because successful communication is a cooperative effort, especially in face-to-face conversation, any improvement in carrying out the listener role can improve communication with an aphasic speaker. Changing the listener can be one goal of family and institutional staff counseling (see Chapter 12). The listener can improve his or her patience in allowing the patient time to speak and can tune in carefully to all available cues to the patient's message. Martin (1981a) stated that we may wish "to improve performance of the clinician before we focus on the performance of the aphasic" (p. 152). He suggested that clinical technique can include "an attempt to understand and to respond to the intent and meaning underlying the aphasic's utterance, defective though it may be" (p. 152).

The aphasic's communication partner can also be improved as a speaker to enhance the patient's comprehension. Common recommendations include using a slow speaking rate and simplified but adult utterances. Pierce's (1981) study of sentence comprehension prompted the following conclusion: "...families should be informed that sentences that are consistent with the subject-verb-object present tense form may be easier for the aphasic patient to understand..." (p. 367). Tense may be recognized more readily with adverbial and auxiliary markers, such as "yesterday" and "has already."

Transfer from within the Clinic

Now we shift from changing the patient's world to bringing the patient's world into the clinic. Clinical procedures can be modified so that they reflect the characteristics of communication in the patient's real-life circumstances. As Florance, et al. (1980) put it, "Without addressing the overall anticipated impact of intervention in the patient's life system, we can spend enormous energy on exercises and drills that may never improve the patient's out-of-clinic interactions" (p. 285). Exercises and drills can be constructed with semantic content and materials which the patient confronts in everyday experience (Holland, 1978). If the patient is to practice following instructions, the instructions can be ones that the patient must follow outside the clinic. The patient can read in the clinic what he or she reads outside the clinic. A telephone can be used for practice in listening and speaking.

Role-playing can be a valuable means of lifting language regained in direct treatment to a more functional level of practice (see Schlanger and Schlanger, 1970). By assuming various roles, the clinician can place real-life demands on the patient's communicative skills. The clinician can be a waitress or waiter, while the patient orders from a menu. The clinician can be a spouse or operator talking to the patient over the phone.

The clinician should have a clear idea of the patient's communicative contexts and demands outside the clinic in order to construct lessons which incorporate these contexts and demands. If the clinician cannot visit the patient's home, for example, then a thorough interview with a family member can provide this information.

One approach to facilitating transfer from the clinic to the patient's living environment is to construct the clinical interaction between clinician and patient so that it is more consistent with real face-to-face conversation. *Promoting Aphasics' Communicative Effectiveness* or PACE therapy was designed to achieve this kind of interaction (Davis and Wilcox, 1981). PACE was developed out of a recognition that the standard direct-stimulation techniques described previously in this chapter do not coincide with the structure of natural conversation as closely as a structured treatment interaction could. Furthermore, a structure of interaction between clinician and patient which is more consistent with natural conversation can take advantage of many of the suggestions made by Wepman, Chapey, Silverman, Holland, Lubinski, and Martin for applying principles of communication to aphasia treatment. PACE focuses the patient and clinician on ideas to be conveyed rather than on the struggle for linguistic accuracy; divergent linguistic behavior is inherent to the interaction; multiple modes of communicating are encouraged; and active participation of the listener in a speaker's effort to convey a message becomes an essential ingredient in the interaction.

Procedures of PACE are derived from four principles, and each principle should be followed so that the interaction conforms to natural conversation. Any one principle might be applied to standard direct treatment, modifying it somewhat in order to achieve a particular goal. Principles 3 and 4 have been recommended frequently in the literature; however, principles 1 and 2 make PACE a relatively unique procedure:

1. *The clinician and patient participate equally as senders and receivers of messages.* The clinician and patient simply take turns conveying messages to each other, alternating as senders and receivers. This role-switching allows a variety of feedback operations to occur, and permits the clinician to model desirable communicative behaviors for the patient. Turn-taking differs from standard direct treatment in which the patient and clinician are focused on one role or the other.

2. *There is an exchange of new information between the clinican and the patient.* This may be the most powerful feature of PACE for creating a truly communicative interaction and for making this procedure different from standard direct treatment (see Davis, 1980). Also, it is the most difficult principle to maintain. In standard direct treatment of verbal expression, the stimulus or referent is usually in view of the clinician and the patient so that the topic of verbalization is shared. However, in natural conversation, some information is shared and part of the message is new to the listener. In PACE, message stimuli such as pictures of objects or actions are kept from view of the receiver. Usually a stack of stimulus cards is face down on the table, and the patient and clinician take turns drawing from the stack. This creates a situation in which the receiver does not already know what the sender is trying to convey, and so the receiver truly must try to figure out the sender's message. The new information principle enables the patient to experience communicative failures and to practice strategies for overcoming them.

The difficulty in maintaining a genuine new information condition lies in the participants' familiarity with the message stimuli. The clinician may select the stimuli and therefore already know what is in the stack of stimulus cards. As a receiver, the clinician may tend to figure out the patient's message by trying to remember what is in the stack of cards rather than by responding to the communicative effectiveness of the patient's behavior. This dilution of the new information condition can be minimized by using a large number of stimuli, changing stimuli at random from session to session, having someone else select the stimuli for a session, and by being aware of the problem and thereby responding to the communicative adequacy of the patient's behavior.

3. *The patient has a free choice as to which communicative channels (modalities) he or she may use to convey new information.* The clinician determines the communicative modalities which the patient can use, such as speech, writing, gesturing, drawing, and pointing to printed words. These are made available to the patient by providing a pencil and paper or a communication notebook. Also, the clinician, when taking a turn as sender, models the use of communicative options, especially in combination. While a patient may possess deficits in speech and symbolic gesturing, the two channels used together may convey a message better than when each channel is tried individually. The crucial feature of this principle is that the clinician *does not instruct or direct* the patient to use a particular strategy. This instruction is best reserved for standard direct treatment. Instead, the clinician allows the patient to discover the value of communicative options, especially when they are needed to overcome obstacles in conveying new information.

4. *Feedback is provided by the clinician, as a receiver, in response to the patient's success in conveying a message.* This contrasts with giving feedback based on how closely the pa-

tient comes to meeting a clinician's criterion for linguistic precision. The contingency for feedback in PACE corresponds to the criterion for best score on the *CADL* (see Chapter 8). A Broca's aphasic may convey a message successfully with one of the adaptive strategies described in Chapter 5, and an anomic aphasic may convey an idea with circumlocution. These behaviors are allowed and encouraged in PACE if they convey messages. Furthermore, communicative success depends not just on what the patient does, but also on the active participation of the clinician as receiver. The patient may give part of a message and the clinician may fill in the rest on the basis of making a good guess which is confirmed by the patient. The patient's success depends in part on the clinician's ability to comprehend, which is consistent with natural communicative interaction.

The content of feedback necessarily differs from the reinforcement and restimulation typical of standard treatment because of the new information condition. In standard direct treatment, the ability to respond to a patient's behavior with a cue to an intended word is derived from the clinician's already knowing what the patient is trying to convey. In PACE, the clinician either should not already know this or should act as if the message were not known beforehand. Feedback can only be given as a reflection of whether the message was understood or of guesses about what the message might be.

GROUP TREATMENT

A great deal of aphasia treatment during and after World War II was conducted with patients in groups (Huber, 1946; Sheehan, 1946, 1948; Wepman, 1951). The large number of aphasic patients in military hospitals made group treatment necessary, but group treatment also quickly came to be viewed as a valu-able supplement to individual treatment. Treatment of patients in groups was seen as having its own goals which could not be achieved in individual treatment, such as socialization, emotional support from peers, and another form of transfer from within the clinic. Wertz, Collins, Weiss, et al. (1981) found that eight hours per week of group discussion and recreation resulted in improved language function between six and eleven months postonset.

Brookshire (1978b) listed four general purposes of group activities: (1) *language treatment,* which in some cases is "clinician-directed, relatively structured, clinician controlled, and task-oriented . . . the kinds of activities which are carried out in individualized single-patient treatment sessions" (p. 156) and in other cases "may emphasize interaction among group members" (p. 157); (2) *transition,* which is to prepare the patient for discharge by providing practice with real-life problems; (3) *maintenance,* for patients who have been discontinued from a schedule of multiple sessions per week so that weekly or monthly meetings might maintain recovered levels of function; and (4) *support,* which was not explained as were the other three but which is probably a purpose associated with each type of group. Brookshire also referred to patient-family and family groups; but these are topics of Chapter 12.

Except for support, Brookshire's categories overlap with the purposes of individual treatment, which is directed toward language skills, transition, and maintenance. However, group treatment has a unique role relative to these categories. As Brookshire pointed out, it provides interactive aspects of language use which are not available in individual treatment; it provides some natural social situations to facilitate transition; and it is a convenient way to schedule a maintenance program. Any group session can provide emotional support and encouragement from other aphasics who understand the problem in ways not attainable by the clinician.

Group treatment has several values, according to Eisenson (1973). The opportunity to socialize provides a relaxed atmosphere for practice of verbal skills. Motivation can come from the special empathy of peers, and the patient feels less isolated. The patient realizes that he or she is not alone in carrying the burdens of aphasia. New appreciation for speech problems may come from observation of others; and one patient may use communicative strategies which another patient may want to try. The patient can respond to styles of language use that differ from the clinician's style, especially when family members are involved in the social period. Eisenson added that a group situation provides an atmosphere for ventilating feelings and airing grievances. These expressions might come forth more readily when listeners are likely to share the same feelings and, therefore, easily accept them.

The advantages vary in their prominence depending on whether the group is structured for practice of language skills, for pure relaxation during a full day of treatment, or for certain psychotherapeutic goals. Group treatment differs depending on the clinician's primary objective and, therefore, should not be considered to be a single entity.

Group treatment does have its risks, and these vary also depending on the purpose and structure of the interaction. Eisenson (1973) cited a few shortcomings; and Schuell, et al. (1964) expressed ambivalent feelings about group situations. Schuell objected strongly to group treatment if it is used as a replacement for individual treatment. The reduced time spent per patient led her to conclude that "we are unable to have confidence in group therapy as a basic method . . ." (p. 343). Because direct treatment of language requires individualized methods and materials, "group therapy is wasteful

and sometimes deleterious" (p. 344). However, Schuell, et al. quickly added that it can be a "good adjunct to individual treatment" (p. 344). Eisenson's list of shortcomings indicate a few risks. Withdrawn and severely impaired patients may be overwhelmed by a group situation. They may inhibit any speaking ability and may feel discouraged in comparison with higher levels of skill and recovery by the others. Group pressure may provoke an individual to talking about personal problems before he or she is ready. Especially when the group consists of members with widely varying abilities, it may bore or slow down the best member and be too demanding for the weakest member.

Although group treatment has been seen as being primarily a social or psychotherapeutic enterprise, it can be an extension of the experiences provided by the clinician for improving communicative skills and for instilling confidence in attained skills. Sociolinguistic skills such as conversational turn-taking can be practiced in a supportive environment where patients are encouraged by the clinician to help each other. The anomic aphasic can help the Broca's expand an utterance; the Broca's can help the anomic think of a word. Aphasic adults congratulate each other, advise each other, and argue with each other—all of which are normal adult communicative activities. Group treatment can be a combination of the two types of language activity described by Brookshire. It can be structured so that interaction among patients is emphasized and clinician-directiveness is minimized, and yet both qualities can be achieved with a task planned by the clinician. Principles of PACE may be incorporated by having patients take turns, convey new information, practice using multiple channels, and provide each other feedback to overcome communicative obstacles. Card games, for example, permit this type of interaction to occur. In this situation the patient becomes an independent communicator at a transitional stage between the security of individual treatment and the demands of real life.

SUMMARY

The idea that aphasia is an interference with language processes, as discussed in Chapter 4, has led to characterization of the clinician as a stimulator or "agent provocateur" for the patient. The clinician stimulates the patient in order to facilitate renewal of weakened processes. Treatment relies on the focal nature of the etiology in that some functions are spared and others are merely reduced in efficiency because of the interconnections among areas of the brain. The goals are to improve the functioning of impaired processes and to enhance the use of remaining functions which can convey messages. The overall goal is to improve the patient's ability to communicate.

This chapter offered a panorama of basic approaches to treating aphasia. Since rehabilitation efforts began in earnest in the mid-1940s, the most widely used form of treatment has been direct stimulation of deficient language functions. Specific goals are shaped in terms of the patient's primary deficits. Direct treatment may involve the exercise of language within one modality or another, or may entail stimulation and response with multiple modalities simultaneously or in sequence. The clinician may provide special instructions and cues which facilitate the recovery processes of intrasystemic and intersystemic reorganization. Indirect approaches consist of conversational interactions which direct the patient away from struggle to retrieve words and of tasks which promote divergent response instead of the convergent response of direct treatment. Also, attention to communication leads to the clinician's encouraging or teaching alternative modes for conveying ideas, reinforcing language which gets the idea across, making adjustments in the patient's communicative environment, and creating clinical activities which reflect real-life communicative demands.

Generally, no matter what task is used in standard direct treatment, the interaction between clinician and patient follows a consistent pattern. The clinician presents a stimulus; the patient makes a response; and the clinician responds with feedback to the patient. The manner in which this is done is a major topic of the following chapter.

11 Treatment Procedures

In the previous chapter, procedures were occasionally cited in order to illustrate general principles and approaches. Chapter 11 is merely an extension of Chapter 10. The early emphasis will be on procedures used for different symptoms and primary deficits. The procedures described here should be considered to be examples of what has been done or what can be done, but should not be taken as examples of what must be done. That is, creative variations of these examples are encouraged so that procedures conform to each patient's version of aphasia as well as to each patient's communicative needs and interests.

AUDITORY COMPREHENSION

Schuell oriented clinicians toward using auditory stimulation as a means of improving all language functions (Schuell, et al., 1964; Duffy, 1981). Subsequently, improving auditory comprehension itself became an important objective of treatment. This objective is particularly crucial for improving the communication capacity of severely impaired patients. It may be the only modality through which they possess some degree of spared natural language

function. Improved auditory comprehension with global aphasia may result at least in more appropriate nonverbal expression in response to the speech of others. Wernicke's aphasics have the additional problem of failing to monitor and control their neologistic fluent output. For most cases, exercising auditory comprehension is a primary emphasis of early treatment; at any linguistic level, the patient should demonstrate comprehension before he or she exercises verbal expression at that level.

Exercises for Auditory Problems

Attention. The patient with severe Wernicke's aphasia soon after onset often has difficulty attending to simple tasks designed to exercise word comprehension. The clinician struggles to get the patient to listen to a word and then to point to a picture. The patient appears not to understand what he is supposed to do and, in addition, tends to talk instead of listen. This problem is included in what Sparks (1978) called a poor "therapeutic set." In addition to distractibility and short attention span, the Wernicke's aphasic may possess "a rather flamboyant personality" and does not acknowledge the need for treatment. This patient does not accept readily what the clinician wants him to do.

Therefore, a therapeutic set needs to be established with the patient who is inattentive and unaware of a language problem. The patient should be trained to listen to a discrete auditory stimulus and to make a differential response relative to two choices. Initial auditory stimuli can be nonverbal, such as environmental sounds, and the patient is directed to point to a picture representing the sound source. The clinician may demonstrate the task and direct the patient to imitate a pointing response. As soon as the patient gets the idea of listening to a sound and then pointing to the related picture, the clinician can begin to insert words into the series of nonverbal simuli. Numbers also may be employed in this fashion, in which response choices are an array of digits and/or quantities arranged in numerical sequence. Numerical sequence is a cue that is inherent to this arrangement. Once the patient points accurately to numbers in response to auditory stimulation, the cue of sequence can be faded by placing the response choices in random order. Also, each auditory stimulus can be presented, first, in numerical sequence, then, in random order. The objective is to establish consistent listening and pointing before utilizing this interaction structure in the exercise of more relevant word and phrase comprehension.

Patients may have occasional flights of inattention which can be corrected with an *alerting signal* prior to stimulus presentation (Marshall, 1978; Martinoff, et al., 1980). Eye contact with the patient should be ensured prior to each stimulus. Alerting signals include saying the patient's name, touching the patient, or simply saying "ready" or "listen."

Severe Comprehension Deficit. Once the patient attends to stimuli and makes appropriate differential responses, the clinician can begin exercises of language comprehension at the single-word level. The basic task is the clinician's saying a word and the patient's pointing to a picture from at least two choices. Instructions are kept simple and, because of the comprehension deficit, often are accompanied by demonstration. Variables for modulating task difficulty are listed in Table 11-1. The easiest task might consist of familiar nouns spoken twice by the clinician. The picture choices would be semantically distant from each other. With severe impairments, a small vocabulary is used so that the patient practices the same item several times. The vocabulary set is enlarged continuously as comprehension improves. Feedback upon error includes repeating the word, repeating with a redundant verbal context, or repeating and showing the printed form of the word. Once correct responding is achieved on 95 to 100 percent of the trials with a large vocabulary, the clinician may put demands on processing rate by speeding up the trials, presenting the next stimulus immediately after the preceding response.

Hopefully, this drill will jar loose the use of language in other modalities. Some

TABLE 11-1. Difficulty of the picture-pointing task for severe comprehension deficit can be modulated by several variables. These variables are considered for creating task hierarchies.

Word Comprehension

Stimulus:	Familiarity (*pillow* vs. *gibbon*)
	Emotionality (spouse's name vs. *man/woman*)
	Word class (*bed* vs. *sleep*)
	Datedness (*refrigerator* vs. *ice box*)
	Repetition (*bed, bed*)
	Context (*You sleep on a bed*)
	Rate of trial presentation
Response:	Number of picture choices
	Relatedness between/among choices
	Picture vs. picture + printed word
	Imposed delay of response

patients may start talking, and so this task becomes applicable for improving verbal expression. Word reading may be detected when stimuli are augmented with printed words; a corresponding task focused on printed word comprehension can be added to the session. The clinician capitalizes on evidence of other renewed skills while closely observing the patient's behavior on any task, especially on the simple tasks with severely impaired patients. However, the most severely impaired patients are not likely to exhibit much sprouting into other language functions during basic auditory stimulation.

Wernicke's aphasia poses a problem when press for speech interferes with attention to the auditory stimulus. Whitney (cited in Holland, 1977) coined the term *stop strategy* for these patients, a strategy in which the clinician wants the patient to stop talking. Neologistic jargon serves little useful purpose and interferes with comprehension. In the context of a word-comprehension task, a raised hand or an alerting signal when the patient starts talking should reduce interference from press for speech. The patient eventually gets the idea that he or she should be listening instead of talking.

Short-Term Memory and Sequencing Deficit. When task planning was explained in Chapter 10, the difference between exercising comprehension and stretching short-term memory capacity illustrated how treatment is focused on a particular process. Taxing STM capacity without involving pressure on comprehension entails selecting a linguistic unit which is comprehended easily and then chaining this unit in a series of two, three, or more. This sequence is presented along with a set of pictures for the patient to show recall of the series. Processing demands can be manipulated in the clinician's instructions regarding the expected response. Capacity is reflected in accurate

retrieval of all units, no matter what order they are recalled. Sequencing is an additional burden when the patient is asked to point to all units in order of presentation.

Recall of sequences of linguistic units has been a common device used to place increasing demands on comprehension, a way of increasing comprehension task difficulty. Martinoff, et al. (1980) provided a large section of tasks involving recall and sequencing, such as the following items from one task: Level 1, "Show me what you sit on and then show me what gives light"; Level 3, "Show me a piece of furniture, a fixture, where you sleep and then where you sit" (p. 68). These "point to" sequences are a common procedure for exercising auditory comprehension in moderately and mildly impaired patients (Marshall, 1981). The example just given would be appropriate for mild impairment, while pointing to a series of objects would be for moderate impairment. Also, once a severely impaired patient becomes successful comprehending single words, it is common for the clinician to heighten difficulty by presenting two words to recall (see Salvatore and Davis, 1979). This increases processing demand without adding new linguistic features to the stimulus. While these tasks become unnatural with respect to the language usually confronted in most everyday situations, they do increase complexity while maintaining a simple, nonverbal pointing response and a requirement to process the entire utterance. Generalization to natural language, however, is achieved better if heightening complexity is based on linguistic features and rate of processing in addition to chaining units together.

STM time of storage demands can be added to a comprehension task by imposed filled and unfilled delays of response (see Chapter 5). Though not requiring a distractor to fill a delay of response may allow for rehearsal of the stimulus, rehearsal may not be invoked by patients with

Broca's aphasia anyway (Rothi and Hutchinson, 1981). Filled delays have been used with Token Test commands and were found to increase difficulty of comprehension (DeRenzi, Faglioni, and Previdi, 1978).

Deficient Sentence Comprehension.

Most patients are given sentence-comprehension exercises at some point in their treatment. Wernicke's aphasics are likely to reach a level of comprehension, at least with simple subject-verb-object sentences. Broca's aphasics find such sentences to be rather undemanding unless they must decide upon a picture based on identifying the order of subject and object in a reversible sentence (see Chapter 5). Published aphasia treatment manuals, however, do not provide materials which hook into the special problems of Broca's aphasia. If agrammatic comprehension is a genuine primary deficit, then the best ideas for exercising the deficient function may be found in such journals as *Brain and Language* and *Cortex*.

The tasks for exercising sentence comprehension are the same as those used for assessing this function: pointing to pictures, following instructions, answering questions, and sentence verification.

While **pointing to pictures** is a frequent experimental procedure, it is a relatively uneconomical treatment procedure when the clinician wants to tune the task to the patient's deficit. This tuning involves constructing picture-choice decisions based on one feature of syntactic structure or on processing the entire sentence. One example involves prepositions where the picture choices would keep semantic content constant and force a decision between two or three spatial or temporal relationships. To accomplish this with a wide variety of semantic content and prepositions requires finding and/or drawing many special pictures. Moreover, if the picture choice involves a change of an actor, object, or action, the patient need only deal

with part of the sentence. If the pictures are totally different, only one part of the sentence need be recognized to make the choice.

These dilemmas are a few reasons for the tendency to deploy **following instructions** as a comprehension activity. The Token Test was a model for stimuli presented by Holland and Sonderman (1974), who found that poor comprehenders did not improve on the task and improvements of others did not generalize to other direction-following tasks. West (1973) and Flowers and Danforth (1979) described programs with the structure of Token Test commands but with objects instead of tokens: "Touch the big yellow comb" or "Put the spoon behind the quarter and the thread under the key." West (1973) found improved Token Test scores following her procedure. Kearns and Hubbard (1977) reported rank order of difficulty of several instructions involving sequences of object manipulations. While many of these auditory stimuli could be described as asking the patient to perform unnatural acts, the patient must exercise auditory skills across the entire instruction without the aid of natural situational contexts. Some patients may scoff at putting spoons behind quarters, especially those with moderate-to-mild impairments, and more sensical tasks should be considered.

Compensatory modes of presenting instructions to severely impaired patients have been investigated. Patients were more accurate comprehending instructions when given in the combined modes of speech and pantomime (Beukelman, Yorkston, and Waugh, 1980). Klor (1980) demonstrated that instructions can be followed by aphasics when presented as line drawings. The treatment in these cases is supplemented with changing communicative behaviors of persons in the patient's environment.

One way of getting at specific features of sentence structure and content without some of the problems of picture pointing is with **sentence verification** tasks. Only one picture is needed per sentence, and false decisions can be based on a variety of differences between the sentence and the picture, including content, word order, and preposition (see Chapter 5).

Answering questions is a common treatment procedure (see Martinoff, et al., 1980; Ross and Spencer, 1980). Questions requiring a yes/no response minimize verbalization; but if answers to questions are within the expressive capability of a patient, then such tasks still focus on comprehension. An advantage of questions is that the clinician does not have to find pounds of pictures or display odd combinations of objects. The clinician need only ask "Does your wife have blond hair?" or "Is grass green?" Another advantage is that content can readily have personal significance for the patient. Memory demands are increased by presenting a statement and asking a question about it: "The bus can pick you up at 1:00 and bring you home at 4:00. When does the bus pick you up?" A question about a statement should be answerable by the patient's understanding the statement rather than from the patient's knowledge. The clinician reads aloud a paragraph to mildly impaired comprehenders, and then asks questions about information in the paragraph. These paragraphs are obtained from reading materials of interest to the patient.

Some of the factors to consider in creating a sentence-comprehension task are summarized in Table 11-2. These variables are manipulated in making a task easier when needed or in planning ahead for more challenging tasks.

Comprehension Programs

A few manuals are available which provide exercises for language comprehension. Each consists of suggested auditory stimuli and pictures for the patient to choose from in making a pointing response.

Marshall's *Clinician Controlled Auditory Stimulation for Aphasic Adults* (1978) was devised because "aphasia clinicians generally devote too little time to designing

TABLE 11-2. Variation in sentence-comprehension exercises is considered in planning a task at the patient's level of success and in planning progression of difficulty. These variables have been shown to make a difference in patients' success (see Chapter 5).

Sentence Comprehension

Task:	Point to pictures
	Follow instructions
	Verify sentences
	Answer questions
Stimulus:	Length
	Structural complexity (affirmative vs. passive)
	Rate, pauses
	Meaningfulness (object names vs. tokens)
	Semantic plausibility (*Pound the nail* vs. *Put the nail in your hat*)
	Reversibility of subject and object
	Redundancy in context (Seron and Deloche, 1981)
	Linguistic cues (Pierce, 1981)
Response:	Number of picture choices
	Relatedness between/among choices
	Picture foils (word change vs. order change)
	Complexity of gestural response
	Complexity of verbal response

and evaluating the effects of auditory stimulation therapy, and often begin work on verbal production tasks too early'' (p. 1). The kit contains 360 object pictures affixed to a binder in three stacks of paired objects so that the patient may choose from two, four, or six pictures in an exercise. Also, the pictures are arranged so that response decisions may involve a semantic, phonemic, or no relationship between words represented by the pictures. A detailed manual provides suggestions for stimuli at different linguistic levels. Marshall gives examples of stimuli rather than complete lists of stimuli, thereby encouraging the clinician to be flexible in planning a task. Guidelines refer to variations in manner of presentation such as rate, pause insertion, and delaying response. Forms assist the clinician in task planning and scoring.

Martinoff, Martinoff, and Stokke's *Language Rehabilitation: Auditory Comprehension* (1980) differs from Marshall's manual in that it contains a greater number of task examples, more complex stimuli, and lists of stimuli that could be presented in an exercise. Another difference is that there are minimal guidelines so that the manual is best employed by a clinician with experience in planning tasks for different types and degrees of aphasia. A booklet contains seven sections, with several exercises in each: answering yes/no questions, following commands, auditory sequencing, auditory discrimination, auditory reasoning (words), auditory reasoning (statements), and auditory reasoning (paragraphs). ''Reasoning'' simply refers to various semantic and syntactic decisions forced by the type of stimuli and responses. The booklet is accompanied by pictures of objects and some situational drawings stuffed with content. Their *probe* technique for planning where to begin each section involves sampling performance on each activity to determine where the patient begins to have difficulty. A valuable feature is the numerous paragraph-level stimuli for mildly impaired patients.

Other manuals of comprehension exercises include Keith's *Graduated Language Training for Patients with Aphasia and Children with Language Deficiencies* (1980) and Baer's *The Aphasic Patient: A Program for Auditory Comprehension and Language Training* (1976). Both offer pictures for pointing tasks and naming tasks, and Baer's program contains semantic content targeted for the hospitalized patient. Ross and Spencer (1980) published a book of exercises for auditory comprehension and expression. Their book contains only a few pictures at three levels of familiarity. Exercises include stimuli based only on these pictures, and so the content of treatment is not varied or tailored to the individual—a limitation of all of these published programs. Therefore, these manuals provide suggestions but not complete individualized treatment programs.

VERBAL EXPRESSION

While treatment of auditory comprehension involves relating linguistic levels and processing demands to severity of deficit, treatment of verbal expression can often be focused on qualitatively different symptoms such as inability to retrieve words, agrammatism, and press for speech. The most basic direction of direct treatment is to stimulate the use of appropriate verbal expression in any way imaginable and at a level which is better than what the patient can do normally without such stimulation. The auditory comprehension activities just mentioned stimulate heightened verbalization in some patients, especially when they are not asked to verbalize. Multimodal stimulation, described in Chapter 10, stimulates word retrieval in some when no other circumstances can. Such stimulation may get the mental gears of expression moving with great enough ease so that they can be put into operation in natural communicative situations where the gears had once stood still. Early in treatment the patient depends on the clinician to lubricate these gears; eventually the patient must do the best he or she can on his or her own.

Global Aphasia

Treatment of the most severe aphasia has had mixed results (DiCarlo, 1980; Sarno, Silverman, and Sands, 1970; Sarno and Levita, 1981). It appears that these patients improve at least in auditory comprehension and use of gestures (see Chapter 9). Direct language treatment is tried with everyone soon after onset; and, when little change of deficient language functions occurs, the clinician emphasizes compensatory communicative strategies. Nonverbal symbol systems have been examined on an experimental basis (see Chapter 5). Nevertheless, treatment begins based on principles and methodologies already reviewed, emphasizing auditory comprehension and retention and watching for any appearance of verbalization.

From the start of treating global aphasia, the hard realities of this disorder should be recognized as Marshall, Tompkins, Rau, et al. (1979) pointed out. They found that while test scores improved after at least two months of treatment, communicative ability did not change in daily life. Marshall, et al. suggested that more than one or two months of standard direct treatment is not warranted for the severely aphasic person, a conclusion which would be of interest to anyone paying for these services. One or two months is necessary because Broca's aphasia may emerge from what only initially appears to be global aphasia.

However, this pessimistic outlook, while correct in many respects, is still based on language-specific goals and not on communicative goals. Marshall acknowledged that perhaps all possibilities

for rehabilitation have not been exhausted. A small number of severely impaired patients have been able to communicate on a limited basis within the structure of PACE by using nonverbal channels. In the previous section on auditory comprehension, the value of combined verbal and nonverbal inputs was suggested. Communication with these patients can be improved by concentrating on people in the patient's environment, enhancing their stimuli to the patient, and refining their interpretation of the patient's nonverbal cues (Towey and Pettit, 1980).

Nancy Helm-Estabrooks has advocated direct training which capitalizes on existing verbal and nonverbal behaviors (Albert, Goodglass, Helm, et al., 1981; Helm and Barresi, 1980). Her Visual Action Therapy (VAT) is a program of finely graded tasks intended to develop gesturing as a substitute communicative channel. Patients must be able to match pictures and objects as a prerequisite skill. The program utilizes a set of eight objects, such as a salt shaker and a hammer, and consists of twelve steps. Nearly 100 percent correctness is required to move from one step to the next. Stimuli include large and small line drawings of the eight objects and eight drawings, called action pictures, of the objects being manipulated. The first six steps are designed to train recognition and production of gestures, using the objects with contextual cues such as a nail and a block of wood with the hammer. The last six steps move the patient toward gesturing without the objects, called "representational gesturing."

Severe Expressive Deficit

Some patients develop or already possess fairly good comprehension but fail to initiate propositional verbalization or struggle desperately to produce a few occasional isolated words. Furthermore, long periods of standard direct stimulation may not change this situation. These patients may be saddled with apraxia of speech on top of a severe agrammatism. A few special procedures have been developed for this problem.

Melodic Intonation Therapy. MIT was introduced in Chapter 10 as an excellent example of programming steps of direct stimulation. It was reported first by Albert, Sparks, and Helm (1973) with three case studies. Sparks, Helm, and Albert (1974) described the procedure in more detail, reported favorable outcomes with respect to the *BDAE,* and listed characteristics of patients who benefited most from the program. In addition to auditory comprehension being better than verbal expression, these patients recognized their own verbal errors, had fairly good emotional stability and attention spans, had the poorest pre-MIT repetition skills of all patients who received the program, and possessed some stereotypic speech. The good candidate is a nonfluent aphasic (Sparks, 1981).

The complete program has been presented elsewhere and, therefore, is not detailed here (Sparks and Holland, 1976; Sparks, 1981). MIT takes advantage of the curious phenomenon in which some severely impaired aphasics can sing the melody and words of familiar songs (Keith and Aronson, 1975). A spared right hemisphere may be responsible for leaving this ability intact.

American Indian Sign Code. Madge Skelly and her colleagues introduced AMERIND as a supplemental communication mode for patients with severe apraxia of speech and aphasia (Skelly, Schinsky, Smith, et al., 1974). A complete training program and illustrations of several signs were subsequently published (Skelly, 1979). Simmons and Zorthian (1979) demonstrated the teaching of these signs to a patient with Wernicke's aphasia. Skelly (1977) has been careful to distinguish between AMERIND and sign languages for the deaf: "Indian Hand Talk was created to provide a universal communication mode among the many tribes who did not share a common language" (p. 746). The signs directly depict concepts and concrete referents and are in many ways like pantomime. A "dialect" was developed so that the signs could be done with one hand.

The first group of patients who learned AMERIND had gestural scores which greatly surpassed their verbal scores on the *PICA,* a pattern similar to patients who were helped by MIT (Skelly, et al., 1974). Five patients had received at least six months of prior language treatment without improvement of verbal scores. Three of these patients, who had at least twelve months of prior treatment, improved at least 6.29 points on the verbal section of the *PICA* during AMERIND training. The gesture system seemed to draw two and three-word phrases out of these patients. One advantage of this system is that it is understood by others without special training. "The motivated viewer with a modicum of visual imagination interprets Indian Sign without any instruction at the 80 to 88 percent level, and in many instances even higher" (Skelly, 1977, p. 746).

Word-Retrieval Deficits

Word retrieval has been the most common target of aphasia treatment. Schuell's multimodal stimulation was designed to elicit words. Other early treatment programs led the patient to this end (Keenan, 1966; Taylor and Marks, 1959). The core activity for training word retrieval has been confrontation naming, and methods for eliciting words in this way have been referred to in Chapters 5 and 10. Cueing procedures to facilitate picture naming may be part of the clinician's initial stimulus or may be augmenting feedback upon occasional retrieval failure. The clinician attempts to elicit words from all patients:

from the Wernicke's aphasic after some comprehension and shutdown of neologistic jargon have been achieved; from the Broca's aphasic in order to increase efficiency; and from the anomic aphasic to improve search accuracy and efficiency. The confrontation-naming procedure is basically the same for all patients, but some respond to supplemental cues better than others.

Treatment of word retrieval varies among patients according to the type of word-retrieval activity which can be managed, especially with respect to auditory input. The main point of this section is that word retrieval can and should be exercised in a wide variety of circumstances in addition to the picture-naming task. Many of these circumstances were surveyed in Chapter 5. Some conditions elicit words better than others for each patient. Variables to be considered in manipulating retrieval difficulty are summarized in Table 11–3.

Activities which can challenge the moderate-to-mildly impaired patient include

TABLE 11-3. Variables in basic word-retrieval activities are considered in planning appropriate tasks. Most of these variables have been demonstrated to make a difference in the patient's ability to retrieve words (see Chapter 5).

Word Retrieval

Stimulus:	Referent (with or without verbal cue)
	Familiarity of referent
	Uncertainty of referent
	Operativity of referent
	Object vs. action
	Verbal (completions, associations, questions)
	Rate of item presentation
	Personal meaningfulness (emotionality)
Response:	Word frequency
	Grammatical class
	Convergent vs. divergent
	Degree of accuracy required
	Number of words required
	Expected latency of response

giving synonyms and opposites, divergent tasks, and answering questions. Demands on the retrieval system are increased with rapid pacing of the tasks. Once accuracy is achieved on any word-retrieval task, the patient should be instructed to respond more quickly to see how fast he or she can come up with a word or several words.

More severely impaired patients may be given retrieval exercises which are built from simple repetition or reading aloud. Retrieval becomes a factor as memory demands are imposed upon repetition. Again, unfilled and filled response delays can be employed to force the patient into more demanding recall. The interval between stimulus presentation and permission to respond can be increased gradually subsequent to success at each interval. Also, systematic hierarchical cueing can be instituted, as described later in this chapter (pages 277–278).

Some skepticism has arisen as to whether confrontation-naming drills have any impact, at least on retrieval of words not practiced in treatment. Brookshire (1975a) found that ten aphasic subjects did not generalize to other words. He wrote "The author's clinical experiences with naming training have generally been unsatisfactory. Prolonged drill on object or picture naming has generally been frustrating for the aphasic individual, and has not appeared to be very effective in improving the individual's general word-retrieval abilities" (p. 64). Brookshire's procedure in this study included imitation as a facilitator (or "prompt"). Wiegel-Crump and Koenigsknecht (1973) administered regular probes of words and semantic categories not included in training. They found generalization to untrained items by four subjects. Two differences between these studies may have contributed to different conclusions: (1) Brookshire's subjects varied in degree of impairment from 28 to 82 percentile points on the *PICA*, while Wiegel-Crump's subjects were anomic aphasics; (2) Brookshire studied only imitative cues in confrontation naming, while Wiegel-Crump employed a variety of cues which supplemented the pictures. Therefore, the effectiveness of confrontation naming may depend on the type of disorder and the type of naming task employed as treatment. The effectiveness of treating the patient with a wide variety of word-retrieval activities, including divergent tasks, has not been studied in this way. Also, "general word retrieval abilities," indicated by a variety of tasks, have not been explored adequately as a criterion for generalization.

Agrammatism

While Whitney advocated a stop strategy for Wernicke's aphasia, she advocated a *go strategy* for Broca's aphasia (cited in Holland, 1977). The thrust of treatment for the latter is to encourage as much verbalization as possible in order to get the verbal formulation mechanism started and to keep it running. When the Broca's aphasic has a severe apraxia of speech, expressive agrammatism is difficult to approach directly, and so this work should be preceded by some treatment for the apraxia (see Rosenbek, 1978).

The most direct route to stimulating verbal output in agrammatic patients is with **verbal repetition,** occasionally supplemented with reading aloud. The objective of any treatment of this symptom is to increase completeness of the patient's spontaneous utterances. While the Wernicke's aphasic is usually unable to repeat, the Broca's aphasic is able to verbalize better in repetition than in spontaneous speech. Repetition can be part of a package of cues, to be explained shortly, which are faded gradually in the direction of best possible spontaneous output. Wiegel-Crump (1976) treated agrammatic patients primarily with repetition to facilitate picture description; she would have the patient repeat an utterance up to ten times or until two complete sentence repetitions were achieved. To maximize success in

practice, utterances are chosen which have been just beyond the reach of the patient's current regular spontaneous production. The patient should be able to repeat most (80 percent) of these utterances, with occasional omission of functors. Hain and Lainer (1977, 1980) described a program of repetition accompanying pictures drawn to depict several grammatical features.

Feedback in response to error on repetition tasks is usually intended to stimulate the patient to fill in missing words. If the patient does not recognize that an omission has occurred, the clinician may repeat back what the patient has actually said. This is considered to be a minimal cue to encourage patient independence through self-correction. The maximum feedback cue is what Wiegel-Crump (1976) called *expansion,* which is retaining the words spoken by the patient and adding the missing functors. She also used *modeling* as feedback, which was a well-formed sentence which did not contain the content in the patient's response. Modeling can be helpful feedback when responses are correct, after the clinician acknowledges the completeness of the response. In this instance, the feedback is a conversational response in order to see if even more verbalization comes forth from the patient. Such exchanges provide the clinician with an opportunity to determine whether additional capabilities are being developed for which other stimuli can be planned.

Picture-description drills without saying a sentence as the initial stimulus can be a next step of treatment and involve the same clinician feedback upon error. Pictures are selected based on the length and complexity of expected response. *Agent + action* sentences are elicited with pictures of simple actions such as an athlete running. Simple actions are contained within pictures depicting *agent + action + object,* for which two articles and one verb auxiliary can be part of the response goal. Instructions to the patient would be to describe each picture in a complete sentence.

In order to follow the general principle of providing the least cueing which ensures success, it has been desirable to cue the patient to say complete sentences without having to present the whole sentence. The clinician wants to escape from repetition as soon as possible at each linguistic level being exercised. Showing the patient a printed version along with the picture at least removes the auditory component of the cue and injects transcoding into the task. These cues can be removed gradually, word by word, from right to left. Also, Luria's (1970b) externalization of inner schemas, introduced in Chapter 10, is another intermediate step between repetition and spontaneous picture description. These nonverbal cues can be paired with printed phrases, and these phrases can be faded first, followed by the nonverbal cues (Davis, 1973). The nonverbal cues described by Luria assist the patient in coming close to spontaneous production of complete sentences. As with any programming, initial stimuli which have been faded can be reused as feedback upon error at more advanced levels.

Specific grammatical structures can be targeted for the patient's response by presenting a different kind of stimulus. Helm-Estabrooks, et al. (1981) has incorporated Gleason and Goodglass' Story Completion Test into a treatment program for agrammatism. At one level, the patient repeats the target sentence after a delay. At the next level, the patient completes the story with an accompanying picture.

The impaired central processor of syntax can be exercised with certain **metalinguistic tasks.** Sorting printed words into sentences which describe a picture (or without a picture) is a derivative of early research on agrammatism (see Shewan, 1976b; Smith, 1974b). Also the patient can be presented with grammatical and subtly ungrammatical sentences and be asked to (1) recognize correct and incorrect sentences and (2) correct the incorrect sentence. Making corrections can be assisted by presenting a printed version of the anomalous sentence (Bliss, Guilford, and Tikofsky, 1976). This could be a step prior to improvement of the patient's ability to correct his or her own errors. It is similar to the previously recommended feedback of repeating the patient's incomplete response and allowing him or her to attempt a correction.

A "verbing strategy" was developed by Loverso, Selinger, and Prescott (1979) to facilitate production of *agent-action-object* sentences. The authors reported performances of two subjects but did not describe the subjects' symptom pattern. They used the "verb as core" by presenting them as "pivot-stimuli" and then asking *who* and *what* questions to elicit complete sentences orally and graphically. Shewan (1976b) gave a Broca's aphasic a printed verb along with a picture and asked him to produce a sentence from these stimuli. Gallaher (1981) studied ten agrammatic subjects by presenting printed verbs and having the subjects place agents and objects on either side.

When the patient is ready to string sentences into a narrative (or discourse), one facilitating structure is the presentation of sequenced pictures which depict a series of connected events. Such "story sequence cards" are common among commercial treatment materials. Performances by Broca's and Wernicke's aphasics were analyzed in detail by Gleason, et al. (1980; see Chapter 5). In the spirit of enhancing communicative adequacy and confidence, it is not necessary to delay administering such stimuli until the patient can describe single pictures fluently. The patient should be encouraged to string incomplete sentences together in discourse which still conveys a theme and a variety of ideas.

Jargon

In the section on treating comprehension, a stop strategy was recommended because jargon, especially neologistic jargon, serves no useful communicative purpose. It is incomprehensible and interferes with auditory processing. To clear the path for comprehension, the patient should establish a therapeutic set and learn to "put a noose around his speech and pull it in." Once this is done and comprehension improves, some of these patients begin to repeat. Getting to this point, however, may take several months. Once repetition is established, the exercising of meaningful speech can begin. However, the focus of early treatment for Wernicke's aphasia is comprehension, which is needed for communication and for controlling press for speech.

This approach differs from the approach Martin (1981a, 1981b) rejected and the approach he recommended. He wrote: "There are two ways to deal with jargon: first, to correct faulty speech itself—the thrust of most speech therapy; and second, to improve the clinician as a listener" (Martin, 1981b, p. 317). Direct modification of neologistic jargon has not been demonstrated, especially because of inability to repeat and poor responsiveness to word-retrieval cues. The stop strategy is useful instead. Martin, however, gave a few examples of how words and phrases in fluent aphasia can be communicative and recommended that clinicians and significant others learn to interpret this speech better. He described interference to communication which is created by trying to correct a word-retrieval error when context conveys the message. The linguistic contexts for his examples were not provided, leaving it unclear as to whether fluent neologistic or semantic jargon was being analyzed. Therefore, Martin's recommendation awaits evidence to support its basic assumption about the communicative adequacy of expression in Wernicke's aphasia.

A communication-oriented strategy is warranted for Wernicke's aphasia. PACE assists the patient in turn-taking, listening to a speaker, and experiencing communicative success when jargon is inhibited and gestures are attempted. This type of therapy may be best applied after a period of direct treatment of comprehension and after some inhibition of jargon has been achieved.

Another consideration in treating Wernicke's aphasia is speculative but is derived from the possibility that a primary deficit is disorganization of semantic memory. The experiments surveyed in Chapter 5, which are suggestive of this deficit, harbor some procedures which could be evaluated as treatment for this syndrome. If semantic constriction or disorganization is a primary deficit, then exercises of sorting pictures into categories ought to be accompanied or followed by changes in language function. This is a question for clinical research.

GENERAL CONSIDERATIONS IN DIRECT TREATMENT

Only a few examples of treatment activities have been given here as an indication of the type of task used for different problems. The following overview focuses on procedural considerations that are applicable to most direct treatment tasks. The literature has established certain consistent rules and guidelines for what the clinician actually does. Most procedures fit within the interaction structure of a task trial: clinician's *stimulus*—patient's *response*—clinician's *feedback*.

Instructions to the Patient

A vital consideration in the administration of treatment activities is task instructions. The clinician begins each task by informing the patient of the type of stimulus to be presented and of the response expected. The purpose of the activity is explained, especially for moderately and mildly impaired patients. Instructions are direct and stated simply. Though they may have to be revised if not understood initially, extended revisions of an instruction become confusing. Therefore, the clinician usually plans the instruction when planning a task in order to avoid extended revisions. Encouraging instructions have been shown to promote better performance than discouraging instructions (Stoicheff, 1960).

Clinician's Stimulus

Several of Schuell's principles of treatment focused on the clinician's stimulation of the patient. Her earliest list of principles (Schuell, Carroll, and Street, 1955) was modified about ten years later (Schuell, et al., 1964), but the central theme continued to be use of intensive and controlled auditory stimulation. It should be an adequate stimulus so that "the stimuli we use get into the brain" and ". . . the patient can perceive it" (Schuell, et al., 1964, p. 339). Also, the stimulus should elicit, not force, a response. That is, the patient's response should come naturally from what the clinician does.

Schuell's principles are consistent with operant conditioning and programmed learning in terms of the general importance of the *antecedent event* in speech-language treatment (Hedrick, Christman, and Augustine, 1973). Instead of focusing on the consequent event to shape responses, the clinician relies on planning the antecedent event so that it achieves the expected response. Bollinger and Stout (1976) used the concept of "stimulus power" to explain programming for aphasics, where power of the stimulus is manipulated with respect to number of modalities, length, complexity, and addition of cues.

One of Schuell, et al.'s (1964) principles can be questioned, namely, "the use of repetitive sensory stimulation" (p. 341). It appears that she was referring both to repeating a stimulus to elicit a response and to repeating the stimulus as a consequence of an inadequate response. Pre-

senting an auditory stimulus at least twice, especially in a comprehension task, should improve perception of that stimulus; La-Pointe, Rothi, and Campanella (1978) found that comprehension of Token Test commands improved when the stimulus was repeated after failure on the first attempt, but comprehension was not helped significantly when the command was presented twice or four times prior to the initial response. For some patients, repeating a linguistic stimulus of some length *prior to a response* may add "noise" to the system and create some confusion. Nicholas and Brookshire (1979) found that repetition of a stimulus after response failure did not result in a better response. This appears to contradict LaPointe, et al. (1978), but Nicholas and Brookshire were examining tasks which included verbal expression as expected responses. Therefore, the value of repetition subsequent to failure may be high for a comprehension task and low for an expression task.

In tasks of verbal expression, the clinician's initial stimulus is often a pictured object to be named, described, or explained. Pictures traditionally have represented common household and personal objects and other things found in the environments of most adults. They have been simple line drawings without context. Background for objects has been said to be distracting to the patient and disruptive to establishing the clinician's control over the verbal response. It makes little difference as to whether real objects, line drawings, or photographs are used. The main reason for having the patient name from pictures is the potential for practice with a wide variety of referents.

Pictures are often supplemented with auditory cues to facilitate word retrieval. Podraza and Darley (1977) found that the first sound and a carrier phrase presented as prestimulation, just prior to the picture (see Chapter 10), elicited more words than indirect prestimulation.

One approach to supplemental cueing

in picture-naming tasks is to present a series of auditory cues, beginning with the most difficult level and proceeding through easier levels until the word is retrieved. Then the clinician moves on to the next trial (picture). This procedure was described by Linebaugh and Lehner (1977). On each naming trial the clinician first presents a picture and asks "What's this called?" and then continues through nine more levels of stimulation, ending with a carrier phrase plus the first two phonemes (ninth level) and a request for repetition (tenth level). This "top-down" procedure is contrasted with the common "bottom-up" strategy of successive cueing per item. In the latter, the clinician starts with the easiest cue and proceeds until the greatest demand is placed on the patient. The bottom-up approach pushes the patient toward independence from the clinician on each item, from maximum stimulation to minimum stimulation in eliciting a word.

Expected Response

Another of Schuell's principles was that every stimulus should elicit a response, partly so that the clinician can determine the adequacy of processing the stimulus. The patient should be responding continuously throughout a session; a large number of responses, especially verbal responses, should be elicited (Brookshire, 1978b; Schuell, et al., 1964). Consistent with the attention to processing and the tendency not to teach specific vocabulary, the several trials of a task should consist of a variety of semantic content. Each task involves practice with many different words and sentences, so that the patient's clinical experience with language is addressed to the variety of possible inputs and outputs to be confronted outside the clinic.

As noted before, each task is defined in terms of the type and level of expected responses. Adequacy of performance is measured according to the closeness of the actual response to the expected response. The patient is successful, however, when the expected response is not normal or linguistically precise but rather is an improvement over the patient's usual verbal behavior without clinical stimulation. From programmed learning, the principle of shaping successive approximations toward a normal response has been applied to aphasia treatment (Holland, 1970). In planning an expressive task, the clinician determines what the patient is capable of producing and begins treatment by stimulating and reinforcing this level of response. The plan includes identification of a target behavior toward which the patient should progress. The clinician's feedback selectively reinforces approximations which come closer and closer to the target. Stimulation is always designed to elicit responses within the patient's capabilities.

Clinician's Feedback

The clinician's response to the patient's behavior is a crucial part of the treatment interaction. Because exercises are structured to elicit successful responses, the clinician's response is positive on most trials per task. Holland (1970) suggested that verbal reinforcement should be used for adults instead of the tangible reinforcers often used for children. The proper feedback when an incorrect or unacceptable response occurs has been studied, but this component of what the clinician does has been ignored to a large degree in manuals of treatment activities. The occurrence of this feedback depends on the clinician's criterion for an acceptable response.

Schuell provided a clue as to what the clinician should do when a patient's response on a trial occasionally does not meet the criterion for an expected acceptable response. She advised that unacceptable responses should usually not be corrected (Schuell, et al., 1955), that the clinician should stimulate rather than correct (Schuell, et al., 1964). This differs from Keith's (1977) instructions to the clinician: the clinician asks "Is this a cup?" with a picture of a glass; if the patient says "yes," the clinician is to reply "No, this is a glass" (p. 4). Because aphasia does not involve a loss of language in most cases, little is gained by teaching patients the relationship between their errors and correct responses. Patients with Broca's and anomic aphasia, especially, recognize the nature of their errors when they occur. Negative consequences of inadequate responses are felt by the Broca's patient with respect to his or her own frustration; additional negative consequences are not needed from the clinician. As Schuell, et al. (1964) stated, "The objective is to get language processes working, not to teach the patient that whatever he says is wrong" (p. 342). Schuell's recommendations indicate that the clinician should continue to stimulate the patient rather than punish or correct an inadequate response.

Brookshire's (1978b) sixth principle of treatment was that the clinician should routinely provide feedback regarding accuracy of responses "where such feedback appears to be beneficial" (p. 144). He described two kinds of feedback. Incentive feedback rewards acceptable responses and punishes unacceptable responses; it may be warranted for only a small proportion of aphasics who will not respond unless they are reinforced for specific responses. Information feedback provides qualitative information about the difference between an unacceptable response and the expected response. Brookshire suggested that information feedback is most useful when self-motivated patients are unaware of the target response or of the relationship between it and the unacceptable response. This may be of value when the patient is working on a subtle detail of grammar. For a third category of patients, Brookshire wrote the following:

"If the patient (a) is motivated to respond, (b) knows the target response, and (c) knows how closely his attempts approximate the target, both qualitatively and quantitatively, then *any* feedback may be trivial" (p. 145).

There is a third type of clinician response to the patient, which may not be consistent with Brookshire's use of the term "feedback" in his discussion of his sixth principle. This third type is the *restimulation* of the patient implied in Schuell's admonition of "stimulate rather than correct."

Before considering the nature of restimulation as feedback, let us examine a study by Brookshire and Nicholas (1978) of how clinicians actually responded to patients' unacceptable responses in forty ten-minute videotaped samples of treatment. Did they follow Schuell's recommendation? The clinicians in these samples exhibited a strong tendency not to provide feedback for unacceptable responses. When feedback for unacceptable responses did occur, in most instances it was either negative or contained a correction. Therefore, contrary to Schuell's principle, these clinicians neither stimulated the patient nor refrained from pointing out error in providing feedback. Because unacceptable responses tended to cluster, these clinicians' strategies may not have been the most effective means of getting the patient back to successful responding.

Nicholas and Brookshire (1979) then examined seventy-five thirty-minute videotaped sessions to determine the effectiveness of clinician behaviors in "breaking up" the tendency for errors to cluster. They found that evaluative feedback on one trial did not tend to result in improved performance on the next trial. This feedback included positive and negative responses, correction, repetition of the patient's response, and elaboration.

Brookshire defined the clinician's feedback as any response which consists of a judgment of the patient's response. That is, it contains an indication of the patient's success. However, the clinician's feedback is viewed more broadly here; the clinician's feedback includes anything that the clinician does based on the patient's response to the initial stimulus. Feedback may consist of restimulation instead of an evaluative behavior. If the patient's response is unacceptable, the clinician can stimulate again in order to improve the response. Nicholas and Brookshire (1979) looked at such clinician responses by examining the trials after unacceptable responses in which the clinician pursued the same expected response from the patient. These instances of restimulation were considered to be another stimulus-response trial in Brookshire's coding system. The restimulation consisted of repeating the same stimulus which had resulted in error, rewording the same type of stimulus, and presenting a different type of stimulus. A different type of stimulus included a sentence completion or first sound cue to elicit the same response expected on the previous trial. None of these strategies were successful in improving the response, though rewording and a different stimulus were more effective than repeating the original stimulus.

Restimulation is similar to pursuit of the same expected response observed by Brookshire. This strategy consists of modifying or augmenting the initial stimulus in order to improve a response. For example, tense markers might be added to a sentence to improve comprehension (Pierce, 1981). Or, cues can be provided as a consequence of failure on a naming task (Love and Webb, 1977; Goodglass and Stuss, 1979; Pease and Goodglass, 1978). These cues include the first sound of a target word, a carrier phrase for sentence completion, a printed word, and a picture supplied after failure to a description of the object to be named. In the cited studies, the first sound cue was most effective, and Broca's aphasics tended to be more responsive to cues than anomic and Wer-

nicke's aphasics. In any case, the clinician can attempt to improve the patient's response on a trial by providing feedback which has been determined to result in more success for the patient. That is, *augmented restimulation* upon failure has the effect of increasing the power of the original stimulus. Brookshire's data do not clearly assess the value of augmented restimulation. Pease and Goodglass (1978) found, for example, that mildly and moderately impaired aphasics responded successfully to first sound cues more than 60 percent of the time after naming failures. Broca's aphasics responded successfully to over 70 percent of these cues. Wernicke's aphasics were successful after only 40 percent of these cues, including the first sound. Therefore, the value of augmented restimulation for improving a response may vary depending on the type of aphasia.

Restimulation can come too quickly. The patient should be allowed time to correct an error on his own or to repair an utterance on his own before the clinician pitches in to help. This is especially important for maximizing the patient's independence from the clinician. Delaying feedback is contingent on the patient's recognition of an error and then on any tendency to continue processing in order to self-correct. These efforts should not be permitted to continue when they near the point of producing frustration. Then, restimulation is warranted. Even with restimulation, patient independence is maximized when the first augmentation consists of minimal cueing. For example, to elicit a word in the feedback phase, a bottom-up approach is taken starting with a semantic cue. If that does not work, then the next cue might be a carrier phrase or the first sound.

The feedback to a patient's response in direct treatment depends on the clinician's criterion for a successful response. This criterion need not be a normal verbal response but, rather, can be an approximation to a standard of linguistic completeness and accuracy. However, a different basis for accepting responses was proposed by Holland (1978) and was later applied to PACE therapy by Davis and Wilcox (1981). Holland suggested that responses in standard direct verbal exercises be reinforced according to their adequacy in getting the message across, rather than according to their degree of linguistic sophistication or accuracy. The clinician may tune into the communicative value of the patient's effort in addition to, and sometimes instead of, its linguistic nuances as one basis for providing positive feedback.

Finally, the patient's mastery of a step in treatment is experienced by the clinician in the feedback component of the interaction. A step has not been mastered when the clinician must frequently augment the stimulus to improve a response. Whenever a response is frequently inaccurate, this is a sign that the task must be changed to a previous and easier step. However, when the clinician finds that augmentation is no longer needed on most trials of a task, then the patient is ready for the next step in the progression of treatment.

In summary, standard direct treatment consists of specific tasks designed to exercise particular language functions. Each function is identified with respect to a primary deficit of the patient, whether it

be auditory comprehension in general or comprehension of complex syntactic relationships in particular. The impaired functions are exercised at a level, determined by initial assessment, where the patient can respond accurately at least 80 percent of the time. For severely impaired patients, this may entail simply imitating the clinician; for less-impaired patients, it may entail practice with word retrieval, while imitation is used sparingly as an augmented restimulation when an occasional failure occurs. The basic interaction between clinician and patient, whether the task exercises comprehension, expression, or both, is summarized in Table 11-4. The clinician stimulates the patient in order to elicit an expected response. When the response is acceptable, the clinician responds with an adult acknowledgment of success and then presents the next stimulus in the task. When the response is unacceptable, the clinician repeats the trial or presents the original stimulus again in a simpler form or with additional cues in order to improve the response. If the response cannot be improved readily, the clinician may choose to provide information feedback in the circumstances suggested by Brookshire. In any case, the clinician should return the patient to successful responding as quickly as possible. Dwelling on incorrect responding fails to exercise the targeted process; spending

TABLE 11-4. The essential clinician-patient interaction in a trial of a standard direct task applies to exercises for comprehension and expression.

Clinician's Stimulus	Patient's Response	Clinician's Feedback
	Acceptable	(1) Acknowledgment and/or praise
		(2) Move on
	Unacceptable	(1) Restimulation repeat modify augment with cues or Inform about accuracy
		(2) Move on

time with failure on a particular item of semantic content, a word or a phrase, ignores the assumption that aphasia is not a loss of particular words but rather is an interference with a process which involves words in general.

A Comment on Style

While a treatment activity may be structured similarly to a test, it is not administered as is a test. A principal difference lies in the feedback phase of each trial. In assessment, feedback is minimal because the objective is to determine how well a patient responds to certain stimuli. In treatment, stimuli should produce adequate responses most of the time; and when responses are inadequate, feedback should improve the response. Furthermore, a treatment activity need not be modulated by measurement criteria such as reliability. Concern for reliable measurement of performance in treatment can stiffen the interaction between clinician and patient and can reduce the clinician's flexibility in creatively responding to the patient's errors and frustrations. The modality-focused activities described in previous discussions lend themselves to measurement, but measurement of improvement need not be taken during the treatment activity. Measurement can be achieved with tasks administered independent of the treatment activity, a topic for later discussion.

In many respects, the structured interactions of treatment are less stressful to the patient than real-life communicative situations. The clinician plans stimulation which is intended to avoid frustrating failures. The clinician gives the patient time to respond where others may be impatient. The clinician understands the patient's anxiety and anger and allows these feelings to be expressed freely. On the one hand, if treatment is to move the patient toward dealing with real life, then perhaps

the clinician should give the patient less time to respond and should create situations where failure is more likely. On the other hand, these conditions may not foster the levels of success desired in treatment. The clinician should strike a balance between these opposing forces, with emphasis on minimal stress during the early phases of treatment.

The administration of structured tasks can be shaped by the patient's personality and changing moods. The clinician should be prepared to adjust to the patient's behavior; the patient should not be forced to adjust to the clinician. If the patient is listless, the clinician may have to become more spirited to raise the frequency and level of responsiveness. If the patient is anxious and excitable, the clinician may have to become soothing and mellow in manner of stimulation in order to accomplish the goals for the session. Discovery of the patient's sense of humor can be capitalized upon in order to enhance enjoyment of any structured activity. However, the clinician does not have to accept or allow a reduction of motivation or a lack of cooperativeness from the patient. The clinician sometimes becomes a leader or a coach and reminds the patient of his or her reasons for being in treatment. Occasionally the clinician will have to shock the patient out of unproductive doldrums in a respectful but forceful manner.

In general, a structured activity can be administered in a conversational tone to heighten naturalness of the interaction and decrease anxiety. A structured interaction can be conducted so that it does not seem structured to the patient. The clinician maintains a concept of task goals and structure in mind in order to analyze the patient's performance, but the structure of the clinician's thought does not have to be apparent in interaction with the patient. If the clinician is scoring responses during a task, this activity should go on "under the table" and not be obvious to the patient.

STIMULUS AND RESPONSE CONTENT

Content, in this text, refers to the semantic *and* syntactic characteristics of the language used in the clinician's stimulation and in definition of the expected response. Semantic characteristics are considered here specifically with respect to the vocabulary selected for practice of comprehension and expression and, more generally, with respect to topics or themes used to generate treatment activities. Syntactic characteristics include sentence structures and morphological components which are selected for practice. Semantic and syntactic features of language are considered in the selection of pictures used as referents.

Semantic Content

Schuell and most other writers have recommended that vocabulary and corresponding pictures should be "meaningful" to the patient in order to provide an adequate stimulus. Aphasics respond to and retrieve best the most frequently used words in a language community. Commercially available treatment materials usually contain pictures of referents which are found in the environments of most people and, therefore, the semantic content of these materials is homogenized across all patients. This content includes common furniture, appliances and utensils, food, clothing, body parts, people, occupations, sports, hobbies, and modes of transportation. These categories are assumed to represent not only elements from the patient's everyday world but also words that are commonly used in communications among the patient and his or her family and friends. This assumption is questionable, considering Goodglass, Hyde, and Blumstein's (1969) observation that aphasics tend not to use picturable nouns in spontaneous speech. While this section focuses on picturable language, the clinician should attend to the stimulation of commonly used abstract nonpicturable words, such as "love," "life," "truth," and "justice." This may be done with question-answering and conversation, sometimes about meaningful and interesting pictures.

A variety of picture stimuli have been published for aphasia treatment. Discrete objects may be either line drawings (Taylor and Marks, 1959; Places and Things by Modern Education Corporation), or photographs (Photo Resource Kit by Modern Education Corporation). These pictures are on individual cards so that the clinician can be flexible in arranging them, while other kits have pictures grouped on a page (Canetta, 1974; Abbate and La Chappelle, 1978). Action pictures have been produced for drill at the sentence level, and these are on individual cards (Hain and Lainer, 1977, 1980; Stryker and Stryker, 1976), or are grouped on a page (Abbate and La Chappelle, 1978). Schlanger (1978, 1980) developed drawings of real-life situations and problems which are intended to promote discussion.

Holland (1978) extended the concept of meaningful stimulus to include the functional value of content, namely, what the patient actually deals with on a daily basis that involves use of language. The clearest examples are daily requirements for reading which include the mail, phone directory (especially emergency numbers), product labels, and occasional forms. Practice in writing one's name and address may be more functional than writing words such as "table," and "fork." In Baer's (1976) comprehension program for hospitalized aphasics, the semantic content is addressed to the hospital context. The patient may attach an importance to certain content that is most likely to be used, which can enhance motivation to engage in the repetitive drill of direct treatment.

The importance of semantic content to the patient is heightened by the *individualization of content* to the patient's context, interests, and background. As semantic content becomes more individualized, commercially available materials become less relevant, because these materials are designed to be meaningful to everyone. Individualization of content has been recommended most frequently with respect to the patient's vocational and avocational interests. Occupational content is especially motivating for moderately and mildly impaired aphasics who may return to work. Words such as "flange" or "caulk" may be used frequently by certain people. A patient wishing to return to work in a warehouse may concentrate on practice in following and giving instructions pertaining to the movement of objects to the left or right, or up or down. Likewise, the clinician would explore the language of the patient's hobbies as a source of content directed toward the patient's return to pursuit of these activities.

Certain common categories of content can be individualized even further when the proper names of people, places, and objects in the patient's context are considered. Aphasics can be more responsive to family names than to the homogenized terms "father" or "son." They can be more responsive to "Snoopy" or "Kilgore" than to "dog" or "cat." A picture of a store is likely to be called "Krogers" or "Sears"; a cigarette might be called a "Camel" and a car called a "Ford." Employing proper names of referents familiar to the patient can increase the likelihood of successful exercise of auditory comprehension, and such vocabulary should be reinforced when retrieved.

Stimulability of pictured referents may be enhanced according to a concept introduced in a unique study by Faber and Aten (1979). Faber and Aten wrote about the degree of arousal of multiple nonverbal and verbal mental images which might be achieved by the pictured stimulus. For example, the success of operative stimuli in Gardner's (1973) study might be attributed to the multimodality arousal of sensory images which is possible with manipulable objects; Goodglass, Barton, Kaplan (1968) had found that objects presented through multiple modalities were named more readily than objects presented in a single modality. Faber and Aten compared verbal performances between presentation of intact objects and objects depicted as broken. Thirteen aphasic subjects were asked to "Tell me what you see" rather than to specifically name the pictures. The two conditions did not differ in their stimulation of object names; they did differ significantly, however, in their elicitation of additional verbalization such as "glasses is cracked" or "the sleeve is torn." This difference occurred for agrammatic patients (Broca's aphasia) but did not occur with the fluent aphasic subjects. The nonfluent aphasics were thought to be more aroused to verbalize to the peculiar features of the broken objects.

This concept of *stimulus arousal* might be extended to the individualization of content with material which is most meaningful to the patient. Family members may assist the patient in bringing photographs to the clinic; these photographs serve to maximize the meaningfulness of stimuli to the patient. The nature of arousal may be to enhance interest and motivation rather than the multiplicity of mental images. Boller, et al. (1979) drew attention to the potential value of emotional arousal in enhancing linguistic performance. Patients have been observed to verbalize better when their messages pertain to topics that are personal and of real consequence to them. Eisenson (1963) observed improved reading in a patient when the topic dealt with his divorce. In a study of verbal fluency in aphasia, some patients said more during emotional speech, while others said less during emotional speech

(Kreindler, Mihailescu, and Fradis, 1980). Helm and Barresi (1980) reported on an unpublished study in which word reading was better with emotional words. These hints about an effect of emotionality should be extended to more formal and extensive research to determine how this factor might be managed in a treatment program.

The historical dimension of the patient is a valuable source of arousing topics and referents (see Davis and Holland, 1981). By searching an almanac, the clinician can discover topics concerning news events and entertainment phenomena which were prominent while the patient was going to school and raising a family. Pictures from books featuring U.S. Presidents, World War II, and famous persons during the rise of sports, radio, and television often excite the patient to recall personal experiences from the earlier periods. One day in our clinic, a severely apraxic and aphasic patient was working on word retrieval using a small print-out machine as an alternate response mode. He was asked to think of a famous golfer, but he could not respond. Then he was asked about golfers who were famous when he was growing up. He typed "Jones" (Bobby Jones).

Recognition of pictures to be named is believed to involve the right cerebral hemisphere because of its role in the mental coding format of visual imagery (see Chapter 3). West (1977, 1978) suggested that verbal performance of aphasics might be enhanced by maximizing the visual-imaging processes of the right hemisphere, just as verbal recall has been heightened by maximizing the visual imagery of normal adults (Paivio and Begg, 1981). Visual imagery in normals has been heightened by the use of "dynamic" pictures (objects in motion) instead of "static" pictures (objects stationary). Myers (1980) argued that mental imagery consists of more than a mere "mental picture" of experiences; it contains "a non-

verbal confluence of emotion, intellect, and sensation" (p. 69). She suggested that right-hemisphere activation can be heightened with pictured referents which include "*inter*actions, rather than simple actions" (p. 71), that is, with pictures which display people and objects in an enriched and meaningful context. Kelly (1981) compared contextually rich pictures with object and simple action pictures as stimuli for word retrieval. There was no difference among these pictures when convergent object naming was required. Contextually rich pictures stimulated more accurate words and a greater number of words when instructions were more open-ended: "Tell me about these pictures." Of course, there is more to talk about in contextually rich pictures. Involving the right hemisphere's cognitive style in the treatment process is an interesting possibility that awaits empirical support.

Syntactic Content

Early specification of treatment procedures was centered on the patient's recognition, imitation, and retrieval of single words. Schuell, et al. (1964) were most specific about content and procedure with respect to training the use of words. When higher levels of language function were considered, recommendations focused on increasing retention span or practicing general activities like reading the newspaper or listening to the radio and then reporting on items of interest. In describing new trends in clinical aphasiology during the 1960's, Holland (1969) observed that "with new information from structural linguistics we are learning that the lexicon does not equal the language" (p. 4). The realization that people speak in sentences and that sentences possess a certain structure was a catalyst for the development of systematic procedures for the practice of sentence comprehension and production. Holland provided an illustration of this influence which was a hint of what was to come in aphasia treatment:

> . . . we all taught aphasics to use nouns, for instance, we taught the word *book*. The appropriate answer to the question, "What is this?" would have been, "Book." Now we see the error in our ways; the utterance "book" is an unreal linguistic event. The noun phrase "a book," as the response to my question "What is this?", is structurally more sound, more appropriate, more apt to help the aphasic generalize, and easier to teach. (Holland, 1969, p. 4)

Syntactic content refers to the grammatical features of language stimuli and expected responses, including arrangement of word order and selection of bound morphemes and function words which signal temporal and spatial relationships. The prominence of Chomsky's generative grammar in the 1960s brought the field of linguistics to the attention of clinical aphasiologists as a means of defining the nuances of language being dealt with in treatment. While programmed learning theorists showed clinicians *how* to manipulate the use of language, linguists demonstrated for clinicians the complexity of *what* was being manipulated, that is, the linguistic content of treatment (Holland, 1969; Sefer and Shaw, 1972). More attention was given to the symptom of agrammatism with descriptions of linguistic elements that are missing and structures that are present. One of the first clinicians to do this was Schuell (Schuell, Shaw, and Brewer, 1969).

The increasing sophistication of clinicians in their awareness of the linguistic parameters of utterances has influenced treatment in two ways: (1) the identification of specific categories of utterances which might be the object of assessment or repeated practice, such as drill with *agent + action + object* constructions or with a certain *question transformation,* and (2) the specification of small differences in the complexity of these sentential categories. These differences contribute to the development of hierarchies of difficulty for specific stimuli and expected responses.

Naeser (1975) selected three simple syntactic structures which were incorporated in a program for the training of picture description with four aphasic patients. These structures were described as *NP + be + Pred. (NP)* ("That is a house"), *NP + V + NP* ("The woman opens the door"), and *NP + V* ("Soldiers march"). The *agent + action + object (NP + V + NP)* construction has been the focus of several treatment strategies including Holland and Levy's (1971) study of programmed instruction and generalization to other syntactic structures with seven aphasic subjects, Luria's (1970b) use of nonverbal cues to facilitate sentence production with his cases of agrammatism, and Culton and Ferguson's (1979) auditory comprehension program with seven subjects. Various combinations of constituents from this basic structure have been the object of training in the use of shorter phrase units, such as *NP* ("the boy") and *NP + V* ("The horse drinks") by Culton and Ferguson (1979). Chapey (1981a) directed attention to various combinations: *action + object* ("Eat lunch"), *agent + object* ("John pipe"), and *attribution + object* ("Dirty table"). Prepositional phrases have received special attention from Luria (1970b) and Smith (1974a) in comprehension training and from Luria in using cues to elicit these phrases.

Some treatment programs are based on a definition of phrase or sentence-level performance in terms of length with minimal consideration given to syntax. Culton and Ferguson (1979), for example, defined levels of comprehension training primarily in terms of number of words in the utterance. Their first level consisted of two-word stimuli such as "the bird," "big fish," and "under bed." These examples illustrate their use of three different syntactic structures in a level of treatment which was initially conceived to be homogeneous. They reported that two-word phrases were difficult for their subjects relative to levels with longer utterances. Though the two-word level seemed as if it would be easy when the program was planned, the empirical test of the program demonstrated that it was not easy. One explanation is the mixture of structures used and the inclusion of prepositional phrases which are of great difficulty for some aphasic patients. Culton and Ferguson also pointed out the unnatural nature of these utterances; "... they do not reflect typical adult speech" (p. 77). Aphasic patients sometimes find it awkward to be practicing comprehension or expression with such utterances as "John pipe" and "under box" (see Chapter 10, pages 247–248).

MEASUREMENT

There are two main objectives associated with measuring a patient's performance during a treatment session: (1) to determine whether useful improvement is taking place and, if so, the amount of improvement, and (2) to determine whether treatment is having an effect on recovery. A common misconception in the way measurement often is discussed is that procedures which meet the first objective are thought of as meeting the second objective. Determining the *effect of* treatment *on* a criterion communicative skill is a difficult task. The necessary comparisons relative to spontaneous recovery were presented in Chapter 9.

Useful Improvement

"Useful improvement" refers to improvements in language function and communicative ability outside the clinical setting, that is, improvements where the patient needs them most. A common term for this change is "carry-over." It has been at least uneconomical and particularly without reliable precedent for a clinician in a typical clinical setting to measure language behavior in the patient's living environment; Holland did so in a research project for validating the *CADL*. Nevertheless, an underlying principle has led to procedures for doing the next-best thing. The principle is that we want to determine whether the patient will show *improvement of language function in circumstances other than the treatment activity itself.* Furthermore, these circumstances should be similar to the natural communicative demands on the patient. We have several tests, including typical aphasia batteries, which approach these circumstances to varying degrees. An overall score from a test battery at least reflects a variety of circumstances, while a variety of linguistic demands is the norm in real life.

The clinician commonly measures performance on the treatment task itself. This measurement is of value for providing an objective basis for selecting a task for treatment (80 percent accuracy) or for advancing to the next step of treatment (95 to 100 percent proficiency, for example). It provides an observation of improvement within boundaries defined by the task. The Base-10 forms developed by LaPointe (1977, 1978a) are of assistance to the clinician in plotting improvement graphically on a task across several sessions. However, these forms were designed to answer additional questions, to be mentioned later.

Improvement on treatment task performance does not necessarily indicate that useful improvement is taking place. Advances in picture pointing, picture naming, sentence completion, and imitation do not mean that the patient is becoming a better talker in the hospital ward, at home, or in any circumstance other than the treatment activity itself. Therefore, clinicians obtain measures of performance with stimulus content and on tasks which are not being utilized as treatment. The clinician looks for whether *generalization* is occurring.

Several studies have included measures of generalization relative to certain treatment activities. Improvement of confrontation naming has been assessed relative to words not included in the treatment (Brookshire, 1975a; Seron, et al., 1979; Wiegel-Crump and Koenigsknecht, 1973). Holland and Levy (1971) investigated whether improvement in use of active sentences would generalize to other syntactic structures. Improvement in following instructions with objects was compared with changes in the Token Test (West, 1973). Changes in the Token Test were compared with measurements on following instructions from the *MTDDA* (Holland and Sonderman, 1974). Generalization measures are not obtained as frequently as treatment administration. They may be obtained once per week, every two weeks, or once per month.

An extended form of generalization measurement addresses improvement relative to the long-range objective of a treatment activity. All treatment activities are a means to an end. Repetition is not done so that a patient will someday be a better repeater but, rather, so that the patient will speak better spontaneously. Confrontation naming and word associations are practiced so that the patient will speak better spontaneously. Therefore, improvement can be assessed regularly in circumstances which may be much more difficult than the treatment. While the patient is performing at 80 percent accuracy on word comprehension, for example, the clinician would occasionally measure the patient's performance on sentence comprehension which may begin at 20 percent accuracy. This strategy affords the opportunity to measure recovery with respect to what the patient confronts outside of treatment, namely, sentences. It permits a wider range of possible recovery to be detected. Therefore, measures of extended generalization are designed to tap into

what the treatment is really supposed to accomplish. Also, as mentioned previously, occasional probing of meaningful behavior frees the clinician to be more natural and flexible during a treatment activity. Measuring everything tends to suppress natural interaction.

Because aphasia is a central disorder, clinicians expect that generalization will extend across language modalities. Kushner and Winitz (1977) studied a patient who exercised only comprehension in treatment, but the investigators took regular measurements of picture naming, which improved during treatment of comprehension.

We cannot be certain that improvement on untreated materials and tasks is an effect of treatment. This is a possibility, however, because generalization to untreated content or tasks has not occurred in some instances (Brookshire, 1975a; Holland and Sonderman, 1974). When the patient does not improve on a range of content and skills, we know that the treatment is not working. However, when a range of improvements does occur, it can be attributed to spontaneous recovery or reconciliation of a faltering marriage rather than to treatment. When we want to demonstrate that treatment has an effect on something, we always look over our shoulders at spontaneous recovery (and, perhaps, ask "How's your marriage these days?")

Effects of Treatment

Effects of treatment are assumed to be determined relative to three criterion levels: (1) the effect of a certain clinician behavior on treatment task performance, (2) the effect of treatment in general on an independent measure such as a test battery, and (3) the effect of treatment on natural communication. Because of the elusiveness of measuring recovery at (3), measures at (2) are assumed to be somewhat valid as an indication of (3). In any case, effects are usually determined by comparing the presence and absence of a specific clinician behavior, such as a phonemic cue, or the presence and absence of an entire treatment program.

The clinician determines daily the effects of specific behaviors at level (1). When interested in the effect of a cue on confrontation naming, the clinician compares naming with the cue present and with the cue absent. The effectiveness of a cue for improving confrontation naming is confirmed when it is consistent over several trials. Inserting pauses improves comprehension of instructions (Liles and Brookshire, 1975); operant procedures improve card sorting (Smith, 1974); and increased syllable duration improves performance on MIT (Laughlin, Naeser, and Gordon, 1979). These effects, measured with respect to treatment task performance, are restricted to this limited circumstance of language function.

A common method for determining the effect of a specific clinician behavior is to obtain a *baseline* of task performance before the treatment activity begins (LaPointe, 1977, 1978a). LaPointe's Base-10 form provides a place for recording a baseline. A baseline is a measurement of task performance without the special cues which are used as part of the initial stimulus or as feedback upon error. It is administered similarly to a test. If the treatment is picture naming, the treatment is preceded by at least three administrations of picture naming without cues. These three measures may indicate a stable performance, but naming may improve when the treatment is added. This is a limited comparison between the absence and then presence of cueing behavior. Principles of alternating-phase single-subject designs suggest that alternating baseline and treatment measures would be a better indicator of effect (see Chapter 9).

The ingredients for determining the effect of treatment, therefore, are (1) a comparison between the presence and absence of a treatment paradigm and (2) a criterion measure reflecting the object of this effect. If we are to say that treatment is beneficial for a patient, we should specify what function(s) received this help. Treatment had an effect on what? Usually we can say only with respect to what was measured that it had an effect, for example, on naming or on the *PICA*. If these tasks are a valid measure of real-life communication, then we can say that treatment helped the patient at criterion level (3).

12 Psychosocial Adjustment by the Patient and Family

The aphasic individual must confront numerous adjustments in his or her life which interact with the treatment process. The individual must learn about a new self, one who looks differently because of hemiparesis, who talks differently, and whose limitations have interminable effects on the details of day-to-day living which are constantly being discovered. Getting dressed, for example, becomes a time-consuming chore. Explaining to the family what transpired in the speech clinic is a time-consuming chore.

The setting of realistic goals and the sustaining of motivation for months of treatment exercises are influenced by the family's adjustment to the upset of family balance, or homeostasis (Webster and Newhoff, 1981). An individual's aphasia is a family problem. Each person who lives with an aphasic person must make unplanned and unwanted changes in his or her life. Communicating with an aphasic husband or wife becomes a chore; and, because of role changes, there are new chores such as monitoring finances or preparing meals. The role stereotypes for males and females of traditional society leave persons ill-prepared for the disruption of these functions in the family unit. It can be frightening for a wife to find herself having to be the one to park the car in a big-city medical center. "The little things become big things." A balance between opposing goals must be achieved: retaining as much of established roles as possible while accepting the necessity of taking over unfamiliar roles.

Does the speech-language pathologist contribute to the patient's and family's overall adjustment to aphasia? The conveying of information about prognosis, treatment, and recovery is a vital service to the family as well as to the patient. The clinician is likely to be the only professional available to the family on a regular basis. His or her responsibilities include recognition of problems which require the services of other professionals such as a social worker or psychologist. The clinician makes many contributions to family adjustment which are consistent with his or her training, experience, and capabilities.

CLINICIAN-CLIENT RELATIONSHIP

The aphasic person's motivation to improve and interest in the treatment program will depend upon the relationship developed with a clinician which may progress over a period of several months. The patient should have confidence in and be comfortable with the clinician. From time to time, the clinician must present the patient with activities which are unfamiliar, awkward or unnatural, and frustrating because of their difficulty. This is especially true of assessment procedures in which the stimuli are standardized, the procedures controlled, and the tasks varied in complexity. Compounding the challenge to the development of rapport is the fact that such procedures are often presented soon after the participants' first meeting. Therefore, a good start in developing a positive atmosphere for therapeutic change is for the clinician and patient to spend some time getting to know each other, as any strangers would upon first meeting.

Also, at the first meeting, the clinician and client should come to a common understanding of the goals of treatment to the greatest extent possible, and to an agreement on the shared responsibility for accomplishing these goals. It is the patient who will be improving his or her language function and developing new strategies for communication, with assistance from the clinician. The patient and family should understand that their attention and energy are necessary if the clinician's planning and procedures are to achieve their maximum effect. It is a joint effort.

Two conditions necessary for a climate which promotes therapeutic change are the clinician's unconditional positive regard and empathy for the patient.

Unconditional positive regard is "an outgoing positive feeling without reservations, without evaluations" (Rogers, 1961, p. 62). The aphasic person usually enters a language treatment program with reduced self-esteem because of changes in appearance due to paralysis as well as because of changes in expressive ability. Inability to get ideas across and impeded mobility produce frustrations which are reflected in anger and depression. Emotions may sometimes be difficult to control. Odd words and profanity may be unwittingly produced. If the patient is to begin to feel comfortable with and develop trust of the clinician, the clinician should present an atmosphere of acceptance of the aphasic condition and the aphasic as a person. Davis and Holland (1981) explained as follows: "The notion of an accepting atmosphere in the clinic should not be misconstrued to mean that 'anything goes,' that there are no boundaries within which the patient must function to achieve the goals of language treatment. It does mean, however, that the patient's depression, frustration, or anger is allowed in the clinical setting without reservation or evaluation by the clinician" (p. 218).

The aphasic person can detect subtle nonverbal cues which are indicative of another's attitude toward him or her. Patients surveyed by Skelly (1975) "cited numerous subtle signs of impatience from those around them which were deeply discouraging—audible sighs, tightening of the mouth muscles, shoulder and eye movements, and drumming fingers" (p. 1141). The novice clinician should be prepared to exercise patience with delayed or inappropriate responses and to present a positive attitude toward the client. Wulf (1979) commented on her first contact with her therapist with the "radiant smile":

And this was the first miracle speech therapy wrought for me. No word was needed—it was the magic of a look—an instantaneous rapport partly because my innermost messenger had told me that it would be that way. Speech therapy's rare talent is this: being able to hop on anybody's wave length and stay there until the aphasic has learned how to climb the unending tortuous crag facing him.[1]

[1] Quoted by permission from Wulf, H. H., *Aphasia, My World Alone* (Detroit: Wayne State University Press, 1979), p. 50.

Empathy is the genuine understanding of another person's thoughts, feelings, and values, or, as defined by Rogers (1961), the capacity to sense the feelings and personal meanings that another person is experiencing at each moment. Rogers (1951) advised that "it is the counselor's function to assume, in so far as he is able, the internal frame of reference of the client . . . to lay aside all perceptions from the external frame of reference while doing so, and to communicate something of this empathic understanding to the client" (p. 29). The external frame of reference to be put aside includes a stereotypic conception defined along some attribute such as sex, age, or race, or, as might be the case with aphasic adults, an image of a parent of the clinician (Davis and Holland, 1981). Also, a generalized or one-dimensional view of aphasia may limit the clinician's perception of the unique characteristics of the patient's disorder. In a survey of clients in speech clinics in the United States, Haynes and Oratio (1978) asked about clinician attributes which were found to have been most helpful in their treatment. Of six factors emerging in an analysis of 162 questionnaires, qualities reflecting "empathetic-genuineness" ranked second in importance to technical skill. When a clinician's understanding of the patient's disorder and feelings about that disorder are conveyed to the patient, he or she recognizes that the clinician indeed may be a person who can help, and trust of the clinician begins to develop.

Experienced clinicians are familiar with the soothing of frustration that comes with statements to the patient like "I know, you know what you want to say but just can't say it." The patient producing a succession of phonemic paraphasias may need to hear "You know the word but are having trouble with the sounds." Just verbalizing frustration for the patient can reduce its interference with the treatment process. One area in which inexperienced clinicians sometimes do not respond to the patient's internal frame of reference is with regard to the reinforcement of certain successes in word retrieval or in any verbal expression at a simplified level. A clinician may express an unbridled joy over hearing a patient say "bread," while the patient at that moment is feeling unhappiness over the fact that he used to say "pass the bread" with ease, without thinking about it. Though the first production of a word after weeks of failure should be acknowledged as a success, the clinician should also acknowledge the patient's understandable lack of exhilaration over what sometimes seems to him to be such a trivial accomplishment. In addition, an aphasic may try to articulate a sense that improvement has occurred, but often the nature or amount of recovery is difficult to identify. Merely saying "The frustration is a little less" probably captures what the patient consciously experiences as recovery.

THE PATIENT

A patient's wife will say, "He's a different person." Brain damage may precipitate certain modifications of personality, though the patient's premorbid personality determines the shape of these modifications. Certain emotional reactions are characteristic; and it is helpful for the clinician, patient, and family to realize that these reactions are natural and likely to be temporary. Family reactions and adjustments are similar to those of the patient; and so the reader should keep the family in mind while reviewing this section. We learn much about persons with aphasia by reading the accounts of well-recovered aphasics or their spouses (Buck, 1968; Cameron, 1959; Dahlberg and Jaffe, 1977; Knox, 1971; McBride, 1969; Moss, 1972; Ritchie, 1961; Sies and Butler, 1963; Wulf, 1979). While individuals and family units differ, the consistency of issues and coping mechanisms is rather remarkable.

Psychological Changes and Reactions

Eisenson (1973) identified several components of personality and behavior which may be modified subsequent to onset of aphasia. These modifications vary in degree and in kind among patients, and are difficult to detect in some. Manifestations of these changes are often most evident to the patient's spouse. *Ego involvement,* or egocentrism, is reflected in a concern for self which reduces premorbid consideration of feelings and needs of others. Eisenson referred to the patient "whose concerns with what he was or might have been get in the way of making adjustments to acquired disabilities . . ." (p. 71). He explained ego involvement as often being coincident with *concretism,* with both being strong in patients who tended to be concrete and ego-involved before onset of aphasia. In fact, Eisenson's discussion of concretism was dominated by discussion of ego involvement. Concretism seems to refer to a heightened attention to the here-and-now and an intense desire for routine and structure. Spouses report that "he seems to ignore me" and "he has to have everything done the same way and put in its proper place."

The patient's disability may result in or be accompanied by *unproductive coping and defense mechanisms.* These methods are a way of shielding the self from the disorder and from the difficult responsibilities of adapting to it. Withdrawal from social contact is a common response which is reinforced by withdrawal by friends and, occasionally, by family members. Spouses sometimes say that it is too difficult for them to explain or argue anymore and so "it is easier to be quiet." Also, patients may deal with their insecurity by developing a constant concern for the health of their spouses. One woman told of her mildly aphasic husband who constantly woke her in the middle of the night to make sure she was "okay." The person with aphasia may not allow the spouse to be out of his or her sight.

Emotional behavior may occur which is due to a neurologically based reduction of inhibitory mechanisms. Some patients exhibit *emotional lability,* which is highly variable emotional behavior such as when a patient appears content one moment and starts crying the next moment for the slightest reason or for no apparent reason. The patient seems unsettled and brittle and shows feelings in frequency and degrees never shown before onset. *Catastrophic reaction* is often an appropriate emotional reaction in kind but is carried out with an intensity that far exceeds what would be expected normally. Frustration may precipitate a ferocious outburst of anger.

Aphasic individuals experience many feelings which are common reactions to crisis and are expressed normally. These emotions and moods may linger for a while and yet are likely to be resolved to some degree with successful adjustment. These natural reactions include anxiety or fear, frustration, anger, depression, guilt, and embarrassment.

Anxiety and *fear* can be early reactions to awareness of having suffered a stroke, for indeed that small episode in the brain may have brought the person very close to death. The patient and family worry about the somewhat increased likelihood that it could happen again. Four years after his stroke, one individual recalled the time when he awoke in a hospital bed and discovered he could not move one arm and leg and could not talk. Being a speech pathologist, he knew immediately what had happened to him. He saw his concerned family in the room, including a son and daughter who, he knew, must have traveled a great distance very quickly to be there. Their presence made him wonder if he was going to die. He could not ask.

Not being able to ask about or ask for things can be frustrating, especially when needs are clearly in mind. *Frustration* comes from continually being blocked from reaching goals that were so easily achieved before, such as ordering food for breakfast or unwrapping a candy bar. It can also come from the slowness of recovery, the small steps of improvement that are imperceptible on a day-to-day basis. People with aphasia have a strong desire to be the way they were before, and some continue for a long time thinking that they can be.

Anger is one way to strike back after an unexpected loss. "Why did this happen to me?" Once regular churchgoers now refuse to go to church. Wives have concluded that their husbands feel as if lightning has struck them, while they have done nothing wrong. Anger also breeds in the aphasic person who is faced with the misunderstandings or insensitivity of others who are not aphasic. Buck (1968) was frequently haunted by memories of remarks and speculations by hospital staff and visitors concerning his condition that were made in his presence. People sometimes assume that because a person cannot talk he or she also cannot comprehend. The patient may detect parts of utterances and the gist of accompanying facial expression; patients interviewed by Skelly (1975) wished more people would realize this.

Buck (1968) concluded that the greatest enemy of the aphasic person is *depression.* Depression drains energy and the motivation to pursue recovery. It can come and go and, then, return again. It may settle in for a while when the patient recognizes the nature of his or her problem or returns to familiar environments in which previously he or she was functioning easily. Robinson and Benson (1981) determined that nonfluent aphasics are more depressed than fluent aphasics several months after onset. Among fluent patients, larger lesions are accompanied by less depression.

The aphasic person is not always depressed, angry, or anxious. Though there may be some common phases of reaction to the condition and to interacting situations, people with aphasia are as different as people in general are different. Moss (1972) described an apparent detachment, "as if the stroke had benumbed any emotional investment in the future and I simply shrugged at my perception of my imminent demise" (p. 4). Dahlberg wrote about his "stroke personality" in which he felt no fear and experienced no anxiety in the few days after onset, "confident I would be cared for, a perfect undemanding patient" (Dahlberg and Jaffe, 1977, p. 20). However, Moss and Dahlberg reported becoming depressed for a period of time after returning home from the hospital. Eisenson (1973) referred to some patients who exhibit *euphoria* as a self-defense. The appearance of a sense of well-being inconsistent with reality is found in Wernicke's aphasia, overlapping with the neurological symptom of anosognosia for the language disorder.

An unusual amount of *fatigue,* though a common symptom of depression, is a common poststroke characteristic in its own right. When the patient has hemiparesis, the simplest activities of daily living require much more effort than before. Once-automatic activities, such as getting dressed, applying makeup, shaving, and eating, demand conscious planning and a healthy dose of patience. Similarly, attempts to communicate can be quite demanding, varying in degree depending on the situation. Dahlberg remarked, "Speech, as it improved, was quite fatiguing and had to be limited to short periods with only one person at a time . . . it was like a telegram where you pay for every word . . ." (Dahlberg and Jaffe, 1977, p. 29).

Eisenson (1973) noted the *guilt* which an aphasic person might feel. Some people may react to a crisis by wondering if they are being punished for doing something wrong. However, a recognition of the adjustments that family members have to make is a more common source of this feeling. The patient may feel a weight of responsibility for a wife having to get a job, a husband having to prepare the meals, or a daughter feeling she has to quit college. Guilt may keep a patient from seeking or accepting help from others.

Embarrassment is another natural reaction to deficits of talking, sensation, and motor function. It can come from a recognition that profanity came out when it was not supposed to. There can be a self-consciousness about appearance changed by facial and limb weakness. One patient, without sensation from the right side of his face, said that he would not smile when people greeted him because, if he did smile, his mouth would be crooked.

An aphasic person's self-image can be shaped by the attitudes of others toward persons with this disorder. Duffy, Boyle, and Plattner's (1980) preliminary inquiry into these attitudes consisted of a variety of judgments by eighty-eight undergraduate students of one fluent, anomic aphasic and one nonfluent aphasic. The students rated both patients as low on composure, viewing the patients as less poised and relaxed than normal controls. Also, the students were unsure as to how they would respond to the nonfluent patient.

While anger, depression, and guilt may be temporary stages of adjustment and may require some counseling, anxiety and fear of communicative situations may be dealt with by behavior-modification techniques (Ince, 1968; Damon, Lesser, and Woods, 1979). A speech-language pathologist and psychologist collaborated in Damon, et al.'s study of a patient with mild aphasia. The goals were to reduce anxiety and fear of failure and to increase social interaction. Procedures included deep muscle relaxation and desensitization. The patient was trained to relax through a hierarchy of real-life social situations. The authors suggested that the roles of psychologist and speech-language pathologist overlap when developing a patient's self-confidence in communication ability.

Role Changes

Aphasia results in weakened abilities to carry out roles with respect to family, occupation, and community. Many men, having satisfied most career goals by age forty-five or fifty, begin developing a renewed interest in family and in community affairs. A stroke will sidetrack retirement plans and remove a person from participation on a school board. The patient may simply be fearful of continuing involvement in a community organization such as the Lions Club or Sertoma. However, the involuntary removal of work from a patient's daily activity can be especially devastating. Many people thrive emotionally on their occupations, and after a stroke there suddenly appears to be nothing to do.

Adjustment to these changes may depend on an interaction between severity of aphasia and the communicative demands of an endeavor. Schuell, et al. (1964) observed that patients in her relatively young simple aphasia group had the most adjustment problems. Many patients with mild aphasia believe that they either possess the capacity to return to work or will attain that capacity, and their success depends on the linguistic and general mental processing demands of the job. This is a serious problem for people with mild head injuries and subtle deficits that tests do not reveal readily. These patients return to work too quickly and often are overwhelmed, developing emotional problems while trying to meet subtle demands of work. Patients with severe aphasia, and particularly with hemiparesis, often adjust more quickly to the absence of work because of obvious incapacitation.

Traditional male and female roles have

maintained a division of everyday responsibilities, so that when one marriage partner is unable to assume them the other must take over. Furthermore, sex-defined responsibilities have been tied to self-concept, so that a reduced capacity infringes upon one's sexual identification. Dahlberg addressed this point: "Since I'd grown up in middle-class America, I was used to taking care of 'masculine' details. I signed into hotels, picked up the bags, gave taxi directions, and ordered in restaurants. I couldn't do any of these things now and Jane managed marvelously" (Dahlberg and Jaffe, 1977, p. 52). His wife added: ". . . I looked forward to the time Clay would be able to do the managing again. It wasn't the physical exertion I minded as much as the loss of my female enjoyment of being 'Taken care of'."

Role changes can be understood with respect to shifts in the balance of ego states as defined in transactional analysis (TA). Porter and Dabul (1977) applied TA to conceptualization of changes resulting from aphasia and to helping spouses understand the situation and return to the balance achieved before onset. The three ego states of Adult, Parent, and Child in the aphasic person are related to shifts in ego states of the spouse: "He acts like a child." In the aphasic, the Adult state is often weakened, resulting in reduced ability to examine options, reduced responsibilities—as "head of household," for example—and reduced communication with the spouse as Adult. "He just sits around all day and does nothing but watch TV." Reciprocally, the Child state is exaggerated, with increased dependency and feelings of helplessness. Ego-involved impulsivity dominates, and the spouse senses a continual attention to "me, me, me." The Parent state may be weakened in some patients, with an inability to act on the socially approved "shoulds" reflected in emotional liability and frequent profanity. The overly-exercised Child dominates over the Parent. Other patients may exhibit an exaggerated Parent "in an effort to provide structure for a world that appears chaotic" (Porter and Dabul, 1977, p. 245). The patient may become overly protective of the spouse, constantly monitoring his or her activities.

The Grieving Process

Tanner (1980) used the grieving process to analyze reaction to the loss of speech, language, and hearing functions. The sense of loss consists of many dimensions. The patient's family feels the "loss of a significant person" the way he or she was before. The patient may experience a "loss of external objects," especially when the disability results in extended hospitalization or a move to a nursing home. The aphasic may grieve over loss of a home and valued objects associated with it. Aphasia may accompany "developmental loss" already experienced as a result of the aging process. There may be the absence of children no longer living at home, the loss of a youthful physical appearance, and in some cases the recent death of the spouse. The "loss of security" comes from diminished physical health, transition in living environment, and fear that the spouse may leave for a better situation. Finally, there is the "loss of some aspect of self" that may include communicative ability, physical attractiveness, and family roles.

Before defining stages of the grieving process, Tanner (1980) explained:

It is important for the speech-language pathologist and audiologist to realize that the process of grieving has application to all patients and their families who are experiencing loss in any dimension. The grieving individual who successfully adjusts to loss may be expected to pass through all of the stages regardless of the dimension. Some may fixate at a particular stage of the process. The order and progress of the stages of grief may vary, but it is suggested that the stages are common to all who grieve. (p. 920).

The stages were derived largely from Kubler-Ross' (1969) account of the grieving process. The first stage is usually *denial:* "I don't believe it." It acts as a buffer for the news of what has happened. Webster and Newhoff (1981), who discussed the family's reaction to crisis, referred to this initial stage as a period of shock characterized by numbness and an inability to think clearly.

The second stage is *anger,* the "Why me" stage. Anger, resentment, and even rage are natural reactions to loss and should not necessarily be interpreted by the clinician as a reaction to the treatment program. It is a difficult period for family and friends to understand. Anger may be acted out as indifference to family and treatment or as a general lack of cooperation with hospital staff. It may result from the initial realization of the disorder (the second phase of reaction to crisis in Webster and Newhoff's discussion).

The third stage is *bargaining,* an attempt to delay loss or reduce the effects of loss. Unrealistic bargaining should be avoided, as Tanner (1980) gave an example of an aphasic's nonverbal cues to the clinician: "If I work hard and do everything you require of me then perhaps I will get all of my speech back . . ." (p. 922).

The fourth stage is *depression,* coming after the disorder no longer can be denied and anger has been vented. "Attempts to cheer-up the patient and to devalue the significance of the loss should be weighed carefully. To reach ultimate acceptance, the patient needs to experience the full pain of the loss" (Tanner, 1980, p. 922).

The final stage is *acceptance,* or acknowledgement of the reality of the situation (Webster and Newhoff, 1981). In this stage the patient and family will be most cooperative in the rehabilitation program. Acceptance includes not only acknowledgement of the disorder but also acknowledgement of its prognosis. As mentioned before, patients with mild disorders can have a more difficult time reaching this final stage than patients with obvious incapacity.

The rate of passage from denial to acceptance will vary from case to case. Tanner suggested that the grieving process for a major loss may last six to twelve months; but if the individual remains in stages one through four more than six months, then the mourning patterns can be suspected to be pathological. In this case, the clinician should refer to or seek advice from a clinical psychologist or psychiatrist. Meanwhile, the speech-language clinician's primary role is to facilitate normal progression of the process.

The Helpful Clinician

According to Tanner (1980), the clinician should avoid certain behaviors which interrupt the grieving process and should employ certain behaviors in order to facilitate the process.

The clinician should avoid the following:

1. Positive reinforcement of denial, a stage which should be replaced as soon as possible. Instead, there should be compassionate discussion of the disorder and of a realistic prognosis. Prognosis should address language functions and communication, and in this distinction there is hope for even the most severely impaired.

2. Avoid *punishing anger,* a necessary reaction which goes away by allowing for its release. By making the patient's living environment a comfortable one in which progress is facilitated, the clinician can advise family and hospital staff that anger is normal and should not be taken as a personal affront.

3. Avoid *bargaining with the patient;* especially avoid creating false hopes by offering more from treatment than can be delivered.

4. Avoid *providing secondary gains* from attention and sympathy received during the grieving process. The clinician should watch out for the possibility that concern for the patient might serve to maintain a stage of the process too long and create excessive dependency on the clinician and the treatment program. Tanner suggested encouraging the patient to be his or her own therapist. As stated in previous chapters, treatment should move the patient toward being an independent communicator.

5. Avoid *displaying anxiety about the patient's depression*. Like anger, depression is a natural and necessary reaction to be experienced in order for acceptance to be achieved.

The clinician can facilitate the process further by doing the following:

1. *Permit the patient control* by allowing the patient to participate in decisions about treatment and family activities.

2. *Provide the patient with perspective* by explaining that the awful pain of adjustment will end eventually, and by simply providing the successful experience of a well-planned treatment program. Also, the opportunity to have contact with other patients who are feeling the same things adds a perspective of not being alone. Contact with well-adjusted patients is proof that there is light at the end of the tunnel. These are among the values of group treatment noted in Chapter 10.

3. *Acknowledge the reality of the loss.* The clinician (and family) should not avoid the difficult issues which the patient may want to express. Whenever the patient expresses a concern during treatment, the activity should be stopped and the clinician should listen and attempt to understand.

4. *Listen to the patient without defending or explaining his or her concerns.* Clinicians do not have all the answers or explanations for what any patient is feeling at any moment. Trying to explain or debate these feelings with the patient can be perceived by the patient as a negation of his or her real feelings (Tanner, 1980). Again, the clinician need only listen and provide the atmosphere of unconditional positive regard and empathy described earlier.

Counseling the Aphasic Patient

So far, the speech-language clinician's role in the patient's psychological adjustment to aphasia has been described as a rather passive one. Like a good friend, but with a somewhat detached objectivity, the clinician listens, offers encouragement and acceptance, and generally refrains from intervening in certain ways which could be disruptive. However, "counseling" implies that the clinician might serve an active role by intervening for the purpose of assisting the patient in solving problems which accompany aphasia. The term counseling or the idea of a more active role in the patient's psychological adjustment bring a mixture of reactions from experienced clinical aphasiologists: from "We aren't trained to do that" or "Where's your data" to "We should become involved in the patient's life system." Some of the apparent difference of orientation comes from different meanings for the term "counseling." For some clinical aphasiologists, it implies clinical or counseling psychology and, therefore, a special field of expertise. For others, it is a word from the dictionary meaning "to give advice," something which everyone does without special training.

This distinction between professional counseling and giving advice is an important one because, relative to the former, the clinician should know when to refer a patient for expert help; and, relative to the latter, the clinician normally plays a direct role. This is not an issue of whether the speech-language clinician becomes a counseling psychologist because the clinician happens to be available. Instead, the issue is one of being inclined to give advice and assist the patient with normal psychological or emotional problems as they arise during speech-language treatment.

We see aphasic patients from time to time who are suffering from psychological stress which disrupts the language-treatment process. These patients may have had premorbid psychological problems which have still not been resolved or have been exacerbated by brain damage. Serious marital problems, for example, probably had their origin years before onset of aphasia. There are people with aphasia who have always had trouble holding a job, forming intimate relationships, and meeting family responsibilities. An aphasic may already have been undergoing difficult adjustments to retirement, death of a spouse, or a move into a nursing home. These problems are likely to require assistance from a marriage counselor, personal counselor, or a counselor specializing in problems of the elderly. As a direct result of brain damage, mild aphasics may confront occupational adjustments which can be facilitated by a rehabilitation counselor. Advice from these professionals about people with a communication disorder may be directed most effectively to the speech-language pathologist; advice may deal with the interplay between psychological problems and conducting an effective language-treatment program. If patients with interfering psychological disturbances do not choose to accept help from or are unable to be helped by professional counselors, effecting a language treatment program may be an unrealistic objective.

While there is this special group of aphasics with special problems, every aphasic individual copes with the day-to-day problems faced by all of us. Also, aphasia produces the occasional frustration, fear, and sadness which were described previously. The patient has an argument with a friend, goes to a restaurant for the first time in six months, is confused about the purpose of a treatment activity, is concerned about his or her progress, wants to try hypnosis for his or her speech, or is getting tired of coming to the clinic. In the middle of a treatment activity the aphasic may become impatient or distracted, and so it is time for the clinician to stop the activity and deal with the problem so that the patient can feel better and so that treatment may continue. It is in this sense that the clinician does some counseling.

Webster (1977; Webster and Newhoff, 1981) specified four counselor functions which can be served by the speech-language pathologist: (1) receive information from the patient; (2) give information to the patient; (3) help the patient clarify ideas, attitudes, and emotions; and (4) provide the patient with options for chang-ing behavior. Information is elicited from the patient concerning needs and interests which shape treatment objectives and concerning progress outside of the clinic. Information is given concerning the purpose of testing and treatment, the prospects for recovery, and the progress being made in treatment. The patient may develop certain attitudes and feelings about treatment which need to be discussed. One issue may surround the introduction of alternative modes of communication which the patient may feel awkward about or may reject outright. Silverman (1980) stressed the importance of gaining acceptance of nonspeech modes from the patient and family. The aphasic may have trouble expressing a feeling that the clinician has given up trying to improve speech or that further improvement is impossible. Finally, if the patient is having difficulties getting along with others in the hospital or at home, the clinician can suggest ways of dealing with the situation. The clinician need not look for these difficulties because the patient will bring them up during regular treatment sessions.

THE FAMILY

The problems of the aphasic individual are inseparable from the changes confronting the patient's family, and so clinical goals for the patient are more attainable with understanding and cooperation from the family. Family members are incorporated into the rehabilitation process in two respects: (1) assisting the patient in his or her recovery and adjustment and (2) obtaining assistance for themselves in adjusting to the sudden and drastic changes in their own lives.

Support for the Patient and Treatment

The patient's living environment is considered in numerous ways. Treatment plans are directed toward preparing the patient to meet communicative demands outside the clinic. The living environment influences the patient's adjustment to aphasia and motivation to work on communication skills. A complete treatment program takes into account modifications in the environment which could make communication more frequent, enjoyable, and successful (Lubinski, 1981a, 1981b). Care-givers and significant others are involved in each of these considerations. Furthermore, they are a valuable source of information concerning generalization of improvements seen in treatment.

Providing a Positive Atmosphere. Making life comfortable for the patient and maximizing communicative success requires an understanding of the patient's disorder. Misunderstandings arise from confusing aphasia with intellectual impairment, thinking of comprehension problems in terms of a hearing loss, and putting demands on the patient which are thought to be helpful but which actually inhibit real communicative capabilities. A few investigators have looked into what family members do know about aphasia and how they perceive the patient's disorder. Helmick, Watamori, and Palmer (1976; 1977) had spouses rate patients' communicative behavior with the *FCP* and concluded that spouses underestimate the patient's communication impairment. Holland (1977a) responded that "acontextual" language tests may underestimate communicative competence and that spouses may actually have a better idea of how well the patient can communicate using nonverbal cues and natural context. This, again, is a matter of distinguishing between communication and language, because family members may still harbor some misconceptions of the patient's language functions. For example, they may not recognize severe auditory comprehension deficits, attributing the patient's behavior to depression, fatigue, or obstinacy (Czvik, 1977). Spouses appear to be very confident in their ratings of aphasic impairment, especially in auditory and verbal modalities (Linebaugh and Young-Charles, 1981). However, spouses of aphasic patients consistently express a need for information about stroke and aphasia (Linebaugh and Young-Charles, 1978; Newhoff and Davis, 1978). Many will search the public library for literature on these topics.

Several booklets contain explanations of stroke and aphasia for the layperson, including Boone (1965), Taylor (1958), and Cohen (1971). The Sister Kenny Institute in Minneapolis, Minnesota, publishes several booklets on problems related to aphasia and stroke, including Cohen's (1977) suggestions regarding nonspeech communication aids for patients with aphasia, apraxia, and dysarthria. Hale (1979) published a beautifully illustrated "guide to easier, more independent living for physically disabled people, their families and friends." Some of the booklets on aphasia include lists of "do's and don'ts" addressing matters such as treating the patient as an adult, making appropriate demands on language, and fostering a positive atmosphere for the patient to find his or her own way to deal with aphasia. J.E. Sarno and Sarno (1979) and Broida (1979) wrote substantial explanations in a question-and-answer format. Bollinger, Waugh, and Zatz (1977) developed a booklet on communication disorders common in an elderly population, aimed primarily at hospital personnel, especially in a nursing-home setting. These guides for hospital personnel can supplement in-service training programs and assist in meeting the goals of environmental management (see Chapter 10).

Spouses can be very sensitive to a patient's reactions to their behavior and often develop, on their own, effective communicative strategies and other behaviors which facilitate the patient's psychosocial adjustment. Common maladaptive behaviors, however, include a tendency to demand a spoken word even though communication has been achieved, and a tendency not to give the patient enough time to talk when talking is possible. Some spouses may be impatient and want to speak for the patient. Depending on circumstances, the patient may feel that this behavior is helpful or may be frustrated by it. Communication is facilitated by the spouse's simplifying and slowing the rate of his or her own utterances and by using gestures to enhance understanding by the patient. Newhoff, Bugbee, and Ferreira (1981) examined PACE as a circumstance in which spouses and other family members might develop communicative strategies with the patient.

The patient's progress toward maximum adjustment may be obstructed by overprotectiveness from family members. Protectiveness becomes harmful when the patient is kept from family decisions and activities which are within the patient's capabilities. The patient may become dependent on the spouse, and this dependency limits the extent of recovery even further. This vicious cycle between protectiveness and dependency can be avoided or reduced by counseling of family members (Malone, 1969).

Participation in Treatment. In numerous ways, the spouse or care-giver is called upon to assist in the communication-treatment process. He or she is asked to reinforce the patient's use of new communicative strategies such as gesturing or pointing to words in a notebook. Furthermore, he or she extends the patient's time for formal language exercises by monitoring homework assignments or by actually administering language drills. This form of participation becomes valuable when the patient is seen by the speech-language pathologist for a brief time each week. Goodkin, Diller, and Shah (1973) trained spouses in behavior-modification techniques, and Flowers and Danforth (1979) enlisted spouses in the administration of sentence-comprehension drills.

Several workbooks are available for the patient to practice language skills at home or in a hospital room, either independently or with assistance from a family member or care-giver. When assistance is required, these workbooks contain instructions for the helper. Sometimes the helper should be present to provide stimulation specified in a task, but more frequently a helper should be available to provide feedback on response adequacy (reviewed in Chapter 11). A patient can practice an exercise in a workbook when the clinician has determined that the patient does not require feedback from another person. The clinician is careful to be sure that each homework assignment is within the patient's capability either without or with feedback from a helper. Most workbooks, especially those intended to provide independent activities, are oriented toward reading and writing modalities. They can be a source of ideas for the clinician's planning of activities to be done in regular treatment.

A sampling of these resources begins with two volumes called *Speech and Language Rehabilitation: A Workbook for the Neurologically Impaired,* developed by Keith (1972, 1977). These were designed for the patient who is "unable to receive continuous therapy from a professional speech pathologist" (1972, p. v). The second volume contains more pictured stimuli and tasks requiring a helper. Some instruction is given for feedback, but this feedback is corrective upon inaccurate response, which is contrary to recommendations reviewed here in Chapter 11. McKeown's (1976) *A Practicebook for Aphasics* contains pictures drawn by a young aphasic veteran of the Vietnam War and is organized according to everyday topics instead of language functions. Kilpatrick and Jones' (1977) *Therapy Guide for the Adult with Language and Speech Disorders* includes activities for practice of gesturing and exercises for dysarthria and apraxia of speech. The last section contains printed words for the patient to use as a communication aid. A second volume provides more exercises focused on verbal expression for the aphasic (Kilpatrick, 1979). Brubaker's (1978) *Workbook for Aphasia* contains reading and writing exercises designed for the higher-level aphasic patient. Traendly's (1979) four volumes for word finding, reading, writing, and math are intended to be used with supervision. The word-finding activities are still oriented toward reading and writing.

There are two somewhat different treatment supplements which were intended primarily to provide independent practice for the patient. Kilpatrick's (1980) *Working with Words* is a source of potentially enjoyable word puzzles and games such as simple but adult crossword puzzles. Bedwinek (1981) developed a set of fifteen audio cassette tapes so that the moderately and mildly impaired patient can stimulate himself using a tape recorder. Pictures are provided, and the activities are centered around repetition for language and speech disorders.

While these workbooks contain activities molded in the tradition of direct stimulation of language and conform to many of the principles outlined here in Chapters 10 and 11, they do not provide information as to how these activities were actually applied to different types of patients. There is minimal description of the extent to which the activities have been employed in the contexts for which they are advertised. The experienced clinician, however, is able to make judgments about the judicious use of these workbooks; and any clinician can ensure that a patient is capable of using these activities independently, without someone to provide feedback or to make subtle adjustments when the patient is fatigued or frustrated. Also, the authors of these guides provide little description of their experience with how well helpers have done in monitoring and administrating these activities. The clinician should prepare hospital personnel or family members for this task so that they will be appropriately responsive to the patient's successes and occasional inadequacies.

The Family's Problems

"I want someone to help *me*" is an appeal likely to be heard from the spouse of a person with aphasia. The aphasic patient is the center of concern in the rehabilitation process, and educating and advising the family is usually viewed as a means toward helping the patient. Most of Broida's (1979) book for families, for example, informs the family about brain damage, aphasia, apraxia, and dysarthria; the last chapter, addressed to changes in the family, still focuses on caring for the aphasic. While this information is requested by the family and is helpful for their own adjustment, the family's own problems seem to be of secondary concern in the traditional rehabilitation scheme. The spouse, in particular, bears the brunt of new responsibilities in caring for the patient and in keeping familial structure afloat. Interest in the family's perspective has been a relatively recent development in the study of aphasia's impact.

There have been a few somewhat formal studies of the special problems of families. Malone, Ptacek, and Malone (1970) administered a questionnaire to thirty spouses in order to determine the extent of different attitudes toward the patient and their own lives. Carpenter (1974) studied the effect of a husband's physical disability on the wife's household roles in a comparison of employed and unemployed wives. Spouses and offspring were interviewed and given questionnaires by Malone (1969), Kinsella and Duffy (1978), and Linebaugh and Young-Charles (1978). Kinsella and Duffy analyzed attitudes and adjustment by three groups in which the patient had aphasia only, aphasia and hemiplegia, and hemiplegia only. Chwat focused on the perspective of sons and daughters with a questionnaire designed for the patient's offspring (Chwat, Chapey, Gurland, et al., 1980; Chwat and Gurland, 1981). In addition, the concerns of spouses have been reported through descriptions of counseling programs (Newhoff and Davis, 1978; Porter and Dabul, 1977).

Before getting into the results of these studies, we can consider the reactions and adjustments of the spouse in terms of models already used here to explain the reactions and adjustments of the patient. Adjustment to disability is especially demanding when the disability is sudden and unexpected. Unprepared, the entire family experiences a deep sense of loss of the patient's role in the family and of each member's life patterns and plans, especially those living with the patient. In one study, "spouses of patients with aphasia indicated an acute sense of loss—in some cases the inability to talk over the mundane events of the day, or in other cases the loss of discussion on more abstract topics, or as one subject commented 'the loss of a speech partner'" (Kinsella and Duffy, 1978, p. 40). Therefore, the grieving process is a natural reaction for family members (Tanner, 1980). Also, with respect to transactional analysis, the spouse may strengthen his or her Parent and Adult ego states and weaken the Child state as the premorbid balance between husband and wife shifts when the patient becomes more dependent (Porter and Dabul, 1977).

The patient's spouse may harbor certain unhealthy attitudes toward the patient which can be a source of anxiety and guilt in the spouse. *Unrealistic expectations* concerning recovery are common (Kinsella and Duffy, 1978). In response to questionnaire items (Malone, et al., 1970), husbands and wives agreed to "if one puts in enough effort any condition can be changed," a statement which can be interpreted as being realistic depending on

what is meant by "change." However, 67 percent agreed that "even the most seriously handicapped person can be made perfect by prayer," and 63 percent agreed that "my spouse will talk as well as anybody." Malone's subjects were questioned at six months to three years post-onset. Much less frequent are feelings of *rejection of the patient* (Kinsella and Duffy, 1978; Malone, et al., 1970).

Overprotection of the patient was mentioned previously as an approach which fosters dependency on the spouse and limits the patient's use of capabilities. It is a frequent attitude among spouses. Malone, et al. (1970) found that 70 percent agreed that "I manage things so my spouse is not put into situations where he might get his feelings hurt" and 63 percent agreed that "I am constantly warning my spouse to be careful." This attitude blends with the spouse's desire to attend to the genuine needs of severely disabled aphasic and hemiplegic partners. The patient's demands are a heavy burden for the spouse, and these demands include an apparent *overprotectiveness of the patient's spouse.* An aphasic husband, becoming dependent, may be fearful of any possible illness in his wife. The wife may become reticent about mentioning any minor aches and pains. The aphasic husband may insist that his wife get help with housework when she does not need or want it. Aphasic husbands may insist that their wives meet them somewhere or return home at a precise time, and become terribly frightened when their wives are a little late. An aphasic wife may keep a constant watch on her husband, not wanting him to leave the house, fearing that he might leave her. The spouse may feel smothered by the patient's dependency and fears.

One wife wrote of her aphasic husband's dependency and of her realization that it should not be encouraged:

> Clay needed nursing and nurturing and I was eager to do whatever I could. As time

went on and he was gradually improving, I occasionally was concerned about his dependency on me, which seemed to be unnecessary. I had no problem about any physical limitations he had, but I wasn't prepared for, nor desirous of, the psychological dependencies. We had always shared chores and responsibilities. . . . With prolonged illness this relationship had changed. I made up my mind that I wouldn't allow him to regress, to lose his independence and responsibility. . . .

Apart from my needs, I basically knew that Clay would not benefit from prolonged overindulgence and childlike dependency.[2]

Most spouses continually analyze their situations and attempt to do what is best for their partners and themselves.

Especially within the context of family structure, the *role adjustments* of the aphasic precipitate role adjustments by other family members. In the study by Linebaugh and Young-Charles (1978), 76 percent of twenty-one spouses reported shifts in responsibilities. Wives become responsible for finances, and husbands become responsible for cooking and general housework. The spouse may develop a feeling of being "swallowed up" by a situation in which he or she is now responsible for activities which once were divided between two people. When assessing the status of role division and change within a family unit, the clinician should keep in mind that these differ among families and that role divisions have been changing in the past couple of decades. With contemporary shifts toward both marriage partners pursuing careers and toward equal division of housework, the impact of aphasia upon family homeostasis may be more varied by the year 2000.

Changes in marital relationships were striking in Kinsella and Duffy's (1978) survey and were more prominent in groups with aphasia than in the group with only hemiplegia. The changes included more friction, lack of communication about major topics, loss of partnership, and diminished sexual activity. Sexual intercourse had ceased altogether in 83 percent of the couples. In another study, 76 percent of spouses reported a change in the marital relationship (Linebaugh and Young-Charles, 1978). In the report of her aphasia, Wulf (1979) noted: "Adapting to aphasia is a dilemma for which there are no easy, magic solutions, and when a marriage has been pummeled and bruised by a stroke with aphasia, the needs of both partners have to be examined minutely, carefully, wisely, and with optimistic realism" (p. 92).

Alteration of relationships extends beyond the family, with *diminished leisure and social activity* (Kinsella and Duffy, 1978). Linebaugh and Young-Charles (1978) found that 67 percent of spouses and 82 percent of children experienced change in social life. Over 70 percent of Malone, et al.'s (1970) subjects "go out for an evening" and "go to parties" less than before. Over 50 percent entertained at home less and took fewer vacations.

These pressures and life changes may affect the mental and physical health of the spouse. Malone (1969) found that some spouses were getting less sleep. In Kinsella and Duffy's (1978) study, 42 percent of spouses exhibited depressive symptoms and 62 percent had an increased liability to minor psychiatric disorder which was more prominent in wives of hemiplegics with aphasia than wives of nonaphasic hemiplegics. Through a questionnaire, 80 percent agreed that "I feel miserable and sad" and 78 percent that "I get tired for no reason."

Offspring of aphasic parents have reported less anxiety and helplessness and less frequent changes of relationships than spouses (Linebaugh and Young-Charles, 1978). Still, 47 percent reported a change. Malone (1969) described some children as feeling neglected. Dahlberg's son discussed the following change: ". . . this was the first year I had spent being comfortable

---

[2] Quoted by permission from Dahlberg, C.C., and Jaffe, J., *Stroke: A Doctor's Personal Story of His Recovery* (New York: W.W. Norton, 1977), p. 64.

and open with my parents. . . . Now I was finally realizing how much I enjoyed my father, and we were just starting to get comfortable and open when—bang!—the stroke threw everything off course" (Dahlberg and Jaffe, 1977, p. 26).

Precedents in Family Services

The surveys cited here indicated not only that families have problems attributed to aphasia in one member, but also that many spouses especially feel the need for help with these problems. Kinsella and Duffy (1978) reported that 57 percent of thirty spouses had one source of help, with the most common sources being children (48 percent) and friends (37 percent). There was no mention of receiving help from spouses of other aphasics or from a rehabilitation specialist such as a counselor or a speech-language pathologist. All twenty-one spouses in Linebaugh and Young-Charles' (1978) study felt that formal counseling should be available for them; and if it were offered, most said they would employ techniques for coping with physical problems (85 percent), emotional problems (95 percent), and facilitating communication (100 percent). Most of these spouses had received some formal counseling, which dealt with communication for 48 percent and with emotional problems for only 10 percent. Nearly all spouses had received some counseling from a speech-language pathologist; 59 percent, from a physician; 53 percent, from a social worker; and 24 percent, from a nurse. Therefore, the speech-language clinician most frequently provides assistance for spouses, but spouses may not receive help with many of their problems. Malone (1969) suggested that the family can become more positive members of the rehabilitation team if the speech-language pathologist becomes involved in assisting the family.

Family members have received counseling in conjunction with speech-language treatment individually and in groups (Webster and Newhoff, 1981) and have been provided with special programs that include the patient and family or family members only (Brookshire, 1978b). Most programs described in the literature are group programs, which are not only the most convenient for the clinician's busy schedule but are also of great value for the family members.

One group program which included the patient was designed to develop more realistic attitudes toward aphasia, provide for ventilation of feelings, decrease feelings of isolation, and provide a different context for speech-language treatment of the patient (Redinger, Forster, Dolphin, et al., 1971). A psychiatrist and clinical psychologist joined the clinical aphasiologist in order to manage the ventilation of feelings between patient and spouse and to provide acting out of conflicts in a controlled manner. When such programs are carried out during the period of language treatment, they can be of maximum benefit to the rehabilitation process. However, a patient-family program, called the "Alumni Reunion," was carried out subsequent to discharge by Mogil, Bloom, Gray, et al. (1978). With assistance from a psychotherapist, the patient and family returned for group meetings on Saturday afternoons. Each meeting consisted of three segments: a reception, which was a social gathering including refreshments; a shared experience, in which the entire group listened to a guest speaker; and sessions with a psychosocial focus, in which patients and family members met separately in small groups.

The American Heart Association (AHA) sponsors a patient-family program that is conducted in communities throughout the United States and is called the *Stroke Club*. The AHA's affiliate in Austin, Texas publishes an organizational manual and sends an adviser to a community to assist in establishing a new club. The program guide of 1974 describes a Stroke Club: "It is an organization of stroke families for the purpose of social and recreational activities through group interrelationships.'' Its stated goal is ''to assist members to retain their individual identities and continue to be contributing members of society.'' Stroke Clubs are managed by members who are elected as officers of the club. Ongoing consultants may come from the local AHA chapter and/or may be a spouse of a patient who has volunteered to become active in community activities for stroke victims. Kinsella and Duffy (1978) were strong advocates of a stroke club format as a means of alleviating many of the family problems revealed in their study.

Several group programs for the family, especially the spouse, have been described (Turnblom and Myers, 1952; Derman and Manaster, 1967; Puts-Zwartjes, 1973; Porter and Dabul, 1977; and Newhoff and Davis, 1978). Porter and Dabul assisted spouses in understanding changes in family dynamics, using the transactional analysis model. The spouses took four steps to reestablish balance in the spouse-patient relationship: (1) recognize and increase the patient's Adult ego state, (2) learn to interpret the patient's attempts to communicate, (3) recognize and increase the patient's nurturing Parent, and (4) find outlets for the spouse's own Child state. Derman and Manaster emphasized the ''co-therapeutic'' role of spouses who are experienced with aphasia and who can help those newly burdened with the disorder. A husband told Newhoff and Davis (1978) of the value of regular meetings with other spouses: ''It's nice to find out you're not alone. You get ideas in here of ways to cope. I've learned to enjoy my wife in spite of her stroke. I feel closer to her now'' (p. 324).

Counselor Functions

The spouses of aphasics have many questions about aphasia and its etiologies which need answers. Understanding improves their ability to cope with this some-times bewildering new situation. Also, they develop strong anxiety-provoking feelings about their own circumstances which are difficult to discuss with other members of the family and are especially difficult to discuss with the patient. In a spouse discussion group which meets regularly, the wife or husband finds a safe place to vent their feelings. The empathy provided by other spouses is a powerful elixir for frustrations that build up from being unable to have maximum communication with the patient and from feeling trapped by the increased demands for nurturing and by their own resentments and guilt.

Webster's (1977) four counselor functions, described earlier, can be employed by the speech-language pathologist serving as an organizer, leader, and facilitator of weekly one-hour spouse/family discussion groups. Conceptual models which contribute to defining goals for family members include Satir's (1967) concept of family homeostasis (or balance) and theories of the stages in reaction to crises or loss (see Webster and Newhoff, 1981). Webster and Newhoff suggested, for example, that the spouse may not be able to use information about aphasia during the initial phase of denial or shock. During the early period, feelings of anxiety and helplessness may be at their maximum. The first meeting of a spouse group begins with introductions which include identification of time since onset of aphasia in each family. Spouses are compelled to compare where they are in their adjustment relative to the others.

Receiving Information. Webster's first counselor function is that the clinician obtains information from the spouse about the patient's communicative environment, family activities and interests that might be suggestive of semantic content for the patient's treatment, the patient's communicative behaviors at home, and the spouse's own concerns. In expressing their concerns and in asking questions, family members are very informative about their perceptions of the patient's problem, the communicative demands placed on the patient, and the effectiveness of previous attempts to provide information to the family. Webster's (1977) guidelines for interviewing parents of communicatively handicapped children are applicable in obtaining information from the spouse of an adult client.

Giving Information.   Schuell, et al. (1964) wrote that the clinician should "... arrange a series of interviews to interpret the patient's language disabilities to a responsible member of the family and to prepare the family to assist, not impede, the patient's recovery" (p. 328). The clinician informs the spouse about aphasia, the purpose and results of tests, the goals and plans of treatment, and the patient's prognosis. Booklets cited earlier in this chapter are convenient for the clinician but should be reviewed with the spouse when he or she is ready to understand. No matter how information is given, the clinician makes sure that it is understood and accepted. Booklets are general and sometimes comprehensive. The clinician helps the spouse in relating this information to the unique patterns of deficit in each patient.

Spouses have questions that should be answered with terms and concepts familiar to the general public and with definitions of aphasiologic terms which cannot be avoided. The need for definitions should be anticipated and provided without the spouse having to ask for them. There are many questions: *Why is my husband always upset after a test? Why does my wife occasionally produce whole sentences without thinking? Why will my husband watch TV but not join in a conversation?* (One aphasic wife switched TV preference after onset from soap operas to sports, which she had refused to watch before.) *How long will it take for my husband to change from being an introvert?* In a spouse group, several members will respond: "My husband does that!" or "My wife is

like that!" and, then, "Well, what do *you* do?" The question-answer books display many of the common questions (Broida, 1979; J. E. Sarno and Sarno, 1979). Of paramount concern are all those questions about recovery dealt with in Chapter 9.

Though we do not have much of the data needed to provide answers to many of the common questions about prognosis, our presentation of prognosis to the family can be more differentiated than vague "wait and see" statements. We can address the functions which are likely to recover at different rates; we can distinguish between language and communication. We can talk positively about the adjustments which can occur in face of the hard realities of aphasia. Encouragement should be tempered by avoiding the creation of false impressions, and so there is often an element of "wait and see" when advising families about what to expect. Spouses will hope that the patient's brain will function as before, and this is impossible. The fact of permanent brain damage becomes a part of the already shocking reality of the disorder.

The clinician regularly reports to the family concerning the patient's recovery. Though the most meaningful recovery occurs in presence of the family, some improvements may not be recognized in day-to-day observation. Objective measures made by the clinician are a source of encouragement. Again, the clinician recognizes that improved performance on a treatment task may not necessarily reflect improvement in real-life communication. A spouse may begin to wonder about a clinician's report of changes which the spouse does not observe at home. Therefore, while the clinician reports changes in clinical performance, he or she must also ask the spouse about changes observed at home.

Clarification.   Spouses develop continuously disturbing feelings about their situation, partly because it occurred suddenly and was not planned. In responses to Linebaugh and Young-Charles' (1978) questionnaire, 90 percent of spouses experienced anxiety, 86 percent frustration, 57 percent helplessness, 52 percent depression, 38 percent hostility, and 33 percent guilt. Of Malone, et al.'s (1970) subjects, 63 percent, at least six months postonset, thought that aphasia was God's punishment for wrongdoing. Especially in a spouse discussion group, where there is genuine understanding and a lot of encouragement, a spouse has the opportunity to have attitudes and feelings clarified. The clinician becomes an active listener, acknowledging and accepting the spouse's concerns. Once the spouse discovers that feelings of resentment and guilt are common and natural, he or she can explore the possible reasons for them. Through expression of and understanding of these feelings, the spouse learns to live with them and then to live without them.

Changing Behavior. The fourth counselor function is to provide family members with options for changing their behavior. One of these options might be receiving counseling from a social worker, psychologist, or psychiatrist. However, a spouse will often embark upon changing his or her behavior once aphasia is understood, once attitudes and feelings are clarified, and once suggestions are freely offered from other spouses who have dealt successfully with the same problems.

By encouraging the spouse or other care-giver to modify behaviors communicatively and socially, we can create an environment which fosters increased confidence and independence in the person with aphasia. The patient may return to a few former activities, may be more willing to venture out to visit friends and enjoy a family outing, and may discover abilities to assist in family decision-making. The spouse and patient begin reversing any trend to withdrawal from each other and from other experiences by making the decision to receive speech-language treatment and by participating in group meetings with people strapped with similar difficulties. The community may provide activities, such as government-supported recreation programs for the handicapped. Public libraries provide information services concerning programs for the handicapped and the elderly. The key objective of language rehabilitation, which is its most gratifying effect, is the reduction of isolation stemming from communication impairment.

Bibliography

ABBATE, M.S., and LaCHAPPELLE, N.B., *Pictures, Please! A Language Supplement.* Tucson, Ariz.: Communication Skill Builders (1979).

ALAJOUANINE, T., Aphasia and artistic realization. *Brain,* 71, 229–241 (1948).

ALAJOUANINE, T., Verbal realization in aphasia. *Brain,* 79, 1–28 (1956).

ALBERT, M.L., Short-term memory and aphasia. *Brain and Language,* 3, 28–33 (1976).

ALBERT, M.L., GOODGLASS, H., HELM, N.A., RUBENS, A.B., and ALEXANDER, M.P., *Clinical Aspects of Dysphasia.* New York: Springer-Verlag (1981).

ALBERT, M.L., and OBLER, L.K., *The Bilingual Brain.* New York: Academic Press (1978).

ALBERT, M.L., SPARKS, R., and HELM, N.A., Melodic intonation therapy for aphasia. *Archives of Neurology,* 29, 130–131 (1973).

AMMON, K.H., MOERMANN, C., and GULEAC, J.D., Aphasics' defective perception of connotative meaning of verbal items which have no denotative meaning. *Cortex,* 8, 453–457 (1977).

AMMONS, R.B., and AMMONS, H.S., *Full-Range Picture Vocabulary Test.* Missoula, Mont.: Psychological Test Specialists (1948).

ANDREEWSKY, E., and SERON, X., Implicit processing of grammatical rules in a classical case of agrammatism. *Cortex,* 11, 379–390 (1975).

ARTES, R., and HOOPS, R., Problems of aphasic and non-aphasic stroke patients as identified and evaluated by patients' wives. In Y. Lebrun and R. Hoops (Eds.), *Recovery in Aphasia.* Amsterdam: Swets & Zeitlinger (1976).

ATEN, J.L., and LYON, J.G., Measures of PICA subtest variance: A preliminary assessment of their value as predictors of language recovery in aphasic patients. In R.H. Brookshire (Ed.), *Clinical Aphasiology Conference Proceedings.* Minneapolis: BRK (1978).

BAER, W.P., *The Aphasic Patient: A Program for Auditory Comprehension and Language Training* (Clinician's Edition). Springfield, Ill.: Charles C. Thomas (1976).

BAKAN, P., Hypnotizability, laterality of eye movement and functional brain asymmetry. *Perceptual and Motor Skills,* 28, 927–932 (1969).

BAKER, E., BERRY, T., GARDNER, H., ZURIF, E., DAVIS, L., and VEROFF, A., Can linguistic competence be dissociated from natural language functions? *Nature,* 254, 509–510 (1975).

BAKER, E., and GOODGLASS, H., Time for auditory processing of object names by aphasics. *Brain and Language,* 8, 355–366 (1979).

BAMBER, L., A retrospective study of language recovery in adult aphasics. Unpublished Master's Thesis, Memphis State University (1980).

BARNS, E.K., SAC, A., and SHORE, H., Guidelines to treatment approaches: Modalities and methods for use with the aged. *Gerontologist,* 13, 513–527 (1973).

BARR, M.L., *The Human Nervous System* (2nd Ed.). Hagerstown, Md.: Harper & Row (1974).

BARTON, M.I., Recall of generic properties of words in aphasic patients. *Cortex,* 7, 73–82 (1971).

BARTON, M.I., MARUSZEWSKI, M., and URREA, D., Variation of stimulus context and its effect on word-finding ability in aphasics. *Cortex,* 5, 351–365 (1969).

BASSO, A., CAPITANI, E., and VIGNOLO, L.A., Influence of rehabilitation on language skills in aphasic patients: A controlled study. *Archives of Neurology,* 36, 190–196 (1979).

BASSO, A., TABORELLI, A., and VIGNOLO, L.A., Dissociated disorders of speaking and writing in aphasia. *Journal of Neurology, Neurosurgery, and Psychiatry,* 41, 556–563 (1978).

BASTIAN, H.C., Some problems in connexion with aphasia and other speech defects. *Lancet,* 1, 933–942, 1005–1017, 1131–1137, 1187–1194 (1897).

BEASLEY, D.S., and DAVIS, G.A. (Eds.), *Aging: Communication Processes and Disorders.* New York: Grune & Stratton (1981).

BEDWINEK, A.P., *Supplemental Audio Cassettes: Speech & Language Stimulation for Adults with Neurogenic Communicative Disorders.* Tucson, Az.: Communication Skill Builders (1981).

BELMONT, I., and HANDLER, A., Delayed information processing and judgment of temporal order following cerebral damage. *Journal of Nervous and Mental Disorders,* 152, 353–361 (1971).

BENSON, D.F., Fluency in aphasia: Correlation with radioactive scan localization. *Cortex,* 3, 373–394 (1967).

BENSON, D.F., *Aphasia, Alexia, and Agraphia.* New York: Churchill Livingstone (1979a).

BENSON, D.F., Aphasia rehabilitation. *Archives of Neurology,* 36, 187–189 (1979b).

BENTON, A.L., Problems of test construction in the field of aphasia. *Cortex,* 3, 32–58 (1967).

BENTON, A.L., Development of a multilingual aphasia battery: Progress and problems. *Journal of Neurological Science,* 9, 39–48 (1969).

BENTON, A.L., and HAMSHER, K., *Multilingual Aphasia Examination.* Iowa City, Iowa: Benton Laboratory of Neuropsychology (1978).

BENTON, A.L., SMITH, K.C., and LANG, M., Stimulus characteristics and object naming in aphasic patients. *Journal of Communication Disorders,* 5, 19–24 (1972).

BERLIN, C.I., On: Melodic Intonation Therapy for aphasia by R.W. Sparks and A.L. Holland. *Journal of Speech and Hearing Disorders,* 41, 298–300 (1976).

BERLIN, C.I., and MCNEIL, M.R., Dichotic listening. In N.J. Lass (Ed.), *Contemporary Issues in Experimental Phonetics.* New York: Academic Press (1976).

BERLIN, I., *The Age of Enlightenment.* New York: Mentor (1956).

BERMAN, M., and PEELLE, L.M., Self-generated cues: A method for aiding aphasic and apractic patients. *Journal of Speech and Hearing Disorders,* 32, 372–376 (1967).

BERNDT, R.S., and CARAMAZZA, A., A redefinition of the syndrome of Broca's aphasia: Implications for a neuropsychological model of language. *Applied Psycholinguistics,* 1, 225–278 (1980).

BERNDT, R.S. and CARAMAZZA, A., Syntactic aspects of aphasia. In M.T. Sarno (Ed.), *Acquired Aphasia.* New York: Academic Press (1981).

BERRY, W.R., A psychometric reconsideration of the Token Test. Paper presented at the Third Annual Clinical Aphasiology Conference, Albuquerque, N.Mex. (1973).

BERRY, W.R., Testing auditory comprehension in aphasia: A clinical alternative to the Token Test. In R.H. Brookshire (Ed.), *Clinical Aphasiology: Collected Proceedings 1972–1976.* Minneapolis: BRK (1978).

BEUKELMAN, D.R., YORKSTON, K.M., and WAUGH, P.F., Communication in severe aphasia: Effectiveness of three instructional modalities. *Archives of Physical Medicine and Rehabilitation,* 61, 248–251 (1980).

BEYN, E.S., and VLASENKO, I.T., Verbal paraphasias of aphasic patients in the course of naming actions. *British Journal of Disorders of Communication,* 9, 24–34 (1974).

BIRCHMEIER, A.K., Feature analysis and the Token Test. *Brain and Language,* 10, 98–110 (1980).

BIRREN, J.E., and SLOANE, R.B. (Eds.), *Handbook of Mental Health and Aging.* Englewood Cliffs, N.J.: Prentice-Hall (1980).

BISIACH, E., Perceptual factors in the pathogenesis of anomia. *Cortex,* 2, 90–95 (1966).

BISIACH, E., Characteristics of visual stimuli and naming performance in aphasic adults: Comments on the paper by Corlew and Nation. *Cortex,* 12, 74–75 (1976).

BISSET, J., and DAVIS, G.A., Spinning off the multiple baseline design in its clinical application. In R.H. Brookshire (Ed.), *Clinical Aphasiology Conference Proceedings.* Minneapolis: BRK (1978).

BJORN-HANSEN, V., Social and emotional aspects of aphasia. *Journal of Speech and Hearing Disorders,* 22, 53–59 (1957).

BLACK, F.W., and STRUB, R.L., Digit repetition performance in patients with focal brain damage. *Cortex,* 14, 12–21 (1978).

BLAKEMORE, C., *Mechanics of the Mind.* Cambridge, England: Cambridge University Press (1977).

BLANCHARD, S.L., and PRESCOTT, T.E., The effects of temporal expansion upon auditory comprehension in aphasic adults. *British Journal of Disorders of Communication,* 15, 115–128 (1980).

BLISS, L.S., GUILFORD, A.M., and TIKOFSKY, R.S., Performance of adult aphasics on a sentence evaluation and revision task. *Journal of Speech and Hearing Research,* 19, 551–560 (1976).

BLISS, L.S., TIKOFSKY, R.S., and GUILFORD, A.M., Aphasics' sentence repetition behavior as a function of grammaticality. *Cortex,* 12, 113–121 (1976).

BLUMSTEIN, S.E., *A Phonological Investigation of Aphasic Speech.* The Hague, Netherlands: Mouton (1973).

BLUMSTEIN, S.E., Phonological aspects of aphasia. In M.T. Sarno (Ed.), *Acquired Aphasia.* New York: Academic Press (1981).

BLUMSTEIN, S.E., BAKER, E., and GOODGLASS, H., Phonological factors in auditory comprehension in aphasia. *Neuropsychologia,* 15, 19–30 (1977).

BLUMSTEIN, S.E., COOPER, W.E., GOODGLASS, H., STATLENDER, S., and GOTTLIEB, J., Production deficits in aphasia: A voice-onset time analysis. *Brain and Language,* 9, 153–170 (1980).

BLUMSTEIN, S.E., COOPER, W.E., ZURIF, E.B., and CARAMAZZA, A., The perception and production of voice-onset time in aphasia. *Neuropsychologia,* 15, 371–383 (1977).

BLUMSTEIN, S.E., and GOODGLASS, H., The perception of stress as a semantic cue in aphasia. *Journal of Speech and Hearing Research,* 15, 800–806 (1972).

BOGEN, J., and GORDON, H., Musical tests for functional lateralization with intracarotid amobarbital. *Nature,* 230, 524 (1971).

BOLLER, F., Latent aphasia: Right and left "non-aphasic" brain-damaged patients compared. *Cortex,* 4, 245–256 (1968).

BOLLER, F., COLE, M., VRTUNSKI, P.B., PATTERSON, M., and KIM, Y., Paralinguistic aspects of auditory comprehension in aphasia. *Brain and Language,* 7, 164–174 (1979).

BOLLER, F., and DENNIS, M. (Eds.), *Auditory Comprehension: Clinical and Experimental Studies with the Token Test.* New York: Academic Press (1979).

BOLLER, F., and GREEN, E., Comprehension in severe aphasics. *Cortex,* 8, 382–394 (1972).

BOLLER, F., and VIGNOLO, L.A., Latent sensory aphasia in hemisphere-damaged patients: An experimental study with the Token Test. *Brain,* 89, 815–830 (1966).

BOLLINGER, R.L., and STOUT, C.E., Response-contingent small-step treatment: Performance-based communication intervention. *Journal of Speech and Hearing Disorders,* 41, 40–51 (1976).

BOLLINGER, R.L., WAUGH, P.F., and ZATZ, A.F., *Communication Management of the Geriatric Patient.* Danville, Ill.: Interstate Printers & Publishers (1977).

BOONE, D.R., *An Adult Has Aphasia.* Danville, Ill.: Interstate Publishers & Printers (1965).

BORKOWSKI, J.G., BENTON, A.L., and SPREEN, O., Word fluency and brain damage. *Neuropsychologia,* 5, 135–140 (1967).

BOROD, J.C., GOODGLASS, H., and KAPLAN, E., Normative data on the Boston Diagnostic Aphasia Examination, Parietal Lobe Battery, and the Boston Naming Test. *Journal of Clinical Neuropsychology,* 2, 209–215 (1980).

BRADLEY, D.C., GARRETT, M.F., and ZURIF, E.B., Syntactic deficits in Broca's aphasia. In D. Caplan (Ed.), *Biological Studies of Mental Processes.* Cambridge, Mass.: MIT Press (1980).

BRAMWELL, B., A series of lectures on aphasia. *Lancet,* 1, 71–78, 351–361, 1671–1674, 1742–1747 (1906).

BRANCH, C., MILNER, B., and RASMUSSEN, T., Intercarotid sodium amytal for the lateralization of cerebral speech dominance. *Journal of Neurosurgery,* 21, 399–405 (1964).

BROADBENT, W.H., A case of peculiar affection of speech, with commentary. *Brain,* 1, 484–503 (1878).

BROCA, P., Remarks on the seat of the faculty of articulate language, followed by an observation of aphemia. In G. von Bonin (Trans.), *Some Papers on the Cerebral Cortex.* Springfield, Ill.: Charles C. Thomas (1960).

BROIDA, H., Language therapy effects in long term aphasia. *Archives of Physical Medicine and Rehabilitation,* 58, 248–253 (1977).

BROIDA, H., *Coping with Stroke.* Houston: College-Hill Press (1979).

BROOKSHIRE, R.H., Speech pathology and the experimental analysis of behavior. *Journal of Speech and Hearing Disorders,* 32, 215–227 (1967).

BROOKSHIRE, R.H., Visual discrimination and response reversal learning by aphasic subjects. *Journal of Speech and Hearing Research,* 11, 677–692 (1968).

BROOKSHIRE, R.H., Probability learning by aphasic subjects. *Journal of Speech and Hearing Research,* 12, 857–864 (1969).

BROOKSHIRE, R.H., Effects of task difficulty on naming by aphasic subjects. *Journal of Speech and Hearing Research,* 15, 551–558 (1972).

BROOKSHIRE, R.H., Differences in responding to auditory verbal materials among aphasic patients. *Acta Symbolica,* 5, 1–18 (1974).

BROOKSHIRE, R.H., Effects of prompting on spontaneous naming of pictures by aphasic subjects. *Human Communication,* Autumn, 63–71 (1975a).

BROOKSHIRE, R.H., Recognition of auditory sequences by aphasic, right-hemisphere-damaged and non-brain-damaged subjects. *Journal of Communication Disorders,* 8, 51–59 (1975b).

BROOKSHIRE, R.H., Effects of task difficulty on sentence comprehension performance of aphasic subjects. *Journal of Communication Disorders,* 9, 167–174 (1976).

BROOKSHIRE, R.H., Auditory comprehension and aphasia. In D.F. Johns (Ed.), *Clinical Management of Neurogenic Communicative Disorders.* Boston: Little, Brown and Company (1978a).

BROOKSHIRE, R.H., *An Introduction to Aphasia* (2nd Ed.). Minneapolis: BRK (1978b).

BROOKSHIRE, R.H., A Token Test battery for testing auditory comprehension in brain-injured adults. *Brain and Language,* 6, 149–157 (1978c).

BROOKSHIRE, R.H., and NICHOLAS, L.E., Effects of clinician request and feedback behavior on responses of aphasic individuals in speech and language treatment sessions. In R.H. Brookshire (Ed.), *Clinical Aphasiology Conference Proceedings.* Minneapolis: BRK (1978).

BROOKSHIRE, R.H., and NICHOLAS, L.E., Verification of active and passive sentences by aphasic and nonaphasic subjects. *Journal of Speech and Hearing Research,* 23, 878–893 (1980).

BROOKSHIRE, R.H., NICHOLAS, L.S., KRUEGER, K.M., and REDMOND, K.J., The Clinical Interaction Analysis System: A system for observational recording of aphasia treatment. *Journal of Speech and Hearing Disorders,* 43, 437–447 (1978).

BROWN, J.R., and SCHUELL, H.M., A preliminary report of a diagnostic test for aphasia. *Journal of Speech and Hearing Disorders,* 15, 21–28 (1950).

BROWN, J.W., The neural organization of language: Aphasia and lateralization. *Brain and Language,* 3, 482–494 (1976).

BROWN, J.W., *Mind, Brain, and Consciousness: The Neuropsychology of Cognition.* New York: Academic Press (1977).

BROWN, J.W., Case reports of semantic jargon. In J.W. Brown (Ed.), *Jargonaphasia.* New York: Academic Press (1981a).

BROWN, J.W. (Ed.), *Jargonaphasia.* New York: Academic Press (1981b).

BROWN, J.W., and JAFFE, J., Hypothesis on cerebral dominance. *Neuropsychologia,* 13, 107–110 (1975).

BRUBAKER, S.H., *Workbook for Aphasia: Exercises for the Redevelopment of Higher Level Language Functioning.* Detroit: Wayne State University Press (1978).

BRUBAKER, S.H., *Aphasia: A Guide to Family Resources and Activities.* Detroit: Wayne State University Press (1981).

BUCK, M., *Dysphasia: Professional Guidance for Family and Patient.* Englewood Cliffs, N.J.: Prentice-Hall (1968).

BUCKINGHAM, H.W., Explanation in apraxia with consequences for the concept of apraxia of speech. *Brain and Language,* 8, 202–226 (1979a).

BUCKINGHAM, H.W., Linguistic aspects of lexical retrieval disturbances in the posterior fluent aphasias. In H. Whitaker and H.A. Whitaker (Eds.), *Studies in Neurolinguistics, Volume 4.* New York: Academic Press (1979b).

BUCKINGHAM, H.W., Explanations for the concept of apraxia of speech. In M.T. Sarno (Ed.), *Acquired Aphasia.* New York: Academic Press (1981a).

BUCKINGHAM, H.W., Lexical and semantic aspects of aphasia. In M.T. Sarno (Ed.), *Acquired Aphasia.* New York: Academic Press (1981b).

BUCKINGHAM, H.W., Where do neologisms come from? In J.W. Brown (Ed.), *Jargonaphasia.* New York: Academic Press (1981c).

BUCKINGHAM, H.W., and KERTESZ, A., *Neologistic Jargon Aphasia.* Amsterdam: Swets and Zeitlinger (1976).

BUCKINGHAM, H.W., and REKART, D. M., Semantic paraphasia. *Journal of Communication Disorders,* 12, 197–209 (1979).

BUCKINGHAM, H.W., WHITAKER, H., and WHITAKER, H.A., On linguistic perseveration. In H. Whitaker and H.A. Whitaker (Eds.), *Studies in Neurolinguistics, Volume 4.* New York: Academic Press (1979).

BURNS, M.S., and CANTER, G.J., Phonemic behavior of aphasic patients with posterior cerebral lesions. *Brain and Language,* 4, 492–507 (1977).

BUTFIELD, E., and ZANGWILL, O.L., Reeducation in aphasia: A review of 70 cases. *Journal of Neurology, Neurosurgery and Psychiatry,* 9, 75–79 (1946).

BUTTERS, N., SAMUELS, I., GOODGLASS, H., and BRODY, B., Short-term visual and auditory memory disorders after parietal and frontal lobe damage. *Cortex,* 6, 440–459 (1970).

BUTTERWORTH, B., Hesitation and the production of verbal paraphasias and neologisms in jargon aphasia. *Brain and Language,* 8, 133–161 (1979).

CAMERON, H., Rationalizing aphasic personality. *American Association of Industrial Nurses Journal,* 7, July, 14–18 (1959).

CAMPBELL, K., *Body and Mind.* Garden City, N.Y.: Anchor Books (1970).

CANETTA, R., *Photo Language Stimulation for Aphasic Patients.* Danville, Ill.: Interstate Printers & Publishers (1974).

CANTER, G.J., Comment on "Objective indices of severity of chronic aphasia in stroke patients." *Journal of Speech and Hearing Disorders,* 37, 140–141 (1972).

CAPLAN, D., On the cerebral localization of linguistic functions: Logical and empirical issues surrounding deficit analysis and functional localization. *Brain and Language,* 14, 120–137 (1981).

CAPLAN, D., MATTHEI, E., and GIGLEY, H., Comprehension of gerundive constructions in Broca's aphasics. *Brain and Language,* 13, 145–160 (1981).

CARAMAZZA, A., BASILI, A.G., KOLLER, J.J., and BERNDT, R.S., An investigation of repetition and language processing in a case of conduction aphasia. *Brain and Language,* 14, 235–271 (1981).

CARAMAZZA, A., and BERNDT, R.S., Semantic and syntactic processes in aphasia: A review of the literature. *Psychological Bulletin,* 85, 898–918 (1978).

CARAMAZZA, A., BERNDT, R.S., and HART, J., "Agrammatic" reading. In F.J. Pirozzolo and M. C. Wittrock (Eds.), *Neuropsychological and Cognitive Processes in Reading.* New York: Academic Press (1981).

CARAMAZZA, A., GORDON, J., ZURIF, E.B., and DE-LUCA, D., Right-hemispheric damage and verbal problem solving behavior. *Brain and Language,* 3, 41–46 (1976).

CARAMAZZA, A., and ZURIF, E.B., Dissociation of algorithmic and heuristic processes in language comprehension: Evidence from aphasia. *Brain and Language,* 3, 572–582 (1976).

CARMON, A., and NACHSHON, I., Effect of unilateral brain damage on perception of temporal order. *Cortex,* 7, 410–418 (1971).

CARPENTER, J.O., Changing roles and disagreement in families with disabled husbands. *Archives of Physical Medicine and Rehabilitation,* 55, 272–274 (1974).

CARPENTER, P.A., and JUST, M.A., Sentence comprehension: A psycholinguistic processing model of verification. *Psychological Review,* 82, 45–73 (1975).

CARPENTER, R.L., and RUTHERFORD, D.R., Acoustic cue discrimination in adult aphasia. *Journal of Speech and Hearing Research,* 16, 534–544 (1973).

CARR, M.S., JACOBSON, T., and BOLLER, F., Crossed aphasia: Analysis of four cases. *Brain and Language,* 14, 190–202 (1981).

CASTRO-CALDAS, A., and BOTELHO, M.A.S., Dichotic listening in the recovery of aphasia after stroke. *Brain and Language,* 10, 145–151 (1980).

CERMAK, L.S., and MOREINES, J., Verbal retention deficits in aphasic and amnesic patients. *Brain and Language,* 3, 16–27 (1976).

CERMAK, L.S., and TARLOW, S., Aphasic and amnesic patients' verbal vs. nonverbal retentive abilities. *Cortex,* 14, 32–40 (1978).

CHAIKA, E., A linguist looks at "schizophrenic" language. *Brain and Language,* 1, 257–276 (1974).

CHAPEY, R., The assessment of language disorders in adults. In R. Chapey (Ed.), *Language Intervention Strategies in Adult Aphasia.* Baltimore: Williams & Wilkins (1981a).

CHAPEY, R., Divergent semantic intervention. In R. Chapey (Ed.), *Language Intervention Strategies in Adult Aphasia.* Baltimore: Williams & Wilkins (1981b).

CHAPEY, R., CHWAT, S., GURLAND, G., and

PIERAS, G., Perspectives in private practice: A nationwide analysis. *Asha,* 23, 335–340 (1981).

CHAPEY, R., and LUBINSKI, R., Semantic judgment ability in adult aphasia. *Cortex,* 15, 247–255 (1979).

CHAPEY, R., LUBINSKI, R., CHAPEY, G., and SALZBURG, A., Survey of speech, language and hearing services in nursing home settings. *Long Term Care and Health Services Administration Quarterly,* 3, 307–316 (1979).

CHAPEY, R., RIGRODSKY, S., and MORRISON, E.B., Divergent semantic behavior in aphasia. *Journal of Speech and Hearing Research,* 19, 664–677 (1976).

CHAPEY, R., RIGRODSKY, S., and MORRISON, E.B., Aphasia: A divergent semantic interpretation. *Journal of Speech and Hearing Disorders,* 42, 287–295 (1977).

CHAPIN, C., BLUMSTEIN, S.E., MEISSNER, B., and BOLLER, F., Speech production mechanisms in aphasia: A delayed auditory feedback study. *Brain and Language,* 14, 106–113 (1981).

CHAPMAN, R.M., McCRARY, J.W., CHAPMAN, J.A., and MARTIN, J.K., Behavioral and neural analyses of connotative meaning: Word classes and rating scales. *Brain and Language,* 11, 319–339 (1980).

CHEN, L.Y., "Talking hand" for aphasic stroke patients. *Geriatrics,* 23, 145–148 (1968).

CHEN, L.Y., Manual communication by combined alphabet and gestures. *Archives of Physical Medicine and Rehabilitation,* 52, 381–384 (1971).

CHOMSKY, N., *Aspects of the Theory of Syntax.* Cambridge, Mass.: MIT Press (1965).

CHUSID, J.G., *Correlative Neuroanatomy and Functional Neurology* (17th Ed.). Los Altos, Calif.: Lange Medical Publications (1979).

CHWAT, S., CHAPEY, R., GURLAND, G., and PIERAS, G., Environment impact of aphasia: The child's perspective. In R.H. Brookshire (Ed.), *Clinical Aphasiology Conference Proceedings.* Minneapolis: BRK (1980).

CHWAT, S., and GURLAND, G.B., Comparative family perspectives on aphasia: Diagnostic, treatment, and counseling implications. In R.H. Brookshire (Ed.), *Clinical Aphasiology Conference Proceedings.* Minneapolis: BRK (1981).

CICONE, M., WAPNER, W., and GARDNER, H., Sensitivity to emotional expressions and situations in organic patients. *Cortex,* 16, 145–158 (1980).

CLARK, C., CROCKETT, D.J., and KLONOFF, H., Empirically derived groups in the assessment of recovery from aphasia. *Brain and Language,* 7, 240–251 (1979a).

CLARK, C., CROCKETT, D.J., and KLONOFF, H., Factor analysis of the Porch Index of Communication Ability. *Brain and Language, 7,* 1-7 (1979b).

CLARK, H.H., and CLARK, E.V., *Psychology and Language.* New York: Harcourt, Brace and Jovanovich (1977).

COHEN, L.K., *Communication Problems after a Stroke.* Minneapolis: Sister Kenny Institute (1971).

COHEN, L.K., *Communication Aids for the Brain Damaged Adult.* Minneapolis: Sister Kenny Institute (1977).

COHEN, R., ENGEL, D., KELTER, S., LIST, G., and STROHNER, H., Validity of the Sklar Aphasia Scale. *Journal of Speech and Hearing Research, 20,* 146-154 (1977).

COHEN, R., KELTER, S., and WOLL, G., Analytical competence and language impairment in aphasia. *Brain and Language, 10,* 331-347 (1980).

COLBY, K.M., CHRISTINAZ, D., PARKISON, R.C., GRAHAM, S., and KARPF, C., A word-finding computer program with a dynamic lexical-semantic memory for patients with anomia using an intelligent speech prosthesis. *Brain and Language, 14,* 272-281 (1981).

COLLINS, A.M., and LOFTUS, E.F., A spreading activation theory of semantic processing. *Psychological Review, 82,* 407-428 (1975).

CORLEW, M.M., and NATION, J.E., Characteristics of visual stimuli and naming performance in aphasic adults. *Cortex, 11,* 186-191 (1975).

COSTELLO, J., Programmed instruction. *Journal of Speech and Hearing Disorders, 42,* 3-28 (1977).

CRITCHLEY, M., Jacksonian ideas and the future, with special reference to aphasia. *British Medical Journal, 6,* 6-11 (1960).

CRITCHLEY, M., *Aphasiology and Other Aspects of Language.* Baltimore: Williams & Wilkins (1970).

CROCKETT, D.J., A comparison of empirically derived groups of aphasic patients on the Neurosensory Center Comprehensive Examination for Aphasia. *Journal of Clinical Psychology, 33,* 194-198 (1977).

CRYSTAL, D., FLETCHER, P., and GARMAN, M., *The Grammatical Analysis of Language Disability.* New York: Elsevier (1976).

CULTON, G.L., Spontaneous recovery from aphasia. *Journal of Speech and Hearing Research, 12,* 825-832 (1969).

CULTON, G.L., Reaction to age as a factor in chronic aphasia in stroke patients. *Journal of Speech and Hearing Disorders, 36,* 563-564 (1971).

CULTON, G.L., and FERGUSON, P.A., Comprehension training with aphasic subjects: The development and application of five automated language programs. *Journal of Communication Disorders, 12,* 69-81 (1979).

CZVIK, P.S., Assessment of family attitude toward aphasic patients with severe auditory processing

disorders. In R.H. Brookshire (Ed.), *Clinical Aphasiology Conference Proceedings.* Minneapolis: BRK (1977).

DAHLBERG, C.C., and JAFFE, J., *Stroke: A Doctor's Personal Story of His Recovery.* New York: W.W. Norton (1977).

DAMASIO, H., Cerebral localization of the aphasias. In M.T. Sarno (Ed.), *Acquired Aphasia.* New York: Academic Press (1981).

DAMASIO, H., and DAMASIO, A.R., Dichotic listening pattern in conduction aphasia. *Brain and Language, 10,* 281-286 (1980).

DAMON, S.G., LESSER, R., and WOODS, R.T., Behavioral treatment of social difficulties with an aphasic woman and a dysarthric man. *British Journal of Disorders of Communication, 14,* 31-38 (1979).

DARLEY, F.L., The efficacy of language rehabilitation in aphasia. *Journal of Speech and Hearing Disorders, 37,* 3-21 (1972).

DARLEY, F.L., A retrospective view: Aphasia. *Journal of Speech and Hearing Disorders, 42,* 161-169 (1977).

DARLEY, F.L., Treat or neglect? *Asha, 21,* 628-631 (1979).

DARLEY, F.L., *Aphasia.* Philadelphia: W.B. Saunders (1982).

DARLEY, F.L., ARONSON, A.E., and BROWN, J.R., *Motor Speech Disorders.* Philadelphia: W.B. Saunders (1975).

DAVIS, G.A., Linguistics and language therapy: The sentence construction board. *Journal of Speech and Hearing Disorders, 38,* 205-214 (1973).

DAVIS, G.A., The clinical application of withdrawal, single-case research designs. In R.H. Brookshire (Ed.), *Clinical Aphasiology Conference Proceedings.* Minneapolis: BRK (1978a).

DAVIS, G.A., Psycholinguistic operations in sentence comprehension: Implications for aphasiology. In R.H. Brookshire (Ed.), *Clinical Aphasiology Collected Proceedings 1972-1976.* Minneapolis: BRK (1978b).

DAVIS, G.A., A critical look at PACE therapy. In R. H. Brookshire (Ed.), *Clinical Aphasiology Conference Proceedings.* Minneapolis: BRK (1980).

DAVIS, G.A., Effects of aging on normal language. In A.L. Holland (Ed.), *Recent Advances: Language Disorders.* San Diego, Ca.: College-Hill Press (Forthcoming).

DAVIS, G.A., and HOLLAND, A.L., Age in understanding and treating aphasia. In D.S. Beasley and G.A. Davis (Eds.), *Aging: Communication Processes and Disorders.* New York: Grune & Stratton (1981).

DAVIS, G.A., and WILCOX, M.J., Incorporating parameters of natural conversation in aphasia treatment. In R. Chapey (Ed.), *Language Inter-*

vention Strategies in Adult Aphasia. Baltimore: Williams & Wilkins (1981).

DAY, M.E., An eye-movement phenomenon relating to attention, thought and anxiety. *Perceptual and Motor Skills*, 19, 443–446 (1964).

DEAL, J.L., and DEAL, L.A., Efficacy of aphasia rehabilitation: Preliminary results. In R.H. Brookshire (Ed.), *Clinical Aphasiology Conference Proceedings*. Minneapolis: BRK (1978).

DEAL, J.L., DEAL, L., WERTZ, R.T., KITSELMAN, K., and DWYER, C., Right hemisphere PICA percentiles: Some speculations about aphasia. In R.H. Brookshire (Ed.), *Clinical Aphasiology Conference Proceedings*. Minneapolis: BRK (1979a).

DEAL, L., DEAL, J.L., WERTZ, R.T., KITSELMAN, K., AND DWYER, C., Statistical prediction of change in aphasia: Clinical application of multiple regression analysis. In R.H. Brookshire (Ed.), *Clinical Aphasiology Conference Proceedings*. Minneapolis: BRK (1979b).

DEKOSKY, S.T., HEILMAN, K.M., BOWERS, D., and VALENSTEIN, E., Recognition and discrimination of emotional faces and pictures. *Brain and Language*, 9, 206–214 (1980).

DELOCHE, G., and SERON, X., Sentence understanding and knowledge of the world. Evidences from a sentence-picture matching task performed by aphasic patients. *Brain and Language*, 14, 57–69 (1981).

DEMEURISSE, G., DEMOL, O., DEROUCK, M., DE BEUCKELAER, R., COEKAERTS, M.-J., and CAPON, A., Quantitative study of the rate of recovery from aphasia due to ischemic stroke. *Stroke*, 11, 455–458 (1980).

DEMYER, W., *Technique of the Neurologic Examination: A Programmed Text* (2nd Ed.). New York: McGraw-Hill (1974).

DENNIS, M., Capacity and strategy for syntactic comprehension after left or right hemidecortication. *Brain and Language*, 10, 287–317 (1980a).

DENNIS, M., Language acquisition in a single hemisphere: Semantic organization. In D. Caplan (Ed.), *Biological Studies of Mental Processes*. Cambridge, Mass.: MIT Press (1980b).

DENNIS, M., Strokes in childhood I: Communicative intent, expression, and comprehension after left hemisphere arteriopathy in a right-handed nine-year-old. In R.W. Rieber (Ed.), *Language Development and Aphasia in Children*. New York: Academic Press (1980c).

DENNIS, M., and KOHN, B., Comprehension of syntax in infantile hemiplegics after cerebral hemidecortication: Left hemisphere superiority. *Brain and Language*, 2, 472–482 (1975).

DENNIS, M., and WHITAKER, H.A., Language acquisition following hemidecortication: Linguistic superiority of the left over the right hemisphere. *Brain and Language*, 3, 404–433 (1976).

DENNIS, M., and WIEGEL-CRUMP, C.A., Aphasic dissolution and language acquisition. In H. Whitaker and H.A. Whitaker (Eds.), *Studies in Neurolinguistics, Volume 4*. New York: Academic Press (1979).

DERENZI, E., A shortened version of the Token Test. In F. Boller and M. Dennis (Eds.), *Auditory Comprehension: Clinical and Experimental Studies with the Token Test*. New York: Academic Press (1979).

DERENZI, E., and FAGLIONI, P., Normative data and screening power of a shortened version of the Token Test. *Cortex*, 14, 41–49 (1978).

DERENZI, E., FAGLIONI, P., and PREVIDI, Increased susceptibility of aphasics to a distractor task in the recall of verbal commands. *Brain and Language*, 6, 14–21 (1978).

DERENZI, E., and FERRARI, C., The Reporter's Test: A sensitive test to detect expressive disturbances in aphasics. *Cortex*, 14, 279–293 (1978).

DERENZI, E., and NICHELLI, P., Verbal and nonverbal short-term memory impairment following hemispheric damage. *Cortex*, 11, 341–354 (1975).

DERENZI, E., and VIGNOLO, L.A., The Token Test: A sensitive test to detect receptive disturbances in aphasics. *Brain*, 85, 665–678 (1962).

DERMAN, S., and MANASTER, H., Family counseling with relatives of aphasic patients at Schwab Rehabilitation Hospital. *Asha*, 9, 175–177 (1967).

DEVILLIERS, J., Quantitative aspects of agrammatism in aphasia. *Cortex*, 10, 36–54 (1974).

DICARLO, L.M., Language recovery in aphasia: Effect of systematic filmed programmed instruction. *Archives of Physical Medicine and Rehabilitation*, 61, 41–44 (1980).

DISIMONI, F.G., Therapies which utilize alternative or augmentative communication systems. In R. Chapey (Ed.), *Language Intervention Strategies in Adult Aphasia*. Baltimore: Williams & Wilkins (1981).

DISIMONI, F.G., DARLEY F.L., and ARONSON, A.E., Patterns of dysfunction in schizophrenic patients on an aphasia test battery. *Journal of Speech and Hearing Disorders*, 42, 498–513 (1977).

DISIMONI, F.G., KEITH, R.L., and DARLEY, F.L., Prediction of PICA overall score by short versions of the test. *Journal of Speech and Hearing Research*, 23, 511–516 (1980).

DISIMONI, F.G., KEITH, R.L., HOLT, D.L., and DARLEY, F.L., Practicality of shortening the Porch Index of Communicative Ability. *Journal of Speech and Hearing Research*, 18, 491–497 (1975).

DOEHRING, D.G., Auditory-visual training of aphasics by programmed instruction. In J.W.

Black and E.G. Jancosek (Eds.), *Proceedings of the Conference on Language Retraining for Aphasics.* Columbus, Ohio: The Ohio State University (1968).

Doehring, D.G., and Swisher, L.P., Disturbances of connotative meaning in aphasia. *Journal of Communication Disorders,* 5, 251–258 (1972).

Duffy, J.R., Schuell's stimulation approach to rehabilitation. In R. Chapey (Ed.), *Language Intervention Strategies in Adult Aphasia.* Baltimore: Williams & Wilkins (1981).

Duffy, J.R., Boyle, M., and Plattner, L., Listener reactions to personal characteristics of fluent and nonfluent aphasic speakers. In R.H. Brookshire (Ed.), *Clinical Aphasiology Conference Proceedings.* Minneapolis: BRK (1980).

Duffy, J.R., and Dale, B.J., The PICA scoring scale: Do its statistical shortcomings cause clinical problems? In R.H. Brookshire (Ed.), *Clinical Aphasiology Conference Proceedings.* Minneapolis: BRK (1977).

Duffy, J.R., Keith, R.L., Shane, H., and Podraza, B.L., Performance of normal (non-brain-injured) adults on the Porch Index of Communicative Ability. In R.H. Brookshire (Ed.), *Clinical Aphasiology Conference Proceedings.* Minneapolis: BRK (1976).

Duffy, J.R., and Liles, B.Z., A translation of Finkelnberg's (1870) lecture on aphasia as "asymbolia" with commentary. *Journal of Speech and Hearing Disorders,* 44, 156–168 (1979).

Duffy, R.J., Aphasia in adults. In A.J. Weston (Ed.), *Communicative Disorders: An Appraisal.* Springfield, Ill.: Charles C. Thomas (1972).

Duffy, R.J., and Duffy, J.R., Three studies of deficits in pantomimic expression and pantomimic recognition in aphasia. *Journal of Speech and Hearing Research,* 24, 70–84 (1981).

Duffy, R.J., Duffy, J.R., and Pearson, K.L., Pantomimic recognition in aphasics. *Journal of Speech and Hearing Research,* 18, 115–132 (1975).

Duffy R.J., and Ulrich, S.R., A comparison of impairments in verbal comprehension, speech, reading, and writing in adult aphasics. *Journal of Speech and Hearing Disorders,* 41, 110–119 (1976).

Duffy, R.J., Ulrich, S.R., and Bisantz, J., A funny thing happened on the way to the conclusion: A reply to Smith. *Journal of Speech and Hearing Disorders,* 42, 133–135 (1977).

Dumas, R., and Morgan, A., EEG asymmetry as a function of occupation, task and task difficulty. *Neuropsychologia,* 13, 219–228 (1975).

Dumond, D.L., Hardy, J.C., and Van Demark, A.A., Presentation by order of difficulty of test tasks to persons with aphasia. *Journal of Speech and Hearing Research,* 21, 350–360 (1978).

Dunn, L.M., *Peabody Picture Vocabulary Test.* Circle Pines, Minn.: American Guidance Service (1965).

Eagleson, H.M., Vaughn, G.R., and Knudson, A.B., Hand signals for dysphasia. *Archives of Physical Medicine and Rehabilitation,* 51, 111–113 (1970).

Ebbin, J.B., and Edwards, A.E., Speech sound discrimination of aphasics when intrasound interval is varied. *Journal of Speech and Hearing Research,* 10, 120–125 (1967).

Eccles, J.C., *The Understanding of the Brain.* New York: McGraw-Hill (1973).

Edwards, A.E., Automated training for a "matching-to-sample" task in aphasia. *Journal of Speech and Hearing Research,* 8, 39–42 (1965).

Edwards, B., *Drawing on the Right Side of the Brain.* Los Angeles: J.P. Tarcher (1979).

Efron, R., Temporal perception, aphasia and *deja vu. Brain,* 86, 403–423 (1963).

Eggert, G.H., *Wernicke's Works on Aphasia: A Sourcebook and Review.* The Hague, Netherlands: Mouton (1977).

Ehrlichman, H., and Weinberger, A., Lateral eye movements and hemispheric asymmetry: A critical review. *Psychological Bulletin,* 85, 1080–1101 (1978).

Eisenson, J., Prognostic factors related to language rehabilitation in aphasic patients. *Journal of Speech and Hearing Disorders,* 14, 262–264 (1949).

Eisenson, J., *Examining for Aphasia.* New York: The Psychological Corporation (1954).

Eisenson, J., Language dysfunctions associated with right brain damage. *Asha,* 1, 107 (1959).

Eisenson, J., Language and intellectual modifications associated with right cerebral damage. *Language and Speech,* 5, 49–53 (1962).

Eisenson, J., Aphasic language modifications as a disruption of cultural verbal habits. *Asha,* 5, 503–506 (1963).

Eisenson, J., *Aphasia in Children.* New York: Harper & Row (1972).

Eisenson, J., *Adult Aphasia: Assessment and Treatment.* New York: Appleton-Century-Crofts (1973).

Elmore-Nicholas, L., and Brookshire, R.H., Effects of pictures and picturability on sentence verification by aphasic and nonaphasic subjects. *Journal of Speech and Hearing Research,* 24, 292–297 (1981).

Emerick, L.L., and Hatten, J.T., *Diagnosis and Evaluation in Speech Pathology* (2nd Ed.). Englewood Cliffs, N.J.: Prentice-Hall (1979).

Faber, M.M., and Aten, J.L., Verbal performance in aphasic patients in response to intact and altered pictorial stimuli. In R.H. Brookshire

(Ed.), *Clinical Aphasiology Conference Proceedings.* Minneapolis: BRK (1979).

FARMER, A., Self-correctional strategies in the conversational speech of aphasic and nonaphasic brain damaged adults. *Cortex,* 13, 327–334 (1977).

FARMER, A., and O'CONNELL, P.F., Neuropsychological processes in adult aphasia: Rationale for treatment. *British Journal of Disorders of Communication,* 14, 39–49 (1980).

FARMER, A., O'CONNELL, P.F., and O'CONNELL, E.J., Sound error self-correction in the conversational speech of nonfluent and fluent aphasics. *Folia Phoniatrica,* 30, 293–302 (1978).

FEDIO, P., and VAN BUREN, J.M., Memory and perceptual deficits during electrical stimulation in left and right thalamus and parietal subcortex. *Brain and Language,* 2, 78–100 (1975).

FILLENBAUM, S., and JONES, L.V., An application of "cloze" technique to the study of aphasic speech. *Journal of Abnormal and Social Psychology,* 65, 183–189 (1962).

FILLENBAUM, S., JONES, L.V., and WEPMAN, J.M., Some linguistic features of speech from aphasic patients. *Language and Speech,* 4, 91–108 (1961).

FILLMORE, C.J., KEMPLER, D., and WANG, W. S-Y. (Eds.), *Individual Differences in Language Ability and Language Behavior.* New York: Academic Press (1979).

FLORANCE, C.L., RABIDOUX, P.C., and Mc-CAUSLIN, L.S., An environmental manipulation approach to treating apraxia of speech. In R.H. Brookshire (Ed.), *Clinical Aphasiology Conference Proceedings.* Minneapolis: BRK (1980).

FLOWERS, C.R., Proactive interference in short-term recall by aphasic, brain-damaged nonaphasic, and normal subjects. *Neuropsychologia,* 13, 59–68 (1975).

FLOWERS, C.R., and DANFORTH, L.C., A stepwise auditory comprehension improvement program administered to aphasic patients by family members. In R.H. Brookshire (Ed.), *Clinical Aphasiology Conference Proceedings.* Minneapolis, BRK (1979).

FOLSOM, J.C., Reality orientation for the elderly mental patient. *Journal of Geriatric Psychiatry,* 1, 291–307 (1968).

FORSTER, K.I., Accessing the mental lexicon. In E. Walker (Ed.), *Explorations in the Biology of Language.* Montgomery, Vt.: Bradford Books (1978).

FOSS, D.J., and HAKES, D.T., *Psycholinguistics: An Introduction to the Psychology of Language.* Englewood Cliffs, N.J.: Prentice-Hall (1978).

FRIEDERICI, A.D., and SCHOENLE, P.W., Computational dissociation of two vocabulary types: Evidence from aphasia. *Neuropsychologia,* 18, 11–20 (1980).

FRIEDERICI, A.D., SCHOENLE, P.W., and GOODGLASS, H., Mechanisms underlying writing and speech in aphasia. *Brain and Language,* 13, 212–222 (1981).

FROMKIN, V.A., A linguist looks at "A linguist looks at 'schizophrenic language'." *Brain and Language,* 2, 498–503 (1975).

FURST, C., *Origins of the Mind: Mind-Brain Connections.* Englewood Cliffs, N.J.: Prentice-Hall (1979).

GADO, M.H., COLEMAN, R.E., MERLIS, A.L., ALDERSON, P.O., and LEE, K.S., Comparison of CT and RN imaging in "stroke." *Stroke,* 7, 109–113 (1976).

GAINOTTI, G., The relationship between semantic impairment in comprehension and naming in aphasic patients. *British Journal of Disorders of Communication,* 11, 57–61 (1976).

GAINOTTI, G., CALTAGIRONE, C., and IBBA, A., Semantic and phonemic aspects of auditory language comprehension in aphasia. *Linguistics,* 154/5, 15–29 (1975).

GAINOTTI, G., CALTAGIRONE, C., MICELI, G., and MASULLO, C., Selective semantic-lexical impairment of language comprehension in right-brain-damaged patients. *Brain and Language,* 13, 201–211 (1981).

GAINOTTI, G., and LEMMO, M.A., Comprehension of symbolic gestures in aphasia. *Brain and Language,* 3, 451–460 (1976).

GALIN, D., Implications for psychiatry of left and right cerebral specialization: A neurophysiological context for unconscious processes. *Archives of General Psychiatry.* 31, 572–583 (1974).

GALIN, D., The two modes of consciousness and the two halves of the brain. In P.R. Lee, R.E. Ornstein, D. Galin, A. Deikman, and C.T. Tart, *Symposium on Consciousness.* New York: Penguin (1976).

GALIN, D., and ELLIS, R.R. Asymmetry in evoked potentials as an index of lateralized cognitive processes: Relation to EEG alpha asymmetry. *Neuropsychologia,* 13, 45–50 (1975).

GALIN, D., and ORNSTEIN, R.E., Lateral specialization of cognitive mode: An EEG study. *Psychophysiology,* 9, 412–418 (1972).

GALIN, D., and ORNSTEIN, R.E., Individual differences in cognitive style—I. Reflective eye movements. *Neuropsychologia,* 12, 367–376 (1974).

GALLAHER, A.J., Temporal reliability of aphasic performance on the Token Test. *Brain and Language,* 7, 34–41 (1979).

GALLAHER, A.J., Syntactic versus semantic performances of agrammatic Broca's aphasics on tests of constituent-element-ordering. *Journal of Speech and Hearing Research,* 24, 217–223 (1981).

GARDNER, H., The contribution of operativity to naming capacity in aphasic patients. *Neuropsychologia,* 11, 213–220 (1973).

GARDNER, H., The naming and recognition of written symbols in aphasic and alexic patients. *Journal of Communication Disorders,* 7, 141–154 (1974a).

GARDNER, H., *The Shattered Mind.* New York: Vintage Books (1974b).

GARDNER, H., and DENES, G., Connotative judgments by aphasic patients on a pictorial adaptation of the semantic differential. *Cortex,* 9, 183–196 (1973).

GARDNER, H., DENES, G., and WEINTRAUB, S., Comprehending a word: The influence of speed and redundancy on auditory comprehension in aphasia. *Cortex,* 11, 155–162 (1975).

GARDNER, H., DENES, G., and ZURIF, E.B., Critical reading at the sentence level in aphasics. *Cortex,* 11, 60–72 (1975).

GARDNER, H., LING, P.K., FLAMM, L., and SILVERMAN, J., Comprehension and appreciation of humorous material following brain damage. *Brain,* 98, 399–412 (1975).

GARDNER, H., and ZURIF, E., *Bee* but not *be:* Oral reading of single words in aphasia and alexia. *Neuropsychologia,* 13, 181–190 (1975).

GARDNER, H., ZURIF, E.B., BERRY, T., and Baker, E., Visual communication in aphasia. *Neuropsychologia,* 14, 275–292 (1976).

GATES, A.I., and MACGINITIE, W.H., *Gates-MacGinitie Reading Tests.* New York: Columbia University Teachers College Press (1965).

GAWLER, J., BULL, J.W.D., DuBOULAY, G.H., and MARSHALL, J., Computerized axial tomography: The normal EMI scan. *Journal of Neurology, Neurosurgery, and Psychiatry,* 38, 935–947 (1975).

GAZZANIGA, M.S., The split brain in man. *Scientific American,* 217(2), 24–29 (1967).

GAZZANIGA, M.S., *The Bisected Brain.* New York: Appleton-Century-Crofts (1970).

GAZZANIGA, M.S., Determinants of cerebral recovery. In D.G. Stein, J.J. Rosen, and N. Butters (Eds.), *Plasticity and Recovery of Function in the Central Nervous System.* New York: Academic Press (1974).

GAZZANIGA, M.S., and HILLYARD, S.A., Language and speech capacity of the right hemisphere. *Neuropsychologia,* 9, 273–280 (1971).

GAZZANIGA, M.S., and SPERRY, R.W., Language after section of the cerebral commissures. *Brain,* 90, 131–148 (1967).

GESCHWIND, N., The varieties of naming errors. *Cortex,* 3, 96–112 (1967).

GESCHWIND, N., The organization of language and the brain. *Science,* 170, 940–944 (1970).

GESCHWIND, N., Specializations of the human brain. *Scientific American,* 241, 180–199 (1979).

GESCHWIND, N., and FUSILLO, M., Color-naming defects in association with alexia. *Archives of Neurology,* 15, 137–146 (1966).

GESCHWIND, N., and LEVITSKY, W., Human brain: Left-right asymmetries in temporal speech region. *Science,* 161, 186–187 (1968).

GLASS, A.L., and HOLYOAK, K.J., Alternative conceptions of semantic memory. *Cognition,* 30, 313–339 (1975).

GLASS, A.V., GAZZANIGA, M.S., and PREMACK, D., Artificial language training in global aphasia. *Neuropsychologia,* 11, 95–103 (1973).

GLASSMAN, R.B., The logic of the lesion experiment and its role in the neural sciences. In S. Finger (Ed.), *Recovery from Brain Damage: Research and Theory.* New York: Plenum Press (1978).

GLEASON, J.B., GOODGLASS, H., GREEN, E., ACKERMAN, N., and HYDE, M.R., The retrieval of syntax in Broca's aphasia. *Brain and Language,* 2, 451–471 (1975).

GLEASON, J.B., GOODGLASS, H., OBLER, L., GREEN, E., HYDE, M.R., and WEINTRAUB, S., Narrative strategies of aphasic and normal-speaking subjects. *Journal of Speech and Hearing Research,* 23, 370–382 (1980).

GLONING, K., TRAPPL, R., HEISS, W., and QUATEMBER, R., Prognosis and speech therapy in aphasia. In Y. Lebrun and R. Hoops, (Eds.), *Recovery in Aphasics.* Amsterdam: Swets & Zeitlinger (1976).

GODFREY, C.M., and DOUGLASS, E., The recovery process in aphasia. *Canadian Medical Association Journal,* 80, 618–624 (1959).

GOLDBLUM, M., and ALBERT, M.L., Phonemic discrimination in sensory aphasia. *International Journal of Mental Health,* 1, 25–29 (1972).

GOLDEN, C.J., HEMMEKE, T.A., and PURISCH, A.D., *The Luria-Nebraska Neuropsychological Battery.* Los Angeles: Western Psychological Services (1980).

GOLDFARB, R., Operant conditioning and programmed instruction in aphasia rehabilitation. In R. Chapey (Ed.), *Language Intervention Strategies in Adult Aphasia.* Baltimore: Williams & Wilkins (1981).

GOLDSTEIN, K., *Language and Language Disturbances.* New York: Grune & Stratton (1948).

GOLDSTEIN, K., Organismic approach to aphasia. In D.A. Barbara (Ed.), *Psychological and Psychiatric Aspects of Speech and Hearing.* Springfield, Ill.: Charles C. Thomas (1960).

GOLDSTEIN, L.P., A case report of an edentulous aphasic laryngectomee. *Journal of Speech and Hearing Disorders,* 29, 86–87 (1964).

GOLPER, L.A.C., A study of verbal behavior in recovery of aphasic and nonaphasic persons. In R.H. Brookshire (Ed.), *Clinical Aphasiology Conference Proceedings*. Minneapolis: BRK (1980).

GOLPER, L.A.C., THORPE, P., TOMPKINS, C., MARSHALL, R.C., and RAU, M.T., Connected language sampling: An expanded index of aphasic language behavior. In R.H. Brookshire (Ed.), *Clinical Aphasiology Conference Proceedings*. Minneapolis: BRK (1980).

GOODENOUGH, C., ZURIF, E.B., WEINTRAUB, S., and VON STOCKERT, T., Aphasics' attention to grammatical morphemes. *Language and Speech*, 20, 11-19 (1977).

GOODGLASS, H., Agrammatism. In H. Whitaker and H.A. Whitaker (Eds.), *Studies in Neurolinguistics* (Vol. 1). New York: Academic Press (1976).

GOODGLASS, H., Phonological factors in aphasia. In R.H. Brookshire (Ed.), *Clinical Aphasiology: Collected Proceedings 1972-1976*. Minneapolis: BRK (1978).

GOODGLASS, H., and BAKER, E., Semantic field, naming, and auditory comprehension in aphasia. *Brain and Language*, 3, 359-374 (1976).

GOODGLASS, H., BARTON, M.I., and KAPLAN, E.F., Sensory modality and object-naming in aphasics. *Journal of Speech and Hearing Research*, 11, 488-496 (1968).

GOODGLASS, H., and BERKO, J., Agrammatism and inflectional morphology in English. *Journal of Speech and Hearing Research*, 3, 257-267 (1960).

GOODGLASS, H., BLUMSTEIN, S.E., GLEASON, J.B., HYDE, M.R., GREEN, E., and STATLENDER, S., The effect of syntactic encoding on sentence comprehension in aphasia. *Brain and Language*, 7, 201-209 (1979).

GOODGLASS, H., DENES, G., and CALDERON, M., The absence of covert verbal mediation in aphasia. *Cortex*, 10, 264-269 (1974).

GOODGLASS, H., FODOR, I.G., and SCHULHOFF, C., Prosodic factors in grammar-evidence from aphasia. *Journal of Speech and Hearing Research*, 10, 5-20 (1967).

GOODGLASS, H., GLEASON, J.B., BERNHOLZ, N.A., and HYDE, M.R., Some linguistic structures in the speech of a Broca's aphasic. *Cortex*, 8, 191-212 (1972).

GOODGLASS, H., GLEASON, J.B., and HYDE, M.R., Some dimensions of auditory language comprehension in aphasia. *Journal of Speech and Hearing Research*, 13, 595-606 (1970).

GOODGLASS, H., and HUNTER, M., A linguistic comparison of speech and writing in two types of aphasia. *Journal of Communication Disorders*, 3, 28-35 (1970).

GOODGLASS, H., HYDE, M.R., and BLUMSTEIN, S., Frequency, picturability and availability of nouns in aphasia. *Cortex*, 5, 104-119 (1969).

GOODGLASS, H., and KAPLAN, E., *The Assessment of Aphasia and Related Disorders*. Philadelphia: Lea & Febiger (1972).

GOODGLASS, H., KAPLAN, E., WEINTRAUB, S., and ACKERMAN, N., The "tip-of-the-tongue" phenomenon in aphasia. *Cortex*, 12, 145-153 (1976).

GOODGLASS, H., KLEIN, B., CAREY, P.W., and JONES, K.J., Specific semantic word categories in aphasia. *Cortex*, 2, 74-89 (1966).

GOODGLASS, H., and MAYER, J., Agrammatism in aphasia. *Journal of Speech and Hearing Disorders*, 23, 99-111 (1958).

GOODGLASS, H., QUADFASEL, F.A., and TIMBERLAKE, W.H., Phrase length and the type and severity of aphasia. *Cortex*, 1, 133-153 (1964).

GOODGLASS, H., and STUSS, D.T., Naming to picture versus description in three aphasic subgroups. *Cortex*, 15, 199-211 (1979).

GOODKIN, R., DILLER, L., and SHAH, N., Training spouses to improve the functional speech of aphasic patients. In B.B. Lahey (Ed.), *The Modification of Language Behaviors*. Springfield, Ill.: Charles C. Thomas (1973).

GORDON, H.W., Right hemisphere comprehension of verbs in patients with complete forebrain commissurotomy: Use of the dichotic method and manual performance. *Brain and Language*, 11, 76-86 (1980).

GREEN, E., Phonological and grammatical aspects of jargon in an aphasic patient. *Language and Speech*, 12, 103-118 (1969a).

GREEN, E., Psycholinguistic approaches to aphasia. *Linguistics*, 53, 30-50 (1969b).

GREEN, E., On the contributions of studies in aphasia to psycholinguistics. *Cortex*, 6, 216-235 (1970).

GREEN, E., Aphasic jargon and the speech acts of naming and judging. In J.W. Brown (Ed.), *Jargonaphasia*. New York: Academic Press (1981).

GREEN, E., and BOLLER, F., Features of auditory comprehension in severely impaired aphasics. *Cortex*, 10, 133-145 (1974).

GREEN, E., and HOWES, D.H., The nature of conduction aphasia: A study of anatomic and clinical features and of underlying mechanisms. In H. Whitaker and H.A. Whitaker (Eds.), *Studies in Neurolinguistics, Volume 3*. New York: Academic Press (1977).

GREIMAS, A.J., JAKOBSON, R., MAYENOWA, M.R., et al. (Eds.), *Sign, Language, Culture*. The Hague, Netherlands: Mouton (1970).

GROBER, E., PERECMAN, E., KELLAR, L., and BROWN, J., Lexical knowledge in anterior and posterior aphasics. *Brain and Language,* 10, 318–330 (1980).

GROHER, M., Language and memory disorders following closed head trauma. *Journal of Speech and Hearing Research,* 20, 212–223 (1977).

GROSSMAN, M., The game of the name: An examination of linguistic reference after brain damage. *Brain and Language,* 6, 112–119 (1978).

GROSSMAN, M., A central processor for hierarchically-structured material: Evidence from Broca's aphasia. *Neuropsychologia,* 18, 299–308 (1980).

GROSSMAN, M., A bird is a bird is a bird: Making reference within and without superordinate categories. *Brain and Language,* 12, 313–331 (1981).

GRUBER, F.A., and SEGALOWITZ, S.J., Some issues and methods in the neuropsychology of language. In S.J. Segalowitz and F.A. Gruber (Eds.), *Language Development and Neurological Theory.* New York: Academic Press (1977).

GUR, R.C., and GUR, R.E., Handedness and individual differences in hemispheric activation. In J. Herron (Ed.), *Neuropsychology of Left-Handedness.* New York: Academic Press (1980).

GUR, R.C., and REIVICH, M., Cognitive task effects on hemispheric blood flow in humans: Evidence for individual differences in hemispheric activation. *Brain and Language,* 9, 78–92 (1980).

GUR, R.E., Conjugate lateral eye movements as an index of hemispheric activation. *Journal of Personality and Social Psychology,* 31, 751–757 (1975).

GUR, R.E., and GUR, R.C., Correlates of conjugate lateral eye movements in man. In S. Harnad, R.W. Doty, L. Goldstein, et al. (Eds.), *Lateralization in the Nervous System.* New York: Academic Press (1977).

HAGEN, C., Communicative abilities in hemiplegia: Effect of speech therapy. *Archives of Physical Medicine and Rehabilitation,* 54, 454–463 (1973).

HAIN, R., and LAINER, H., *Language Rehabilitation Program, Level 1.* Hingham, Mass.: Teaching Resources Corporation (1977).

HAIN, R., and LAINER, H., *Language Rehabilitation Program, Level 2.* Hingham, Mass.: Teaching Resources Corporation (1980).

HALE, G. (Ed.), *The Source Book for the Disabled.* New York: Bantam Books (1979).

HALPERN, H., DARLEY, F.L., and BROWN, J.R., Differential language and neurologic characteristics in cerebral involvement. *Journal of Speech and Hearing Disorders,* 38, 162–173 (1973).

HALPERN, H., KEITH, R.L., and DARLEY, F.L., Phonemic behavior of aphasic subjects without dysarthria or apraxia of speech. *Cortex,* 12, 365–372 (1976).

HALSEY, J.H., BLAUENSTEIN, U.W., WILSON, E.M., and WILLS, E.L., Brain activation in the presence of brain damage. *Brain and Language,* 9, 47–60 (1980).

HALSTEAD, W.C., and WEPMAN, J.M., The Halstead-Wepman aphasia screening test. *Journal of Speech and Hearing Disorders,* 14, 9–15 (1949).

HAND, C.R., TONKOVICH, J.D., and AITCHISON, J., Abnormal syntactic compensations utilized by a patient with chronic Broca's aphasia: Implications for treatment. In R.H. Brookshire (Ed.), *Clinical Aphasiology Conference Proceedings.* Minneapolis: BRK (1979).

HANNAY, H.J., Asymmetry in reception and retention of colors. *Brain and Language,* 8, 191–201 (1979).

HANSON, W.R., and CICCIARELLI, A.W., The time, amount, and pattern of language improvement in adult aphasics. *British Journal of Disorders of Communication,* 13, 59–63 (1978).

HARASYMIW, S.J., HALPER, A., and SUTHERLAND, B., Sex, age, and aphasia type. *Brain and Language,* 12, 190–198 (1981).

HARDYCK, C., A model of individual differences in hemispheric functioning. In H. Whitaker and H.A. Whitaker (Eds.), *Studies in Neurolinguistics, Volume 3.* New York: Academic Press (1977).

HARRIS, L.J., Sex differences in spatial ability: Possible environmental, genetic, and neurological factors. In M. Kinsbourne (Ed.), *Asymmetrical Function of the Brain.* London: Cambridge University Press (1978).

HARTJE, W., KERSCHENSTEINER, M., POECK, K., and ORGASS, B., A cross-validation study on the Token Test. *Neuropsychologia,* 11, 119–121 (1973).

HAYNES, W.O., and GREENBERG, B.R., *Understanding aphasia: A Guide for Medical and Paramedical Professionals.* Danville, Ill.: Interstate Printers & Publishers (1976).

HAYNES, W.O., and ORATIO, A.R., A study of clients' perceptions of therapeutic effectiveness. *Journal of Speech and Hearing Disorders,* 43, 21–33 (1978).

HAYWARD, R.W., NAESER, M.A., and ZATZ, L.M., Cranial computed tomography in aphasia: Correlation of anatomical lesions with functional deficits. *Radiology,* 123, 653–660 (1977).

HEAD, H., Hughlings Jackson on aphasia and kindred affections of speech. *Brain,* 38, 1–90 (1915).

HEAD, H., Aphasia and kindred disorders of speech. *Brain,* 43, 87–165 (1920).

HEAD, H., Disorders of symbolic thinking and expression. *British Journal of Psychology,* 11, 179–193 (1921).

HEAD, H., *Aphasia and Kindred Disorders of Speech* (2 Vols.). London: Cambridge University Press (1926).

HECAEN, H., and ALBERT, M.L., *Human Neuropsychology.* New York: John Wiley & Sons (1978).

HECAEN, H., and ANGELERGUES, R., Localization of symptoms in aphasia. In A. DeReuck, and M. O'Connor (Eds.), *Disorders of Language.* London: Churchill (1964).

HECAEN, H., and SAUGUET, J., Cerebral dominance in left-handed subjects. *Cortex,* 7, 19–48, (1971).

HEDRICK, D.L., CHRISTMAN, M.A., and AUGUSTINE, L., Programming for the antecedent event in therapy. *Journal of Speech and Hearing Disorders,* 38, 339–344 (1973).

HEESCHEN, C., Strategies of decoding actor-object relations by aphasic patients. *Cortex,* 16, 5–19 (1980).

HEESCHEN, C., and JURGENS, R., Pragmatic-semantic and syntactic factors influencing ear differences in dichotic listening. *Cortex,* 13, 74–84 (1977).

HEILMAN, K.M., ROTHI, L., CAMPANELLA, D., and WOLFSON, S., Wernicke's and global aphasia without alexia. *Archives of Neurology,* 36, 129–133 (1979).

HEILMAN, K.M., SAFRAN, A., and GESCHWIND, N., Closed head trauma and aphasia. *Journal of Neurology, Neurosurgery and Psychiatry,* 34, 265–269 (1971).

HEILMAN, K.M., and SCHOLES, R.J., The nature of comprehension errors in Broca's, Conduction and Wernicke's aphasics. *Cortex,* 12, 258–265 (1976).

HEILMAN, K.M., SCHOLES, R.J., and WATSON, R.T., Defects of immediate memory in Broca's and conduction aphasia. *Brain and Language,* 3, 201–208 (1976).

HEILMAN, K.M., and WATSON, R.T., The neglect syndrome—a unilateral defect of the orienting response. In S. Harnad, R.W. Doty, L. Goldstein, et al. (Eds.), *Lateralization in the Nervous System.* New York: Academic Press (1977).

HELM, N.A., and BARRESI, B., Voluntary control of involuntary utterances: A treatment approach for severe aphasia. In R.H. Brookshire (Ed.), *Clinical Aphasiology Conference Proceedings.* Minneapolis: BRK (1980).

HELM-ESTABROOKS, N., FITZPATRICK, P.M., and BARRESI, B., Response of an agrammatic patient to a syntax stimulation program for aphasia. *Journal of Speech and Hearing Disorders,* 46, 422–427 (1981).

HELMICK, J.W., WATAMORI, T.S., and PALMER, J.M., Spouses' understanding of the communication disabilities of aphasic patients. *Journal of Speech and Hearing Disorders,* 41, 238–243 (1976).

HELMICK, J.W., WATAMORI, T.S., and PALMER, J.M., Reply to Holland's comment on "Spouses' understanding of the communication

disabilities of aphasic patients." *Journal of Speech and Hearing Disorders,* 42, 308–310 (1977).

HERSEN, M., and BARLOW, D.H., *Single Case Experimental Designs: Strategies for Studying Behavior Change.* New York: Pergamon Press (1976).

HICKS, R.E., BRADSHAW, G.J., KINSBOURNE, M., and FEIGIN, D.S., Vocal-manual trade-offs in hemisphere sharing of performance control in normal adult humans. *Journal of Motor Behavior,* 10, 1–6 (1978).

HIER, D.B., and KAPLAN, J., Verbal comprehension deficits after right hemisphere damage. *Applied Psycholinguistics,* 1, 279–294 (1980).

HIER, D.B., and MOHR, J.P., Incongruous oral and written naming: Evidence for a subdivision of the Syndrome of Wernicke's aphasia. *Brain and Language,* 4, 115–126 (1977).

HINES, D., Recognition of verbs, abstract nouns, and concrete nouns from the left and right visual half-fields. *Neuropsychologia,* 14, 211–216 (1976).

HISCOCK, M., Effects of examiner's location and subject's anxiety on gaze laterality. *Neuropsychologia,* 15, 409–416 (1977).

HOLLAND, A.L., Current trends in aphasia rehabilitation. *Asha,* 11, 3–7 (1969).

HOLLAND, A.L., Case studies in aphasia rehabilitation using programmed instruction. *Journal of Speech and Hearing Disorders,* 35, 377–390 (1970).

HOLLAND, A.L., Comment on "Spouses' understanding of the communication abilities of aphasic patients." *Journal of Speech and Hearing Disorders,* 42, 307–310 (1977a).

HOLLAND, A.L., Some practical considerations in aphasia rehabilitation. In M. Sullivan and M.S. Kommers (Eds.), *Rationale for Adult Aphasia Therapy.* University of Nebraska Medical Center (1977b).

HOLLAND, A.L., Functional communication in the treatment of aphasia. In L.J. Bradford (Ed.), *Communicative Disorders: An Audio Journal for Continuing Education.* New York: Grune & Stratton (1978).

HOLLAND, A.L., *Communicative Abilities in Daily Living.* Baltimore: University Park Press (1980a).

HOLLAND, A.L., The usefulness of treatment for aphasia: A serendipitous study. In R.H. Brookshire (Ed.), *Clinical Aphasiology Conference Proceedings.* Minneapolis: BRK (1980b).

HOLLAND, A.L., and LEVY, C.B. Syntactic generalization in aphasics as a function of relearning an active sentence. *Acta Symbolica,* 2(2), 34–41 (1971).

HOLLAND, A.L., and SONDERMAN, J.C., Effects of a program based on the Token Test for teaching comprehension skills to aphasics. *Journal of Speech and Hearing Research,* 17, 589–598 (1974).

HORNER, J., and LAPOINTE, L.L., Evaluation of learning potential of a severe aphasic adult through analysis of five performance variables. In R.H. Brookshire (Ed.), *Clinical Aphasiology Conference Proceedings.* Minneapolis: BRK (1979).

HORNER, J., and NAILLING, K., Raven's *Coloured Progressive Matrices:* Interpreting results through analysis of problem-type and error-type. In R.H. Brookshire (Ed.), *Clinical Aphasiology Conference Proceedings.* Minneapolis: BRK (1980).

HOWES, D.H., Application of the word-frequency concept to aphasia. In A.V.S. de Reuck and M. O'Conner (Eds.), *Disorders of Language.* London: Churchill (1964).

HOWES, D.H., Hypotheses concerning the functions of the language mechanism. In K. Salzinger and S. Salzinger (Eds.), *Research in Verbal Behavior and Some Neurological Implications.* New York: Academic Press (1967).

HUBER, M., Re-education of aphasics. *Journal of Speech and Hearing Disorders,* 7, 289–293 (1942).

HUBER, M., Linguistic problems of brain-injured servicemen. *Journal of Speech and Hearing Disorders,* 11, 143–147 (1946).

HUMPHREY, M.E., and ZANGWILL, O.L., Dysphasia in left-handed patients with unilateral lesions. *Journal of Neurology, Neurosurgery and Psychiatry,* 15, 184–193 (1952).

INCE, L.P., Desensitization with an aphasic patient. *Behavior Research and Therapy,* 6, 235–237 (1968).

JACKSON, J.H., On affections of speech from disease of the brain. *Brain,* 1, 304–330 (1879).

JAKOBSON, R., Aphasia as a linguistic problem. In H. Werner (Ed.), *On Expressive Language.* Worcester, Mass.: Clark University Press (1955).

JAKOBSON, R., *Child Language, Aphasia, and Phonological Universals.* The Hague, Netherlands: Mouton (1968).

JAKOBSON, R., Two aspects of language and two types of aphasic disturbances. In R. Jakobson and M. Halle, *Fundamentals of Language* (2nd Ed.). The Hague, Netherlands: Mouton (1971).

JAUHIAINEN, T., and NUUTILA, A., Auditory perception of speech and speech sounds in recent and recovered cases of aphasia. *Brain and Language,* 4, 572–579 (1977).

JAYNES, J., *The Origin of Consciousness and the Breakdown of the Bicameral Mind.* Boston: Houghton Mifflin (1976).

JENKINS, J.J., JIMENEZ-PABON, E., SHAW, R.E., and SEFER, J.W., *Schuell's Aphasia in Adults: Diagnosis, Prognosis, and Treatment* (2nd Ed.). Hagerstown, Md.: Harper & Row (1975).

JENKINS, J.J., and SCHUELL, H.M., Further work on language deficit in aphasia. *Psychological Review,* 71, 87–93 (1964).

JENNETT, B., and TEASDALE, G., *Management of Head Injuries.* Philadelphia: F.A. Davis (1981).

JOANETTE, Y., KELLER, E., and LECOURS, A.R., Sequences of phonemic approximations in aphasia. *Brain and Language,* 11, 30–44 (1980).

JOHNS, D.F., and LAPOINTE, L.L., Neurogenic disorders of output processing: Apraxia of speech. In H. Whitaker and H.A. Whitaker (Eds.), *Studies in Neurolinguistics, Volume 1.* New York: Academic Press (1976).

JOHNSON, J.P., SOMMERS, R.K., and WEIDNER, W.E., Dichotic ear preference in aphasia. *Journal of Speech and Hearing Research,* 20, 116–129 (1977).

JOHNSON, R.C., COLE, R.E., BOWERS, J.K., FOILES, S.V., NIKAIDO, A.M., PATRICK, J.W., and WOLIVER, R.E., Hemispheric efficiency in middle and later adulthood. *Cortex,* 15, 109–119 (1979).

JONES, L.V., GOODMAN, M.F., and WEPMAN, J.M., The classification of parts of speech for the characterization of aphasia. *Language and Speech,* 6, 94–107 (1963).

JONES, L.V., and WEPMAN, J.M., Dimensions of language performance in aphasia. *Journal of Speech and Hearing Research,* 4, 220–232 (1961).

JONES, L.V., and WEPMAN, J.M., Grammatical indicants of speaking style in normal and aphasic speakers. In K. Salzinger and S. Salzinger (Eds.), *Research in Verbal Behavior and Some Neurological Implications.* New York: Academic Press (1967).

JUST, M.A., DAVIS, G.A., and CARPENTER, P.A., A comparison of aphasic and normal adults in a sentence-verification task. *Cortex,* 13, 402–423 (1977).

KAIL, R.V., and SIEGEL, A.W., Sex and hemispheric differences in the recall of verbal and spatial information. *Cortex,* 14, 557–563 (1978).

KAPLAN, N.R., and DREYER, D.E., The effect of self-awareness training on student speech pathologist-client relationships. *Journal of Communication Disorders,* 7, 329–342 (1974).

KARIS, R., and HORENSTEIN, S., Localization of speech parameters by brain scan. *Neurology,* 26, 226–230 (1976).

KEAN, M.L., The linguistic interpretation of aphasic syndromes. In E. Walker (Ed.), *Explorations in the Biology of Language.* Montgomery, Vt.: Bradford Books (1978).

KEAN, M.L., Agrammatism: A phonological deficit? *Cognition,* 7, 69–84 (1979).

KEAN, M.L., Grammatical representations and the description of language processing. In D. Caplan (Ed.), *Biological Studies of Mental Processes.* Cambridge, Mass.: MIT Press (1980).

KEARNS, K., and HUBBARD, D.J., A comparison of auditory comprehension tasks in aphasia. In

R.H. Brookshire (Ed.), *Clinical Aphasiology Conference Proceedings*. Minneapolis: BRK (1977).

KEENAN, J.S., A method for eliciting naming behavior from aphasic patients. *Journal of Speech and Hearing Disorders,* 31, 261-266 (1966).

KEENAN, J.S., The detection of minimal dysphasia. *Archives of Physical Medicine and Rehabilitation,* 52, 227-232 (1971).

KEENAN, J.S., *The Procedure Manual in Speech Pathology with Brain-damaged Adults*. Danville, Ill.: Interstate Printers & Publishers (1975).

KEENAN, J.S., *Programming Therapy for Aphasia*. Murfreesboro, Tenn.: Pinnacle Press (1977).

KEENAN, J.S., and BRASSELL, E.G., A study of factors related to prognosis for individual aphasic patients. *Journal of Speech and Hearing Disorders,* 39, 257-269 (1974).

KEENAN, J.S., and BRASSELL, E.G., *Aphasia Language Performance Scales*. Murfreesboro, Tenn.: Pinnacle Press (1975).

KEITH, R.L., *Speech and Language Rehabilitation: A Workbook for the Neurologically Impaired*. Danville, Ill.: Interstate Printers & Publishers (1972).

KEITH, R.L., *Speech and Language Rehabilitation: A Workbook for the Neurologically Impaired. Volume 2.* Danville, Ill.: Interstate Printers & Publishers (1977).

KEITH, R.L., *Graduated Language Training for Patients with Aphasia and Children with Language Deficiencies*. Houston: College-Hill Press (1980).

KEITH, R.L., and ARONSON, A.E., Singing as therapy for apraxia of speech and aphasia: Report of a case. *Brain and Language,* 2, 483-488 (1975).

KELLAR, L.A., and BEVER, T.G., Hemispheric asymmetries in the perception of musical intervals as a function of musical experience and family handedness background. *Brain and Language,* 10, 24-38 (1980).

KELLY, J., The effect of new information and imagery stimulation on the word retrieval abilities of aphasic adults. Unpublished Master's Thesis, Memphis State University (1981).

KENIN, M., and SWISHER, L.P., A study of pattern of recovery in aphasia. *Cortex,* 8, 56-68 (1972).

KERSCHENSTEINER, M., POECK, K., and BRUNNER, E., The fluency-nonfluency dimension in the classification of aphasic speech. *Cortex,* 8, 233-247 (1972).

KERTESZ, A., Classification of aphasic phenomena. *Canadian Journal of Neurological Sciences,* 3, 135-139 (1976).

KERTESZ, A., *Aphasia and Associated Disorders: Taxonomy, Localization, and Recovery*. New York: Grune & Stratton (1979).

KERTESZ, A., The anatomy of jargon. In J.W. Brown (Ed.), *Jargonaphasia*. New York: Academic Press (1981).

KERTESZ, A., and BENSON, D.F., Neologistic jargon: A clinicopathological study. *Cortex,* 6, 362-396 (1970).

KERTESZ, A., HARLOCK, W., and COATES, R., Computer tomographic localization, lesion size, and prognosis in aphasia and nonverbal impairment. *Brain and Language,* 8, 34-50 (1979).

KERTESZ, A., and MCCABE, P., Intelligence and aphasia: Performance of aphasics on Raven's *Coloured Progressive Matrices* (RCPM). *Brain and Language,* 2, 387-395 (1975).

KERTESZ, A., and MCCABE, P., Recovery patterns and prognosis in aphasia. *Brain,* 100, 1-18 (1977).

KERTESZ, A., and POOLE, E., The aphasia quotient: The taxonomic approach to measurement of aphasic disability. *Canadian Journal of Neurological Sciences,* 1, 7-16 (1974).

KERTESZ, A., and SHEPPARD, A., The epidemiology of aphasic and cognitive impairment in stroke: Age, sex, aphasia type and laterality differences. *Brain,* 104, 117-128 (1981).

KILPATRICK, K., *Therapy Guide for the Adult with Language and Speech Disorders: Volume 2. Advanced Stimulus Materials*. Akron, Ohio: Visiting Nurse Service (1979).

KILPATRICK, K., *Working with Words*. Akron, Ohio: Visiting Nurse Service (1980).

KILPATRICK, K., JONES, C.L., and RELLER, J., *Therapy Guide for the Adult with Language and Speech Disorders: Volume 1. A Selection of Stimulus Materials*. Akron, Ohio: Visiting Nurse Service (1977).

KIM, Y.C., Deficits in temporal sequencing of verbal material: The effect of laterality of lesion. *Brain and Language,* 3, 507-515 (1976).

KIMMEL, D.C., *Adulthood and Aging*. New York: John Wiley & Sons (1974).

KIMURA, D., Cerebral dominance and the perception of verbal stimuli. *Canadian Journal of Psychology,* 15, 166-171 (1961).

KIMURA, D., Left-right differences in the perception of melodies. *Quarterly Journal of Experimental Psychology,* 16, 355-358 (1964).

KIMURA, D., Functional asymmetry of the brain in dichotic listening. *Cortex,* 3, 163-178 (1967).

KIMURA, D., The neural basis of language qua gesture. In H. Whitaker and H.A. Whitaker (Eds.), *Studies in Neurolinguistics, Volume 2*. New York: Academic Press (1976).

KINSBOURNE, M., The minor cerebral hemisphere as a source of aphasic speech. *Archives of Neurology,* 25, 302-306 (1971).

KINSBOURNE, M., Eye and head turning indicates cerebral lateralization. *Science,* 176, 539–541 (1972).

KINSBOURNE, M., Minor hemisphere language and cerebral maturation. In E.H. Lenneberg and E. Lenneberg (Eds.), *Foundations of Language Development: A Multidisciplinary Approach, Volume 2.* New York: Academic Press (1975).

KINSBOURNE, M., and COOK, J., Generalized and lateralized effect of concurrent verbalization on a unimanual skill. *Quarterly Journal of Experimental Psychology,* 23, 341–345 (1971).

KINSBOURNE, M., and HISCOCK, M., Does cerebral dominance develop? In S.J. Segalowitz and F.A. Gruber (Eds.), *Language Development and Neurological Theory.* New York: Academic Press (1977).

KINSBOURNE, M., and WARRINGTON, E.K., Jargon aphasia. *Neuropsychologia,* 1, 27–37 (1963).

KINSELLA, G., and DUFFY, F., The spouse of the aphasic patient. In Y. Lebrun and R. Hoops (Eds.), *The Management of Aphasia.* Amsterdam: Swets & Zeitlinger (1978).

KIRSHNER, H.S., and WEBB, W., Selective involvement of the auditory-verbal modality in an acquired communication disorder: Benefit from sign language therapy. *Brain and Language,* 13, 161–170 (1981).

KLOR, B.M., A comparison of auditory-verbal, visual-verbal, and visual-nonverbal presentation of commands to aphasic adults. In R.H. Brookshire (Ed.), *Clinical Aphasiology Conference Proceedings.* Minneapolis: BRK (1980).

KNOX, D.R., *Portrait of Aphasia.* Detroit: Wayne State University Press (1971).

KOCEL, K.M., Age-related changes in cognitive abilities and hemispheric specialization. In J. Herron (Ed.), *Neuropsychology of Left-Handedness.* New York: Academic Press (1980).

KOCEL, K.M., GALIN, D., ORNSTEIN, R., and MERRIN, E.L., Lateral eye movement and cognitive mode. *Psychonomic Science,* 27, 223–224 (1972).

KOFF, E., and RIEDERER, S.A., Hemispheric specialization for syntactic form. *Brain and Language,* 14, 138–143 (1981).

KOHLMEYER, K., Aphasia due to focal disorders of cerebral circulation: Some aspects of localization and of spontaneous recovery. In Y. Lebrun and R. Hoops (Eds.), *Recovery in Aphasics.* Amsterdam: Swets & Zeitlinger (1976).

KOLK, H.H.L., Judgment of sentence structure in Broca's aphasia. *Neuropsychologia,* 16, 617–625 (1978).

KRASHEN, S.D., Cerebral asymmetry. In H. Whitaker and H.A. Whitaker (Eds.), *Studies in Neurolinguistics, Volume 2.* New York: Academic Press (1976).

KRATOCHWILL, T.R. (Ed.), *Single Subject Research: Strategies for Evaluating Change.* New York: Academic Press (1978).

KREINDLER, A., GHEORGHITA, N., and VOINESCU, I., Analysis of verbal reception of a complex order with three elements in aphasics. *Brain,* 94, 375–386 (1971).

KREINDLER, A., MIHAILESCU, L., and FRADIS, A., Speech fluency in aphasics. *Brain and Language,* 9, 199–205 (1980).

KUBLER-ROSS, E.K., *On Death and Dying.* New York: Macmillan (1969).

KUSHNER, D., and WINITZ, H., Extended comprehension practice applied to an aphasic patient. *Journal of Speech and Hearing Disorders,* 42, 296–305 (1977).

KUSSMAUL, A., Disturbances of speech. In H. von Ziemssen (Ed.), *Cyclopedia of Medicine,* J.A. McCreery (Trans.). New York: William Wood (1877).

KUTAS, M., and HILLYARD, S.A., Reading between the lines: Event-related brain potentials during natural sentence processing. *Brain and Language,* 11, 354–373 (1980).

LACKNER, J.R., and TEUBER, H.L., Alternations in auditory fusion thresholds after cerebral injury in man. *Neuropsychologia,* 11, 409–415 (1973).

LAMENDELLA, J.T., The limbic system in human communication. In H. Whitaker and H.A. Whitaker (Eds.), *Studies in Neurolinguistics, Volume 3.* New York: Academic Press (1977).

LAPOINTE, L.L., Base-10 programmed stimulation: Task specification, scoring, and plotting performance in aphasia therapy. *Journal of Speech and Hearing Disorders,* 42, 90–105 (1977).

LAPOINTE, L.L., Aphasia therapy: Some principles and strategies for treatment. In D.F. Johns (Ed.), *Clinical Management of Neurogenic Communicative Disorders.* Boston: Little, Brown (1978a).

LAPOINTE, L.L., Multiple baseline designs. In R.H. Brookshire (Ed.), *Clinical Aphasiology Conference Proceedings.* Minneapolis: BRK (1978b).

LAPOINTE, L.L., and HORNER, J., *Reading Comprehension Battery for Aphasia.* Tigard, Oreg.: C.C. Publications (1979).

LAPOINTE, L.L., HORNER, J., and LIEBERMAN, R.J., Effects of ear presentation and delayed response on the processing of Token Test commands by aphasic adults. In R.H. Brookshire (Ed.), *Clinical Aphasiology Conference Proceedings.* Minneapolis: BRK (1977).

LAPOINTE, L.L., ROTHI, L.J., and CAMPANELLA, D.J., The effects of repetition of Token Test commands on auditory comprehension. In R.H. Brookshire (Ed.), *Clinical Aphasiology Conference Proceedings*. Minneapolis: BRK (1978).

LASKY, E.Z., WEIDNER, W.E., and JOHNSON, J.P., Influence of linguistic complexity, rate of presentation, and interphrase pause time on auditory-verbal comprehension of adult aphasic patients. *Brain and Language*, 3, 386–395 (1976).

LASSEN, N.A., INGVAR, D.H., and SKINHOJ, E., Brain function and blood flow. *Scientific American*, 239, 62–71 (1978).

LAUGHLIN, S.A., NAESER, M.A., and GORDON, W.P., Effects of three syllable durations using the Melodic Intonation Therapy Technique. *Journal of Speech and Hearing Research*, 22, 311–320 (1979).

LAURENCE, S., and STEIN, D.G., Recovery after brain damage and the concept of localization of function. In S. Finger (Ed.), *Recovery from Brain Damage: Research and Theory*. New York: Plenum Press (1978).

LEBRUN, Y., and HOOPS, R., *Intelligence and Aphasia*. Amsterdam: Swets & Zeitlinger (1974).

LECOURS, A.R., and VANIER-CLEMENT, M., Schizophasia and jargonaphasia. *Brain and Language*, 3, 516–565 (1976).

LECOURS, A.R., and ROUILLON, F., Neurolinguistic analysis of jargonaphasia and jargonagraphia. In H. Whitaker and H.A. Whitaker (Eds.), *Studies in Neurolinguistics, Volume 2*. New York: Academic Press (1976).

LENNEBERG, E., *Biological Foundations of Language*. New York: Wiley (1967).

LESSER, R., Word association and the availability of response in an aphasic subject. *Journal of Psycholinguistic Research*, 2, 355–367 (1973).

LESSER, R., Verbal and non-verbal memory components in the Token Test. *Neuropsychologia*, 14, 79–85 (1976).

LESSER, R., *Linguistic Investigations of Aphasia*. London: Edward Arnold (1978).

LESSER, R., Turning tokens into things: Linguistic and mnestic aspects of the initial sections of the Token Test. In F. Boller and M. Dennis (Eds.), *Auditory Comprehension: Clinical and Experimental Studies with the Token Test*. New York: Academic Press (1979).

LEVIN, H.S., Aphasia in closed head injury. In M.T. Sarno (Ed.), *Acquired Aphasia*. New York: Academic Press (1981).

LEVIN, H.S., GROSSMAN, R.G., and KELLY, P.J., Aphasic disorder in patients with closed head injury. *Journal of Neurology, Neurosurgery, and Psychiatry*, 39, 1062–1070 (1976).

LEVIN, H.S., GROSSMAN, R.G., ROSE, J.E., and TEASDALE, G., Long term neuropsychological outcome of closed head injury. *Journal of Neurosurgery*, 50, 412–422 (1979).

LEVIN, H.S., GROSSMAN, R.G., SARWAR, M., and MEYERS, C.A., Linguistic recovery after closed head injury. *Brain and Language*, 12, 360–374 (1981).

LEVY, J., and GUR, R.C., Individual differences in psychoneurological organization. In J. Herron (Ed.), *Neuropsychology of Left-Handedness*. New York: Academic Press (1980).

LEVY, J., and REID, M., Variations in writing posture with cerebral organization. *Science*, 194, 337–339 (1976).

LEZAK, M.D., Recovery of memory and learning functions following traumatic brain injury. *Cortex*, 15, 63–72 (1979).

LICHTHEIM, L., On aphasia. *Brain*, 7, 433–484 (1885).

LILES, B.Z., and BROOKSHIRE, R.H., The effects of pause time on auditory comprehension of aphasic subjects. *Journal of Communication Disorders*, 8, 221–236 (1975).

LINCOLN, N.B., and ELLS, P., A shortened version of the PICA. *British Journal of Disorders of Communication*, 15, 183–187 (1980).

LINDSAY, P.H., and NORMAN, D.A., *Human Information Processing: An Introduction to Psychology* (2nd Ed.). New York: Academic Press (1977).

LINEBAUGH, C.W., and LEHNER, L., Cueing hierarchies and word retrieval: A therapy program. In R.H. Brookshire (Ed.), *Clinical Aphasiology Conference Proceedings*. Minneapolis: BRK (1977).

LINEBAUGH, C.W., and YOUNG-CHARLES, H.Y., The counseling needs of the families of aphasic patients. In R.H. Brookshire (Ed.), *Clinical Aphasiology Conference Proceedings*. Minneapolis: BRK (1978).

LINEBAUGH, C.W., and YOUNG-CHARLES, H.Y., Confidence ratings of aphasics' functional communication: Spouses and speech-language pathologists. In R.H. Brookshire (Ed.), *Clinical Aphasiology Conference Proceedings*. Minneapolis: BRK (1981).

LOCKE, J.L., and DECK, J.W., Retrieval failure, rehearsal deficiency, and short-term memory loss in the aphasic adult. *Brain and Language*, 5. 227–235 (1978).

LOHMANN, L., and PRESCOTT, T.E., The effects of substituting "objects" for "forms" on the Revised Token Test (RTT) performance of aphasic subjects. In R.H. Brookshire (Ed.), *Clinical Aphasiology Conference Proceedings*. Minneapolis: BRK (1978).

LOMAS, J., and KERTESZ, A., Patterns of spontaneous recovery in aphasic groups: A study of adult stroke patients. *Brain and Language,* 5, 388–401 (1978).

LOVE, R.J., and WEBB, W.J., The efficacy of cueing techniques in Broca's aphasia. *Journal of Speech and Hearing Disorders,* 42, 170–178 (1977).

LOVERSO, F.L., SELINGER, M., and PRESCOTT, T.E., Application of verbing strategies to aphasia treatment. In R.H. Brookshire (Ed.), *Clinical Aphasiology Conference Proceedings.* Minneapolis: BRK (1979).

LOZANO, R.A., and GAETH, J.H., Application of a programmable auditory evaluation system (PAVES) to aphasia rehabilitation. In R.H. Brookshire (Ed.), *Clinical Aphasiology Conference Proceedings.* Minneapolis: BRK (1977).

LUBINSKI, R., Environmental language intervention. In R. Chapey (Ed.), *Language Intervention Strategies in Adult Aphasia.* Baltimore: Williams & Wilkins (1981a).

LUBINSKI, R., Speech, language, and audiology programs in home health care agencies and nursing homes. In D.S. Beasley and G.A. Davis (Eds.), *Aging: Communication Processes and Disorders.* New York: Grune & Stratton (1981b).

LUBINSKI, R., and CHAPEY, R., Communication services in home health care agencies: Availability and scope. *Asha,* 22, 929–934 (1980).

LUDLOW, C., Recovery from aphasia: A foundation for treatment. In M. Sullivan and M.S. Kommers (Eds.), *Rationale for Adult Aphasia Therapy.* University of Nebraska Medical Center (1977).

LURIA, A.R., Brain disorders and language analysis. *Language and Speech,* 1, 14–34 (1958).

LURIA, A.R., Factors and forms of aphasia. In A.V.S. de Reuck and M. O'Conner (Eds.), *Disorders of Language.* London: Churchill (1964).

LURIA, A.R., *Higher Cortical Functions in Man.* New York: Basic Books (1966).

LURIA, A.R., The functional organization of the brain. *Scientific American,* 222(3), 66–78 (1970a).

LURIA, A.R., *Traumatic Aphasia.* The Hague, Netherlands: Mouton (1970b).

LURIA, A.R., Language and brain. *Brain and Language,* 1, 1–14 (1974).

LURIA, A.R., On quasi-aphasic speech disturbances in lesions of the deep structures of the brain. *Brain and Language,* 4, 432–459 (1977).

LURIA, A.R., and TSVETKOVA, L.S., The mechanism of "dynamic aphasia." *Foundations of Language,* 4, 296–307 (1968).

MACK, J.L., The comprehension of locative prepositions in nonfluent and fluent aphasia. *Brain and Language,* 14, 81–92 (1981).

MACK. J.L., and BOLLER, F., Components of auditory comprehension: Analysis of errors in a Revised Token Test. In F. Boller and M. Dennis

(Eds.), *Auditory Comprehension: Clinical and Experimental Studies with the Token Test.* New York: Academic Press (1979).

MALONE, P.E., A preliminary investigation of changes in sexual relations following stroke. In R.H. Brookshire (Ed.), *Clinical Aphasiology Conference Proceedings.* Minneapolis: BRK (1975).

MALONE, R.L., Expressed attitudes of families of aphasics. *Journal of Speech and Hearing Disorders,* 34, 146–151 (1969).

MALONE, R., PTACEK, P., and MALONE, M., Attitudes expressed by families of aphasics. *British Journal of Disorders of Communication,* 5, 174–179 (1970).

MALY, J., TURNHEIM, M., HEISS, W.D., and GLONING, K., Brain perfusion and neuropsychological test scores: A correlation study in aphasics. *Brain and Language,* 4, 78–94 (1977).

MARKS, M.M., TAYLOR, M., and RUSK, H.A., Rehabilitation of the aphasic patient: A survey of three years' experience in a rehabilitation setting. *Neurology,* 7, 837–843 (1957).

MARSHALL, J.C., and NEWCOMBE, F., Patterns of paralexia: A psycholinguistic approach. *Journal of Psycholinguistic Research,* 2, 175–199 (1973).

MARSHALL, J.C., and NEWCOMBE, F., Variability and constraint in acquired dyslexia. In H. Whitaker and H.A. Whitaker (Eds.), *Studies in Neurolinguistics, Volume 3.* New York: Academic Press (1977).

MARSHALL, R.C., Word retrieval behavior of aphasic adults. *Journal of Speech and Hearing Disorders,* 41, 444–451 (1976).

MARSHALL, R.C., *Clinician Controlled Auditory Stimulation for Aphasic Adults.* Tigard, Oreg.: C.C. Publications (1978).

MARSHALL, R.C., Heightening auditory comprehension for aphasic patients. In R. Chapey (Ed.), *Language Intervention Strategies in Adult Aphasia.* Baltimore: Williams & Wilkins (1981).

MARSHALL, R.C., JEFFERIES, E.C., RAU, M.T., GOLPER, L.C., and THOMAS, J.C., Intermittent auditory imperception: Clinical characteristics and implications for treatment. In R.H. Brookshire (Ed.), *Clinical Aphasiology Collected Proceedings 1972–1976.* Minneapolis: BRK (1978).

MARSHALL, R.C., TOMPKINS, C.A., RAU, M.T., PHILLIPS, D.S., and GOLPER, L.A., Speech and language services for severely aphasic patients: Some professional considerations. In R.H. Brookshire (Ed.), *Clinical Aphasiology Conference Proceedings.* Minneapolis: BRK (1979).

MARSHALL, R.C., TOMPKINS, C.A., RAU, M.T., PHILLIPS, D.S., GOLPER, L.A., and LAMBRECHT, K.J., Verbal self-correction behavior of aphasic subjects for single word tasks. In R.H.

Brookshire (Ed.), *Clinical Aphasiology Conference Proceedings.* Minneapolis: BRK (1980).

MARTIN, A.D., Some objections to the term *apraxia of speech. Journal of Speech and Hearing Disorders*, 39, 53–64 (1974).

MARTIN, A.D., Aphasia testing: A second look at the Porch Index of Communicative Ability. *Journal of Speech and Hearing Disorders*, 42, 547–562 (1977).

MARTIN, A.D., A critical evaluation of therapeutic approaches to aphasia. In R.H. Brookshire (Ed.), *Clinical Aphasiology Collected Proceedings 1972–1976.* Minneapolis: BRK (1978).

MARTIN, A.D., An examination of Wepman's thought centered therapy. In R. Chapey (Ed.), *Language Intervention Strategies in Adult Aphasia.* Baltimore: Williams & Wilkins (1981a).

MARTIN, A.D., Therapy with the jargonaphasic. In J.W. Brown (Ed.), *Jargonaphasia.* New York: Academic Press (1981b).

MARTIN, A.D., and RIGRODSKY, S., An investigation of phonological impairment in aphasia, part 1. *Cortex*, 10, 317–328 (1974a).

MARTIN, A.D., and RIGRODSKY, S., An investigation of phonological impairment in aphasia, part 2: Distinctive feature analysis of phonemic commutation errors in aphasia. *Cortex*, 10, 329–346 (1974b).

MARTINO, A.A., PIZZAMIGLIO, L., and RAZZANO, C., A new version of the "Token Test" for aphasics: A concrete objects form. *Journal of Communication Disorders*, 9, 1–5 (1976).

MARTINOFF, J.T., MARTINOFF, R., and STOKKE, V., *Language Rehabilitation: Auditory Comprehension.* Tigard, Oreg.: C.C. Publications (1980).

MATEER, C., Impairments of nonverbal oral movements after left hemisphere damage: A followup analysis of errors. *Brain and Language*, 6, 334–341 (1978).

MAZZOCCHI, F., and VIGNOLO, L.A., Computer assisted tomography in neuropsychological research: A simple procedure for lesion mapping. *Cortex*, 14, 136–144 (1978).

MAZZOCCHI, F., and VIGNOLO, L.A., Localisation of lesions in aphasia: Clinical-CT scan correlations in stroke patients. *Cortex*, 15, 627–654 (1979).

MCADAM, D.W., and WHITAKER, H.A., Language production: Electroencephalographic localization in the normal human brain. *Science*, 172, 499–502 (1971).

MCBRIDE, C., *Silent Victory.* Chicago: Nebon-Hall (1969).

MCFIE, J., *Assessment of Organic Intellectual Impairment.* New York: Academic Press (1975).

MCGLONE, J., Sex differences in the cerebral organization of verbal functions in patients with unilateral brain lesions. *Brain*, 100, 775–793 (1977).

MCKEE, G., HUMPHREY, B., and MCADAM, D.W., Scaled lateralization of alpha activity during linguistic and musical tasks. *Psychophysiology*, 10, 441–443 (1973).

MCKEEVER, W.F., and HULING, M.D., Lateral dominance in tachistoscopic word recognition performances obtained with simultaneous bilateral input. *Neuropsychologia*, 9, 15–20 (1971).

MCKEOWN, M.R., *A Practicebook for Aphasics.* Springfield, Ill.: Charles C. Thomas (1976).

MCNEIL, M.R., and KOZMINSKY, L., The efficacy of five self-generated strategies for facilitating auditory processing. In R.H. Brookshire (Ed.), *Clinical Aphasiology Conference Proceedings.* Minneapolis: BRK (1980).

MCNEIL, M.R., and PRESCOTT, T.E., *Revised Token Test.* Baltimore: University Park Press (1978).

MCNEIL, M.R., PRESCOTT, T.E., and CHANG, E.C., A measure of PICA ordinality. In R.H. Brookshire (Ed.), *Clinical Aphasiology Collected Proceedings 1972–1976.* Minneapolis: BRK (1978).

MCREYNOLDS, L.V., and KEARNS, K.P., *Single Subject Experimental Designs for Intervention Research in Communicative Disorders.* Baltimore: University Park Press (In Press).

MERCER, B., WAPNER, W., GARDNER, H., and BENSON, D.F., A study of confabulation. *Archives of Neurology*, 34, 346–348 (1977).

MESSERLI, P., TISSOT, A., and RODRIGUEZ, J., Recovery from aphasia: Some factors of prognosis. In Y. Lebrun and R. Hoops (Eds.), *Recovery in Aphasics.* Amsterdam: Swets & Zeitlinger (1976).

MESSINA, A.V., Cranial computerized tomography. *Archives of Neurology*, 34, 602–607 (1977).

MEYER, J.S., KANDA, T., FUKUUCHI, Y., SHIMAZU, K., DENNIS, E.W., and ERICSSON, A.D., Clinical prognosis correlated with hemispheric blood flow in cerebral infarction. *Stroke*, 2, 383–394 (1971).

MEYER, J.S., SAKAI, F., YAMAGUCHI, F., YAMAMOTO, M., and SHAW, T., Regional changes in cerebral blood flow during standard behavioral activation in patients with disorders of speech and mentation compared to normal volunteers. *Brain and Language*, 9, 61–77 (1980).

MEYER, J.S., SHINOHARA, Y., KANDA, T., FUKUUCHI, Y., ERICSSON, A.D., and KOK, N.K., Diaschisis resulting from acute unilateral cerebral infarction. *Archives of Neurology*, 23, 241–247 (1970).

MICELI, G., CALTAGIRONE, C., GAINOTTI, G., and PAYER-RIGO, P., Discrimination of voice versus place consonants in aphasia. *Brain and Language*, 6, 47–51 (1978).

MICELI, G., GAINOTTI, G., CALTAGIRONE, C., and MASULO, C., Some aspects of phonological impairment in aphasia. *Brain and Language*, 11, 159–170 (1980).

MILBERG, W., and BLUMSTEIN, S.E., Lexical decision and aphasia: Evidence for semantic processing. *Brain and Language*, 14, 371–385 (1981).

MILLER, E., Psychological intervention in the management and rehabilitation of neuropsychological impairments. *Behavior Research and Therapy*, 18, 527–535 (1980).

MILLS, C., Treatment of aphasia by training. *Journal of the American Medical Association*, 43, 1940–1949 (1904).

MILLS, R.H., KNOX, A.W., JUOLA, J.F., and McFARLAND, W.H., Cognitive loci of impairments of picture naming by aphasic subjects. *Journal of Speech and Hearing Research*, 22, 73–87 (1979).

MILNER, B., Brain mechanisms suggested by studies of temporal lobes. In C.H. Millikan and F.L. Darley (Eds.), *Brain Mechanisms Underlying Speech and Language*. New York: Grune and Stratton (1967).

MODERN EDUCATION CORPORATION, *Photo Resource Kit*. Tulsa, Oklahoma.

MODERN EDUCATION CORPORATION, *Places & Things*. Tulsa, Oklahoma.

MOGIL, S., BLOOM, D., GRAY, L., and LEFKOWITZ, N., A unique method for the follow-up of aphasic patients. In R.H. Brookshire (Ed.), *Clinical Aphasiology Conference Proceedings*. Minneapolis: BRK (1978).

MOHR, J.P., Broca's area and Broca's aphasia. In H. Whitaker and H.A. Whitaker (Eds.), *Studies in Neurolinguistics, Volume 1*. New York: Academic Press (1976).

MOHR, J.P., Revision of Broca aphasia and the syndrome of Broca's area infarction and its implications in aphasia theory. In R.H. Brookshire (Ed.), *Clinical Aphasiology Conference Proceedings*. Minneapolis: BRK (1980).

MOHR, J.P., PESSIN, M.S., FINKELSTEIN, S., FUNKENSTEIN, H.H., DUNCAN, G.W., and DAVIS, K.R., Broca aphasia: Pathologic and clinical aspects. *Neurology*, 28, 311–324 (1978).

MOHR, J.P., WATTERS, W.C., and DUNCAN, G.W., Thalamic hemorrhage and aphasia. *Brain and Language*, 2, 3–17 (1975).

MOLFESE, D.L., Infant cerebral asymmetry. In S.J. Segalowitz and F.A. Gruber (Eds.), *Language Development and Neurological Theory*. New York: Academic Press (1977).

MOORE, W.H., and HAYNES, W.O., Alpha hemispheric asymmetry and stuttering: Some support for a segmentation dysfunction hypothesis. *Journal of Speech and Hearing Research*, 23, 229–248 (1980a).

MOORE, W.H., and HAYNES, W.O., A study of alpha hemispheric asymmetries for verbal and nonverbal stimuli in males and females. *Brain and Language*, 9, 338–349 (1980b).

MORGAN, A.H., MacDONALD, H., and HILGARD, E.R., EEG alpha: Lateral asymmtery related to task, and hypnotizability. *Psychophysiology*, 11, 275–282 (1974).

MORLEY, G.K., LUNDGREN, S., and HAXBY, J., Comparison and clinical applicability of auditory comprehension scores on the Behavioral Neurology Deficit Evaluation, Boston Diagnostic Aphasia Examination, Porch Index of Communicative Ability and Token Test. *Journal of Clinical Neuropsychology*, 1, 249–258 (1979).

MORSE, H.N., Aberrational man—tour de force of legal psychiatry. *Journal of Forensic Science*, 13, 1–32, 177–222, 340–375, 470–497 (1968).

MOSCOVITCH, M., On the representation of language in the right hemisphere of right-handed people. *Brain and Language*, 3, 47–71 (1976a).

MOSCOVITCH, M., On interpreting data regarding the linguistic competence and performance of the right hemisphere: A reply to Selnes. *Brain and Language*, 3, 590–599 (1976b).

MOSS, C.S., *Recovery with Aphasia: The Aftermath of My Stroke*. Urbana, Ill.: University of Illinois Press (1972).

MOSSMAN, P.L., *A Problem-Oriented Approach to Stroke Rehabilitation*. Springfield, Ill.: Charles C. Thomas, 1976.

MURRAY, H.A., *Thematic Apperception Test*. Cambridge, Mass.: Harvard University Press (1943).

MYERS, P.S., Profiles of communication deficits in patients with right cerebral hemisphere damage: Implications for diagnosis and treatment. In R.H. Brookshire (Ed.), *Clinical Aphasiology Conference Proceedings*. Minneapolis: BRK (1979).

MYERS, P.S., Visual imagery in aphasia treatment: A new look. In R.H. Brookshire (Ed.), *Clinical Aphasiology Conference Proceedings*. Minneapolis: BRK (1980).

MYERS, P.S., and WEST, J.F., The speech pathologist's role with right hemisphere damaged patients. In R.H. Brookshire (Ed.), *Clinical Aphasiology Conference Proceedings*. Minneapolis: BRK (1977).

MYERSON, R., and GOODGLASS, H., Transformational grammars of aphasic patients. *Language and Speech*, 15, 40–50 (1972).

MYSAK, E.D., *Pathologies of Speech Systems*. Baltimore: Williams & Wilkins (1976).

MYSAK, E.D., and GUARINO, C.G., Self-adjusting therapy. In R. Chapey (Ed.), *Language Interven-*

tion Strategies in Adult Aphasia. Baltimore: Williams & Wilkins (1981).

NAESER, M.A., A structured approach to teaching aphasics basic sentence types. *British Journal of Disorders of Communication,* 10, 70–76 (1975).

NAESER, M.A., and HAYWARD, R.W., Lesion localization in aphasia with cranial computer tomography and the Boston Diagnostic Aphasia Exam. *Neurology,* 28, 545–551 (1978).

NAESER, M.A., and HAYWARD, R.W., The resolving stroke and aphasia: A case study with computerized tomography. *Archives of Neurology,* 36, 233–235 (1979).

NAESER, M.A., HAYWARD, R.W., LAUGHLIN, S.A., BECKER, J.M.T., JERNIGAN, T.L., and ZATZ, L.M., Quantitative CT scan studies in aphasia. II. Comparison of the right and left hemispheres. *Brain and Language,* 12, 165–189 (1981).

NEEDHAM, E.C., and BLACK, J.W., The relative ability of aphasic persons to judge the duration and intensity of pure tones. *Journal of Speech and Hearing Research,* 13, 725–730 (1970).

NEEDHAM, L.S., and SWISHER, L.P., A comparison of three tests of auditory comprehension for adult aphasics. *Journal of Speech and Hearing Disorders,* 37, 123–131 (1972).

NELSON, M.J., *The Nelson Reading Test.* New York: Houghton Mifflin (1962).

NEVILLE, H.J., Event-related potentials in neuro-psychological studies of language. *Brain and Language,* 11, 300–318 (1980).

NEWCOMBE, F., OLDFIELD, R.C., RATCLIFF, G.G., and WINGFIELD, A., Recognition and naming of object-drawings by men with focal brain wounds. *Journal of Neurology, Neurosurgery and Psychiatry,* 34, 329–340 (1971).

NEWHOFF, M., BUGBEE, J.K., and FERREIRA, A., A change of PACE: Spouses as treatment targets. In R.H. Brookshire (Ed.), *Clinical Aphasiology Conference Proceedings.* Minneapolis: BRK (1981).

NEWHOFF, M.N., and DAVIS, G.A., A spouse intervention program: Planning, implementation and problems of evaluation. In R.H. Brookshire (Ed.), *Clinical Aphasiology Conference Proceedings.* Minneapolis: BRK (1978).

NICHOLAS, L.E., and BROOKSHIRE, R.H., An analysis of how clinicians respond to unacceptable patient responses in aphasia treatment sessions. In R.H. Brookshire (Ed.), *Clinical Aphasiology Conference Proceedings.* Minneapolis: BRK (1979).

NILSSON, J., GLENCROSS, D., and GEFFEN, G., The effects of familial sinistrality and preferred hand on dichaptic and dichotic tasks. *Brain and Language,* 10, 390–404 (1980).

NOLL, J.D., and RANDOLPH, S.R., Auditory semantic, syntactic, and retention errors made by aphasic subjects on the Token Test. *Journal of Communication Disorders,* 11, 543–553 (1978).

NORMAN, D.A., *Memory and Attention: An Introduction to Human Information Processing* (2nd Ed.). New York: John Wiley & Sons (1976).

OBLER, L.K., and ALBERT, M.L., Influence of aging on recovery from aphasia in polyglots. *Brain and Language,* 4, 460–463 (1977).

OBLER, L.K., and ALBERT, M.L., Language in the elderly aphasic and the dementing patient. In M.T. Sarno (Ed.), *Acquired Aphasia.* New York: Academic Press (1981).

OBLER, L.K., ALBERT, M.L., GOODGLASS, H., and BENSON, D.F., Aging and aphasia type. *Brain and Language,* 6, 318–322 (1978).

OJEMANN, G.A., Language and the thalamus: Object naming and recall during and after thalamic stimulation. *Brain and Language,* 2, 101–120 (1975).

OJEMANN, G.A., Subcortical language mechanisms. In H. Whitaker and H.A. Whitaker (Eds), *Studies in Neurolinguistics, Volume 1.* New York: Academic Press (1976).

OJEMANN, G.A., Organization of short-term verbal memory in language areas of human cortex: Evidence from electrical stimulation. *Brain and Language,* 5, 331–340 (1978).

OJEMANN, G.A., and WHITAKER, H.A., Language localization and variability. *Brain and Language,* 6, 239–260 (1978).

OLDENDORF, W.H., The quest for an image of brain: A brief historical and technical review of brain imaging techniques. *Neurology,* 28, 517–533 (1978).

OLSON, D.R., and FILBY, N., On comprehension of active and passive sentences. *Cognitive Psychology,* 3, 361–381 (1972).

ORGASS, B., and POECK, K., Clinical validation of a new test for aphasia: An experimental study of the Token Test. *Cortex,* 2, 222–243 (1966).

ORNSTEIN, R.E., *The Psychology of Consciousness.* New York: Penguin Books (1972).

ORNSTEIN, R.E., and GALIN, D., Physiological studies of consciousness. In P.R. Lee, R.E. Ornstein, D. Galin, A. Deikman, and C.T. Tart, *Symposium on Consciousness.* New York: Penguin Books (1976).

OSGOOD, C.E., and MIRON, M.S. (Eds.), *Approaches to the Study of Aphasia.* Urbana, Ill.: University of Illinois Press (1963).

OTTESON, J.P., Stylistic and personality correlates of lateral eye movements: A factor analytic study. *Perceptual and Motor Skills,* 50, 995–1010 (1980).

PAIVIO, A., and BEGG, I., *Psychology of Language.* Englewood Cliffs, N.J.: Prentice-Hall (1981).

PANNBACKER, M., Aphasia according to an expert. *Rehabilitation Literature,* 32, 295–298, 307 (1971).

PANNBACKER, M., Re: Martin and the PICA. *Journal of Speech and Hearing Disorders,* 44, 247–248 (1979).

PARADIS, M., Bilingualism and aphasia. In H. Whitaker and H.A. Whitaker (Eds.), *Studies in Neurolinguistics, Volume 3.* New York: Academic Press (1977).

PARISI, D., and PIZZAMIGLIO, L., Syntactic comprehension in aphasia. *Cortex,* 6, 204–215 (1970).

PATTERSON, K.E., What is right with "deep" dyslexic patients? *Brain and Language,* 8, 111–129 (1979).

PATTERSON, K.E., and MARCEL, A.J., Aphasia, dyslexia and the phonological coding of written words. *Quarterly Journal of Experimental Psychology,* 29, 307–318 (1977).

PEASE, D.M., and GOODGLASS, H., The effects of cuing on picture naming in aphasia. *Cortex,* 14, 178–189 (1978).

PENFIELD, W., and ROBERTS, L., *Speech and Brain Mechanisms.* Princeton, N.J.: Princeton University Press (1959).

PERECMAN, E., and BROWN, J.W., Phonemic jargon: A case report. In J.W. Brown (Ed.), *Jargonaphasia.* New York: Academic Press (1981).

PETERSON, L.N., and KIRSHNER, H.S., Gestural impairment and gestural ability in aphasia: A review. *Brain and Language,* 14, 333–348 (1981).

PETERSON, L.R., and PETERSON, M., Short-term retention of individual items. *Journal of Experimental Psychology,* 58, 193–198 (1959).

PETTIT, J.M., and NOLL, J.D., Cerebral dominance in aphasia recovery. *Brain and Language,* 7, 191–200 (1979).

PEUSER, G., and SCHRIEFERS, H., Sentence comprehension in aphasics: Results of administration of the "Three-Figures-Test" (DFT). *British Journal of Disorders of Communication,* 15, 157–173 (1980).

PHILLIPS, P.P., and HALPIN, G., Language impairment evaluation in aphasic patients. *Archives of Physical Medicine and Rehabilitation,* 59, 327–329 (1978).

PICHOT, P., Language disturbances in cerebral disease. *Archives of Neurology and Psychiatry,* 74, 92–96 (1955).

PIERCE, R.S., A study of sentence comprehension of aphasic subjects. In R.H. Brookshire (Ed.), *Clinical Aphasiology Conference Proceedings.* Minneapolis: BRK (1979).

PIERCE, R.S., Facilitating the comprehension of tense related sentences in aphasia. *Journal of Speech and Hearing Disorders,* 46, 364–368 (1981).

PINSKY, S.D., and McADAM, D.W., Electroencephalographic and dichotic indices of cerebral laterality in stutterers. *Brain and Language,* 11, 374–397 (1980).

PIZZAMIGLIO, L., and APPICCIAFUOCO, A., Semantic comprehension in aphasia. *Journal of Communication Disorders,* 3, 280–288 (1971).

PIZZAMIGLIO, L., and PARISI, D., Studies on verbal comprehension in aphasia. In G.B. D'Arcais and W.J.M. Levelt (Eds.), *Advances in Psycholinguistics.* Amsterdam: North-Holland (1970).

PODRAZA, B.L., and DARLEY, F.L., Effect of auditory prestimulation on naming in aphasia. *Journal of Speech and Hearing Research,* 20, 669–683 (1977).

POECK, K., and HARTJE, W., Performance of aphasic patients in visual versus auditory presentation of the Token Test: Demonstration of a supramodal deficit. In F. Boller and M. Dennis (Eds.), *Auditory Comprehension: Clinical and Experimental Studies with the Token Test.* New York: Academic Press (1979).

POECK, K., KERSCHENSTEINER, M., and HARTJE, W., A quantitative study on language understanding in fluent and nonfluent aphasia. *Cortex,* 8, 299–304 (1972).

POECK, K., ORGASS, B., KERSCHENSTEINER, M., and HARTJE, W., A qualitative study on Token Test performance in aphasic and non-aphasic brain damaged patients. *Neuropsychologia,* 12, 49–54 (1974).

PORCH, B.E., *Porch Index of Communicative Ability, Volume I: Theory and Development.* Palo Alto, Calif.: Consulting Psychologists Press (1967).

PORCH, B.E., *Porch Index of Communicative Ability, Volume II: Administration, Scoring, and Interpretation* (Revised Ed.). Palo Alto, Calif.: Consulting Psychologists Press (1971a).

PORCH, B.E., Multidimensional scoring in aphasia testing. *Journal of Speech and Hearing Research,* 14, 776–792 (1971b).

PORCH, B.E., Comments on Silverman's "Psychometric problem." *Journal of Speech and Hearing Disorders,* 39, 226–227 (1974).

PORCH, B.E., Profiles of aphasia: Test interpretation regarding the localization of lesions. In R.H. Brookshire (Ed.), *Clinical Aphasiology Conference Proceedings.* Minneapolis: BRK (1978).

PORCH, B.E., Response to Pannbacker. *Journal of Speech and Hearing Disorders,* 44, 248–250 (1979).

PORCH, B.E., *Porch Index of Communicative Ability, Volume II: Administration, Scoring, and Interpretation* (3rd Ed.). Palo Alto, Calif.: Consulting Psychologists Press (1981a).

PORCH, B.E., Therapy subsequent to the PICA. In R. Chapey (Ed.), *Language Intervention Strategies in*

Adult Aphasia. Baltimore: Williams & Wilkins (1981b).

PORCH, B.E., and CALLAGHAN, S., Making predictions about recovery: Is there HOAP? In R.H. Brookshire (Ed.), *Clinical Aphasiology Conference Proceedings*. Minneapolis: BRK (1981).

PORCH, B.E., COLLINS, M., WERTZ, R.T., and FRIDEN, T.P., Statistical prediction of change in aphasia. *Journal of Speech and Hearing Research*, 23, 312–321 (1980).

PORCH, B.E., and POREC, J.P., Medical-legal application of PICA results. In R.H. Brookshire (Ed.), *Clinical Aphasiology Conference Proceedings*. Minneapolis: BRK (1977).

PORCH, B.E., WERTZ, R.T., and COLLINS, M.J., A statistical procedure for predicting recovery from aphasia. In B.E. Porch (Ed.), *Proceedings of the Conference in Clinical Aphasiology*. New Orleans, April (1974).

POREC, J.P., and PORCH, B.E., The behavioral characteristics of "simulated" aphasia. In R.H. Brookshire (Ed.), *Clinical Aphasiology Conference Proceedings*. Minneapolis: BRK (1977).

PORRAZZO, S.A., Evaluation and treatment of reading deficits in aphasic patients. In R.H. Brookshire (Ed.), *Clinical Aphasiology Collected Proceedings 1972–1976*. Minneapolis: BRK (1978).

PORTER, J.L., and DABUL, B., The application of transactional analysis to therapy with wives of adult aphasic patients. *Asha*, 19, 244–248 (1977).

POWELL, G.E., BAILEY, S., and CLARK, E., A very short form of the Minnesota Aphasia Test. *British Journal of Social and Clinical Psychology*, 19, 189–194 (1980).

POWELL, G.E., CLARK, E., and BAILEY, S., Categories of aphasia: A cluster-analysis of Schuell test profiles. *British Journal of Disorders of Communication*, 14, 111–122 (1979).

PRIBRAM, K.H., *Languages of the Brain*. Englewood Cliffs, N.J.: Prentice-Hall (1971).

PRINS, R.S., SNOW, C.E., and WAGENAAR, E., Recovery from aphasia: Spontaneous speech versus language comprehension. *Brain and Language*, 6, 192–211 (1978).

PUTS-ZWARTJES, R.A., Group therapy with the husbands or wives of aphasics. *Logopaedie en Foniatrie*, 45, 93–97 (1973).

RABIDOUX, P.C., FLORANCE, C.L., and McCAUSLIN, L.S., The use of a Handi Voice in the treatment of a severely apractic, non-verbal patient. In R.H. Brookshire (Ed.), *Clinical Aphasiology Conference Proceedings*. Minneapolis: BRK (1980).

RAO, P.R., and HORNER, J., Gesture as a deblocking modality in a severe aphasic patient. In R.H. Brookshire (Ed.), *Clinical Aphasiology Conference Proceedings*. Minneapolis: BRK (1978).

RATCLIFF, G., DILA, C., TAYLOR, L., and MILNER, B., The morphological asymmetry of the hemispheres and cerebral dominance for speech: A possible relationship. *Brain and Language*, 11, 87–98 (1980).

RAVEN, J.C., *Coloured Progressive Matrices, Sets A, Ab, B*. London: H.K. Lewis (1962).

RAVEN, J.C., COURT, J.H., and RAVEN, J., *Manual for Raven's Progressive Matrices and Vocabulary Scales, Section 1: General Overview*. London: H.K. Lewis (1976).

RAVEN, J.C., COURT, J.H., and RAVEN, J., *Manual for Raven's Progressive Matrices and Vocabulary Scales, Section 2: Design and Use*. London: H.K. Lewis (1977).

READ, D.E., Solving deductive-reasoning problems after unilateral temporal lobectomy. *Brain and Language*, 12, 116–127 (1981).

REDINGER, R.A., FORSTER, S., DOLPHIN, M.K., GODDUHN, J., and WEISINGER, J., Group therapy in the rehabilitation of the severely aphasic and hemiplegic in the late stages. *Scandanavian Journal of Rehabilitation Medicine*, 3, 89–91 (1971).

RESTAK, R.M., *The Brain: The Last Frontier*. Garden City, N.Y.: Doubleday (1979).

RICHARDSON, J., The effect of word imageability in acquired dyslexia. *Neuropsychologia*, 13, 281–288 (1975).

RIEGE, W.H., METTER, E.J., and HANSON, W.R., Verbal and nonverbal recognition memory in aphasic and nonaphasic stroke patients. *Brain and Language*, 10, 60–70 (1980).

RINNERT, C., and WHITAKER, H.A, Semantic confusions by aphasic patients. *Cortex*, 9, 56–81 (1973).

RISBERG, J., Regional cerebral blood flow measures by 133Xe-Inhalation: Methodology and applications in neuropsychology and psychiatry. *Brain and Language*, 9, 9–34 (1980).

RITCHIE, D., *Stroke: A Study of Recovery*. Garden City, N.Y.: Doubleday (1961).

RIVERS, D.L., and LOVE, R.J., Language performance on visual processing tasks in right hemisphere lesion cases. *Brain and Language*, 10, 348–366 (1980).

ROBBINS, S.D., Examination and re-education of aphasics. *Journal of Speech and Hearing Disorders*, 4, 15–24 (1939).

ROBINSON, R.G., and BENSON, D.F., Depression in aphasic patients: Frequency, severity, and clinical-pathological correlations. *Brain and Language*, 14, 282–291 (1981).

ROCHESTER, S.R., MARTIN, J.R., and THURSON, S., Thought-process disorder in schizophrenia: The listener's task. *Brain and Language*, 4, 95–114 (1977).

ROCHFORD, G., A study of naming errors in dysphasic and in demented patients. *Neuropsychologia, 9,* 437–443 (1971).

ROCHFORD, G., and WILLIAMS, M., Studies in the development and breakdown of the use of names, IV: The effects of word frequency. *Journal of Neurology, Neurosurgery and Psychiatry,* 28, 407–413 (1965).

ROGERS, C.R., *Client-Centered Therapy.* Boston: Houghton Mifflin (1951).

ROGERS, C.R., *On Becoming a Person.* Boston: Houghton Mifflin (1961).

ROLLIN, W.J., Oral responses of aphasics under different syntactical conditions. *Language and Speech,* 7, 167–175 (1964).

ROLNICK, M., and HOOPS, H.R., Aphasia as seen by the aphasic. *Journal of Speech and Hearing Disorders,* 34, 48–53 (1969).

ROSE, C., BOBY, V., and CAPILDEO, R., A retrospective survey of speech disorders following stroke, with particular reference to the value of speech therapy. In Y. Lebrun and R. Hoops (Eds.), *Recovery in Aphasics.* Amsterdam: Swets & Zeitlinger (1976).

ROSENBEK, J.C., Treating apraxia of speech. In D.F. Johns (Ed.), *Clinical Management of Neurogenic Communicative Disorders.* Boston: Little, Brown (1978).

ROSENBEK, J.C., BECHER, B., SHAUGHNESSY, A., and COLLINS, M., Other uses of single-case designs. In R.H. Brookshire (Ed.), *Clinical Aphasiology Conference Proceedings.* Minneapolis: BRK (1979).

ROSENBEK, J.C., GREEN, E.F., FLYNN, M., WERTZ, R.T., and COLLINS, M., Anomia: A clinical experiment. In R.H. Brookshire (Ed.), *Clinical Aphasiology Conference Proceedings.* Minneapolis: BRK (1977).

ROSENBEK, J.C., and LAPOINTE, L.L., The dysarthrias: Description, diagnosis and treatment. In D.F. Johns (Ed.), *Clinical Management of Neurogenic Communicative Disorders.* Boston: Little, Brown (1978).

ROSENBERG, B., The performance of aphasics on automated visuo-perceptual discrimination, training and transfer tasks. *Journal of Speech and Hearing Research,* 8, 165–181 (1965).

ROSENBERG, B., and EDWARDS, A.E., An automated multiple response alternative training program for use with aphasics. *Journal of Speech and Hearing Research,* 8, 415–419 (1965).

ROSS, A.J., A study of the application of Blissymbolics as a means of communication for a young brain damaged adult. *British Journal of Disorders of Communication,* 14, 103–109 (1979).

ROSS, D., and SPENCER, S., *Aphasia Rehabilitation: An Auditory and Verbal Task Hierarchy.* Springfield, Ill.: Charles C. Thomas (1980).

ROTHI, L.J., and HUTCHINSON, E.C., Retention of verbal information by rehearsal in relation to the fluency of verbal output in aphasia. *Brain and Language,* 12, 347–359 (1981).

RUBENS, A.B., Anatomical asymmetries of human cerebral cortex. In S. Harnad, R.W. Doty, L. Goldstein, et al. (Eds.), *Lateralization in the Nervous System.* New York: Academic Press (1977a).

RUBENS, A.B., The role of changes within the central nervous system during recovery from aphasia. In M. Sullivan and M.S. Kommers (Eds.), *Rationale for Adult Aphasia Therapy.* University of Nebraska Medical Center (1977b).

RUBENS, A.B., What neurologists expect of clinical aphasiologists. In R.H. Brookshire (Ed.), *Clinical Aphasiology Conference Proceedings.* Minneapolis: BRK (1977c).

RUSSELL, W.R., and ESPIR, M.L.E., *Traumatic Aphasia.* London: Oxford University Press (1961).

SAFFRAN, E.M., and MARIN, O.S., Immediate memory for word lists and sentences in a patient with deficient auditory short-term memory. *Brain and Language,* 2, 420–433 (1975).

SAFFRAN, E.M., and MARIN, O.S., Reading without phonology: Evidence from aphasia. *Quarterly Journal of Experimental Psychology,* 29, 515–525 (1977).

SAFFRAN, E.M., SCHWARTZ, M.F., and MARIN, O.S.M., Semantic mechanism in paralexia. *Brain and Language,* 3, 255–265 (1976).

SAFFRAN, E.M., SCHWARTZ, M.F., and MARIN, O.S.M., The word order problem in agrammatism. II. Production. *Brain and Language,* 10, 263–280 (1980).

SAGAN, C., *The Dragons of Eden: Speculations on the Evolution of Human Intelligence.* New York: Ballantine Books (1977).

SAHS, A.L., HARTMAN, E.C., and ARONSON, S.M. (Eds.), *Guidelines for Stroke Care* (DHEW Publication No. (HRA) 76-14017). Washington, D.C.: U.S. Government Printing Office (1976).

SALVATORE, A.P., Use of a baseline probe technique to monitor the test responses of aphasic patients. *Journal of Speech and Hearing Disorders,* 37, 471–475 (1972).

SALVATORE, A.P., and DAVIS, K.D., Treatment of auditory comprehension deficits in acute and chronic aphasic adults by manipulating within-message pause duration. In R.H. Brookshire (Ed.), *Clinical Aphasiology Conference Proceedings.* Minneapolis: BRK (1979).

SALVATORE, A.P., STRAIT, M., and BROOKSHIRE, R.H., Effects of patient characteristics on delivery of Token Test commands by experienced and inexperienced examiners. *Journal of Communication Disorders,* 11, 325–333 (1978).

SAMUELS, I., BUTTERS, N., and FEDIO, P., Short term memory disorders following temporal lobe removals in humans. *Cortex,* 8, 283–298 (1972).

SAMUELS, I., BUTTERS, N., GOODGLASS, H., and BRODY, B., A comparison of subcortical and cortical damage on short-term visual and auditory memory. *Neuropsychologia,* 9, 293–306 (1971).

SAMUELS, J.A., and BENSON, D.F., Some aspects of language comprehension in anterior aphasia. *Brain and Language,* 8, 275–286 (1979).

SANDERS, S.B., and DAVIS, G.A., A comparison of the Porch Index of Communicative Ability and the Western Aphasia Battery. In R.H. Brookshire (Ed.), *Clinical Aphasiology Conference Proceedings.* Minneapolis: BRK (1978).

SANDS, E., SARNO, M.T., and SHANKWEILER, D., Long-term assessment of language function in aphasia due to stroke. *Archives of Physical Medicine and Rehabilitation,* 50, 202–207 (1969).

SARNO, J.E., and SARNO, M.T., *Stroke: A Guide for Patients and Their Families.* New York: McGraw-Hill (1979).

SARNO, J.E., SARNO, M.T., and LEVITA, E., Evaluating language improvement after completed stroke. *Archives of Physical Medicine and Rehabilitation,* 52, 73–78 (1971).

SARNO, M.T., *The Functional Communication Profile Manual of Directions.* Rehabilitation Monograph 42, New York University Medical Center (1969).

SARNO, M.T., (Ed.), *Aphasia: Selected Readings.* New York: Appleton-Century-Crofts (1972).

SARNO, M.T., Disorders of communication in stroke. In S. Licht (Ed.), *Stroke and Its Rehabilitation.* Baltimore, Md.: Waverly Press (1975).

SARNO, M.T., The nature of verbal impairment after closed head injury. *Journal of Nervous and Mental Disease,* 168, 685–692 (1980).

SARNO, M.T., Recovery and rehabilitation in aphasia. In M.T. Sarno (Ed.), *Acquired Aphasia.* New York: Academic Press (1981).

SARNO, M.T., and LEVITA, E., Natural course of recovery in severe aphasia. *Archives of Physical Medicine and Rehabilitation,* 52, 175–178, 186 (1971).

SARNO, M.T., and LEVITA, E., Recovery in treated aphasia during the first year post-stroke. *Stroke,* 10, 663–670 (1979).

SARNO, M.T., and LEVITA, E., Some observations on the nature of recovery in global aphasia after stroke. *Brain and Language,* 13, 1–12 (1981).

SARNO, M.T., SILVERMAN, M., and SANDS, E., Speech therapy and language recovery in severe aphasia. *Journal of Speech and Hearing Research,* 13, 607–623 (1970).

SATIR, V., *Conjoint Family Therapy.* Palo Alto, Calif.: Science and Behavior Books (1967).

SATZ, P., Incidence of aphasia in left-handers: A test of some hypothetical models of cerebral speech organization. In J. Herron (Ed.), *Neuropsychology of Left-Handedness.* New York: Academic Press (1980).

SCHLANGER, B.B., SCHLANGER, P., and GERSTMAN, L.J., The perception of emotionally toned sentences by right hemisphere-damaged and aphasic subjects. *Brain and Language,* 3, 396–403 (1976).

SCHLANGER, P.H., *Picture Communication Cards.* Tucson, Ariz.: Communication Skill Builders (1978).

SCHLANGER, P.H., *What's the Solution?* Tucson, Ariz.: Communication Skill Builders (1980).

SCHLANGER, P.H., and SCHLANGER, B.B., Adapting role playing activities with aphasic patients. *Journal of Speech and Hearing Disorders,* 35, 229–235 (1970).

SCHMULLER, J., and GOODMAN, R., Bilateral tachistoscopic perception, handedness, and laterality. *Brain and Language,* 8, 81–91 (1979).

SCHMULLER, J., and GOODMAN, R., Bilateral tachistoscopic perception, handedness, and laterality. II. Nonverbal stimuli. *Brain and Language,* 11, 12–18 (1980).

SCHNITZER, M.L., Toward a neurolinguistic theory of language. *Brain and Language,* 6, 342–361 (1978).

SCHUELL, H.M., Paraphasia and paralexia. *Journal of Speech and Hearing Disorders,* 15, 291–306 (1950).

SCHUELL, H.M., Aphasic difficulties understanding spoken language. *Neurology,* 3, 176–184 (1953a).

SCHUELL, H.M., Auditory impairment and aphasia: Significance and retraining techniques. *Journal of Speech and Hearing Disorders,* 18, 14–21 (1953b).

SCHUELL, H.M., A short examination for aphasia. *Neurology,* 7, 625–634 (1957).

SCHUELL, H.M., *Differential Diagnosis of Aphasia with the Minnesota Test.* Minneapolis: University of Minnesota Press (1965a).

SCHUELL, H.M., *Minnesota Test for Differential Diagnosis of Aphasia.* Minneapolis: University of Minnesota Press (1965b).

SCHUELL, H.M., A re-evaluation of the short examination for aphasia. *Journal of Speech and Hearing Disorders,* 31, 137–147 (1966).

SCHUELL, H.M., Aphasia in adults. In *Human Communication and Its Disorders—An Overview.* Bethesda, Md.: U.S. Department of Health, Education, and Welfare (1969).

SCHUELL, H.M., *Minnesota Test for Differential Diagnosis of Aphasia* (Revised Ed.). Minneapolis: University of Minnesota Press (1972).

SCHUELL, H.M., *Differential Diagnosis of Aphasia with the Minnesota Test* (2nd Ed., revised by Sefer, J.W.). Minneapolis: University of Minnesota Press (1973).

SCHUELL, H.M., CARROLL, V., and STREET, B.S., Clinical treatment of aphasia. *Journal of Speech and Hearing Disorders,* 20, 43–53 (1955).

SCHUELL, H.M., and JENKINS, J.J., The nature of language deficit in aphasia. *Psychological Review,* 66, 45–67 (1959).

SCHUELL, H.M., and JENKINS, J.J., Comment on "Dimensions of language performance in aphasia." *Journal of Speech and Hearing Research,* 4, 295–299 (1961a).

SCHUELL, H.M., and JENKINS, J.J., Reduction of vocabulary in aphasia. *Brain,* 84, 243–261 (1961b).

SCHUELL, H.M., JENKINS, J.J., and Carroll, J.B., A factor analysis of the Minnesota Test for the Differential Diagnosis of Aphasia. *Journal of Speech and Hearing Research,* 5, 349–369 (1962).

SCHUELL, H.M., JENKINS, J.J., and JIMENEZ-PABON, E., *Aphasia in Adults.* New York: Harper and Row (1964).

SCHUELL, H.M., JENKINS, J.J., and LANDIS, L., Relationships between auditory comprehension and word frequency in aphasia. *Journal of Speech and Hearing Research,* 4, 30–36 (1961).

SCHUELL, H.M., SHAW, R., and BREWER, W., A psycholinguistic approach to study of the language deficit in aphasia. *Journal of Speech and Hearing Research,* 12, 794–806 (1969).

SCHWARTZ, G.E., DAVIDSON, R.J., and MAER, F., Right hemisphere lateralization for emotion in the human brain: Interactions with cognition. *Science,* 190, 286–288 (1975).

SCHWARTZ, M.F., MARIN, O.S.M., and SAFFRAN, E.M., Dissociations of language function in dementia: A case study. *Brain and Language,* 7, 277–306 (1979).

SCHWARTZ, M.F., SAFFRAN, E.M., and MARIN, O.S.M., The word order problem in agrammatism. I. Comprehension. *Brain and Language,* 10, 249–262 (1980).

SEAMON, J.G., and GAZZANIGA, M.S., Coding strategies and cerebral laterality effects. *Cognitive Psychology,* 5, 249–256 (1973).

SEARLE, J.R., *Speech Acts.* London: Cambridge University Press (1969).

SEARLEMAN, A., A review of right hemisphere linguistic capabilities. *Psychological Bulletin,* 84, 503–528 (1977).

SEARLEMAN, A., TWEEDY, J., and SPRINGER, S.P., Interrelationships among subject variables believed to predict cerebral organization. *Brain and Language,* 7, 267–276 (1979).

SEFER, J.W., and HENRIKSON, E.H., The relationship between word association and grammatical classes in aphasia. *Journal of Speech and Hearing Research,* 9, 529–541 (1966).

SEFER, J.W., and SHAW, R., The use of psycholinguistic principles in the treatment of aphasics. *British Journal of Disorders of Communication,* 7, 87–89 (1972).

SEGALOWITZ, N., and HANSSON, P., Hemispheric functions in the processing of agent-patient information. *Brain and Language,* 8, 51–61 (1979).

SEGALOWITZ, S.J., and CHAPMAN, J.S., Cerebral asymmetry for speech in neonates: A behavioral measure. *Brain and Language,* 9, 281–288 (1980).

SEITZ, M.R., WEBER, B.A., JACOBSON, J.T., and MOREHOUSE, R., The use of averaged electroencephalic response techniques in the study of auditory processing related to speech and language. *Brain and Language,* 11, 261–284 (1980).

SELNES, O.A., A note on "On the representation of language in the right hemisphere of right-handed people." *Brain and Language,* 3, 583–589 (1976).

SELNES, O.A., and WHITAKER, H.A., Neurological substrates of language and speech production. In S. Rosenberg (Ed.), *Sentence Production: Developments in Research and Theory.* Hillsdale, N.J.: Lawrence Erlbaum (1977).

SEMENZA, C., DENES, G., LUCCHESE, D., and BISIACCHI, P., Selective deficit of conceptual structures in aphasia: Class versus thematic relations. *Brain and Language,* 10, 243–248 (1980).

SERON, X., and DELOCHE, G., Processing of locatives "in," "on," and "under" by aphasic patients: An analysis of the regression hypothesis. *Brain and Language,* 14, 70–80 (1981).

SERON, X., DELOCHE, G., BASTARD, V., CHASSIN, G., and HERMAND, N., Word-finding difficulties and learning transfer in aphasic patients. *Cortex,* 15, 149–155 (1979).

SERON, X., VAN DER LINDEN, M., and VAN DER KAA-DELVENNE, M., The operant school of aphasia rehabilitation. In Y. Lebrun and R. Hoops (Eds.), *The Management of Aphasia.* Amsterdam: Swets & Zeitlinger (1978).

SHALLICE, T., and BUTTERWORTH, B., Short-term memory impairment and spontaneous speech. *Neuropsychologia,* 15, 729–735 (1977).

SHALLICE, T., and WARRINGTON, E.K., Word recognition in a phonemic dyslexic patient. *Quarterly Journal of Experimental Psychology,* 27, 187–199 (1975).

SHALLICE, T., and WARRINGTON, E.K., Auditory-verbal short-term memory impairment and conduction aphasia. *Brain and Language,* 4, 479–491 (1977).

SHANON, B., Classification and identification in an aphasic patient. *Brain and Language,* 5, 188–194 (1978).

SHEEHAN, J.G., ASELTINE, S., and EDWARDS, A.E., Aphasic comprehension of time spacing. *Journal of Speech and Hearing Research,* 16, 650–657 (1973).

SHEEHAN, V.M., Rehabilitation of aphasics in an army hospital. *Journal of Speech and Hearing Disorders,* 11, 149–157 (1946).

SHEEHAN, V.M., Techniques in the management of aphasia. *Journal of Speech and Hearing Disorders,* 13, 241–246 (1948).

SHEWAN, C.M., Error patterns in auditory comprehension of adult aphasics. *Cortex,* 12, 325–336 (1976a).

SHEWAN, C.M., Facilitating sentence formulation: A case study. *Journal of Communication Disorders,* 9, 191–197 (1976b).

SHEWAN, C.M., *Auditory Comprehension Test for Sentences.* Chicago: Biolinguistics Clinical Institutes (1979).

SHEWAN, C.M., and CANTER, G.J., Effects of vocabulary, syntax, and sentence length on auditory comprehension in aphasic patients. *Cortex,* 7, 209–226 (1971).

SHEWAN, C.M., and KERTESZ, A., Reliability and validity characteristics of the Western Aphasia Battery (WAB). *Journal of Speech and Hearing Disorders,* 45, 308–324 (1980).

SHILL, M.A., Motivational factors in aphasia therapy: Research suggestions. *Journal of Communication Disorders,* 12, 503–517 (1979).

SIDMAN, M., STODDARD, L.T., MOHR, J.P., and LEICESTER, J., Behavioral studies of aphasia: Methods of investigation and analysis. *Neuropsychologia,* 9, 119–140 (1971).

SIES, L.F., and BUTLER, R., A personal account of dysphasia. *Journal of Speech and Hearing Disorders,* 28, 261–266 (1963).

SILVERMAN, F.H., PICA: A psychometric problem and its solution. *Journal of Speech and Hearing Disorders,* 39, 225–226 (1974).

SILVERMAN, F.H., *Communication for the Speechless.* Englewood Cliffs, N.J.: Prentice-Hall (1980).

SIMMONS, N.N., and ZORTHIAN, A., Use of symbolic gestures in a case of fluent aphasia. In R.H. Brookshire (Ed.), *Clinical Aphasiology Conference Proceedings.* Minneapolis: BRK (1979).

SISTER KENNY INSTITUTE, *Self-Care for the Hemiplegic* (Revised Ed.). Minneapolis: Abbott-Northwestern Hospital (1977).

SKELLY, M., Aphasic patients talk back. *American Journal of Nursing,* 75, 1140–1142 (1975).

SKELLY, M., Amerind clarified. *Asha,* 19, 746–747 (1977).

SKELLY, M., *Ameri-Ind Gestural Code.* New York: Elsevier (1979).

SKELLY, M., SCHINSKY, L., SMITH, R., DONALDSON, R., and GRIFFIN, J., American Indian Sign: A gestural communication system for the speechless. *Archives of Physical Medicine and Rehabilitation,* 56, 156–160 (1975).

SKELLY, M., SCHINSKY, L., SMITH, R.W., and FUST, R.S., American Indian Sign (AMERIND) as a facilitator of verbalization for the oral verbal apraxic. *Journal of Speech and Hearing Disorders,* 39, 445–456 (1974).

SKLAR, M., Relation of psychological and language test scores and autopsy findings in aphasia. *Journal of Speech and Hearing Research,* 6, 84–90 (1963).

SKLAR, M., *Sklar Aphasia Scale* (Revised Ed.). Los Angeles: Western Psychological Services (1973).

SMITH, A., Objective indices of severity of chronic aphasia in stroke patients. *Journal of Speech and Hearing Disorders,* 36, 167–207 (1971).

SMITH, A., Replies to two comments on "Objective indices of severity of chronic aphasia in stroke patients." *Journal of Speech and Hearing Disorders,* 37, 274–278 (1972).

SMITH, A., Some more "remarkable" aspects of "A comparison of impairments in verbal comprehension, speech, reading, and writing in adult aphasics." *Journal of Speech and Hearing Disorders,* 42, 130–132 (1977).

SMITH, A., and FULLERTON, A.M., Age differences in episodic and semantic memory: Implications for language and cognition. In D.S. Beasley and G.A. Davis (Eds.), *Aging: Communication Processes and Disorders.* New York: Grune & Stratton (1981).

SMITH, E.E., SHOBEN, E.J., and RIPS, L.J., Structure and process in semantic memory: A featural model for semantic decision. *Psychological Review,* 81, 214–241 (1974).

SMITH, M.D., On the understanding of some relational words in aphasia. *Neuropsychologia,* 12, 377–384 (1974a).

SMITH, M.D., Operant conditioning of syntax in aphasia. *Neuropsychologia,* 12, 403–405 (1974b).

SMOKLER, I.A., and SHEVRIN, I., Cerebral lateralization and personality style. *Archives of General Psychiatry,* 36, 949–954 (1979).

SOLOMON, G.E., and PLUM, F., *Clinical Management of Seizures: A Guide for the Physician.* Philadelphia: W.B. Saunders (1976).

SPARKS, R.W., Parastandardized examination guidelines for adult aphasia. *British Journal of Disorders of Communication,* 13, 135–146 (1978).

SPARKS, R.W., Melodic Intonation Therapy. In R. Chapey (Ed.), *Language Intervention Strategies in*

Adult Aphasia. Baltimore: Williams & Wilkins (1981).

SPARKS, R., GOODGLASS, H., and NICKEL, B., Ipsilateral versus contralateral extinction in dichotic listening resulting from hemipshere lesions. *Cortex,* 6, 249–260 (1970).

SPARKS, R., HELM, N.A., and ALBERT, M.L., Aphasia rehabilitation resulting from melodic intonation therapy. *Cortex,* 10, 303–316 (1974).

SPARKS, R., and HOLLAND, A.L., Method: Melodic intonation therapy for aphasia. *Journal of Speech and Hearing Disorders,* 41, 287–297 (1976).

SPELLACY, F.J., and SPREEN, O., A short form of the Token Test. *Cortex,* 5, 390–397 (1969).

SPIEGEL, D.K., JONES, L.V., and WEPMAN, J.M., Test responses as predictors of free-speech characteristics in aphasia patients. *Journal of Speech and Hearing Research,* 8, 349–362 (1965).

SPREEN, O., and BENTON, A.L., *Neurosensory Center Comprehensive Examination for Aphasia (NCCEA),* 1977 Revision. Victoria, British Columbia: Neuropsychology Laboratory, University of Victoria (1969).

SPREEN, O., BENTON, A.L., and VAN ALLEN, M.W., Dissociation of visual and tactile naming in amnesic aphasia. *Neurology,* 16, 807–814 (1966).

SPREEN, O., and RISSER, A., Assessment of aphasia. In M.T. Sarno (Ed.), *Acquired Aphasia.* New York: Academic Press (1981).

SPREEN, O., and WACHAL, R.S., Psycholinguistic analysis of aphasic language: Theoretical formulations and procedures. *Language and Speech,* 16, 130–146 (1973).

SPRINGER, S.P., and DEUTSCH, G., *Left Brain, Right Brain.* San Francisco: W.H. Freeman (1981).

STACHOWIAK, F.J., HUBER, W., POECK, K., and KERSCHENSTEINER, M., Text comprehension in aphasia. *Brain and Language,* 4, 177–195 (1977).

STARK, J., Aphasia in children. In R.W. Rieber (Ed.), *Language Development and Aphasia in Children.* New York: Academic Press (1980).

STEIN, S.C., Medical management of cerebrovascular accidents. In R. Chapey (Ed.), *Language Intervention Strategies in Adult Aphasia.* Baltimore: Williams & Wilkins (1981).

STERNBERG, S., Memory scanning: New findings and current controversies. In D. Deutsch and J.A. Deutsch (Eds.), *Short-Term Memory.* New York: Academic Press (1975).

STOICHEFF, M.L., Motivating instructions and language performance of dysphasic subjects. *Journal of Speech and Hearing Research,* 3, 75–85 (1960).

STRAUSS, E., and MOSCOVITCH, M., Perception of facial expressions. *Brain and Language,* 13, 308–332 (1981).

STROHNER, H., COHEN, R., KELTER, S., and WOLL, G., "Semantic" and "acoustic" errors of aphasic and schizophrenic patients in a sound-picture matching task. *Cortex,* 14, 391–403 (1978).

STRUB, R.L., and BLACK, F.W., *Organic Brain Syndromes: An Introduction to Neurobehavioral Disorders.* Philadelphia: F.A. Davis (1981).

STRUB, R.L., and GARDNER, H., The repetition deficit in conduction aphasia: Mnestic or linguistic? *Brain and Language,* 1, 241–256 (1974).

STRYKER, D., and STRYKER, S., *Speech Illustrated Cards.* Miami Beach, Fla.: Stryker Illustrations (1976).

STUMP, D.A., and WILLIAMS, R., The noninvasive measurement of regional cerebral circulation. *Brain and Language,* 9, 35–46 (1980).

SUBIRANA, H., The prognosis in aphasia in relation to the factor of cerebral dominance and handedness. *Brain,* 8, 415–425 (1958).

SWINNEY, D.A., and TAYLOR, O.L., Short-term memory recognition search in aphasics. *Journal of Speech and Hearing Research,* 14, 578–588 (1971).

SWINNEY, D.A., ZURIF, E.G., and CUTLER, A., Effects of sentential stress and word class upon comprehension in Broca's aphasics. *Brain and Language,* 10, 132–144 (1980).

SWISHER, L., and HIRSCH, I.J., Brain damage and the ordering of two temporally successive stimuli. *Neuropsychologia,* 10, 137–152 (1972).

SWISHER, L.P., and SARNO, M.T., Token Test scores of three matched patient groups: Left brain-damaged with aphasia; right brain-damaged without aphasia; non-brain damaged. *Cortex,* 5, 264–273 (1969).

TALLAL, P., and NEWCOMBE, F., Impairment of auditory perception and language comprehension in dysphasia. *Brain and Language,* 5, 13–24 (1978).

TANNER, D.C., Loss and grief: Implications for the speech-language pathologist and audiologist. *Asha,* 22, 916–928 (1980).

TAYLOR, M.L., *Understanding Aphasia.* New York: New York University Medical Center, Institute of Rehabilitation Medicine (1958).

TAYLOR, M.L., A measurement of functional communication in aphasia. *Archives of Physical Medicine and Rehabilitation,* 46, 101–107 (1965).

TAYLOR, M.L., and MARKS, M.M., Aphasia Rehabilitation Manual and Therapy Kit. New York: McGraw-Hill (1959).

TAYLOR, O.L., and ANDERSON, C.B., Neuropsycholinguistics and language retraining. In J.W. Black and E.G. Jancosek (Eds.), *Proceedings of the Conference on Language Retraining for Aphasics.* Columbus, Ohio: The Ohio State University Research Foundation (1968).

TERR, M.A., GOETZINGER, C.P., and ROUSEY, C.L., A study of hearing acuity in adult aphasic and cerebral palsied subjects. *Archives of Otolaryngology*, 67, 447–455 (1958).

THATCHER, R.W., and APRIL, R.S., Evoked potential correlates of semantic information processing in normals and aphasics. In R.W. Rieber (Ed.), *The Neuropsychology of Language*. New York: Plenum Press (1976).

THOMPSON, J., and ENDERBY, P., Is all your Schuell really necessary? *British Journal of Disorders of Communication*, 14, 195–201 (1979).

THOMSEN, I.V., Evaluation and outcome of aphasia in patients with severe closed head trauma. *Journal of Neurology, Neurosurgery, and Psychiatry*, 38, 713–718 (1975).

TIKOFSKY, R.S., Halstead Aphasia Test, Form M. In F.L. Darley (Ed.), *Evaluation of Appraisal Techniques in Speech and Language Pathology*. Reading, Mass.: Addison-Wesley (1979).

TOMPKINS, C.A., MARSHALL, R.C., and PHILLIPS, D.S., Aphasic patients in a rehabilitation program: Scheduling speech and language services. *Archives of Physical Medicine and Rehabilitation*, 61, 252–254 (1980).

TOMPKINS, C.A., RAU, M.T., MARSHALL, R.C., LAMBRECHT, K.J., GOLPER, L.A.C., and PHILLIPS, D.S., Analysis of a battery assessing mild auditory comprehension involvement in aphasia. In R.H. Brookshire (Ed.), *Clinical Aphasiology Conference Proceedings*. Minneapolis: BRK (1980).

TONKOVICH, J.D., Case relations in Broca's aphasia: Some considerations regarding treatment. In R.H. Brookshire (Ed.), *Clinical Aphasiology Conference Proceedings*. Minneapolis: BRK (1979).

TOPPIN, C.J., and BROOKSHIRE, R.H., Effects of response delay and token relocation on Token Test performance of aphasic subjects. *Journal of Communication Disorders*, 11, 65–78 (1978).

TOWEY, M.P., and PETTIT, J.M., Improving communication competence in global aphasia. In R.H. Brookshire (Ed.), *Clinical Aphasiology Conference Proceedings*. Minneapolis: BRK (1980).

TRAENDLY, C.A., *Aphasia Rehabilitation: Word Finding*. Tigard, Oreg.: C.C. Publications (1979).

TROST, J., and CANTER, G.J., Apraxia of speech in patients with Broca's aphasia: A study of phoneme production accuracy and error patterns. *Brain and Language*, 1, 63–80 (1974).

TUCKER, D.M., Lateral brain function, emotion, and conceptualization. *Psychological Bulletin*, 89, 19–46 (1981).

TUCKER, D.M., ROTH, R.S., ARNESON, B.A., and BUCKINGHAM, V., Right hemisphere activation during stress. *Neuropsychologia*, 15, 697–700 (1977).

TURNBLOM, M., and MYERS, J.S., A group discussion program with families of aphasic patients. *Journal of Speech and Hearing Disorders*, 17, 393–396 (1952).

TZORTZIS, C., and ALBERT, M.L., Impairment of memory for sequences in conduction aphasia. *Neuropsychologia*, 12, 355–366 (1974).

UDELL, R., SULLIVAN, R.A., and SCHLANGER, P.H., Legal competency of aphasic patients: Role of speech-language pathologists. *Archives of Physical Medicine and Rehabilitation*, 61, 374–375 (1980).

ULATOWSKA, H.K., Application of linguistics to treatment of aphasia. In R.H. Brookshire (Ed.), *Clinical Aphasiology Conference Proceedings*. Minneapolis: BRK (1979).

ULATOWSKA, H.K., BAKER, T., and STERN, R.F., Disruption of written language in aphasia. In H. Whitaker and H.A. Whitaker (Eds.), *Studies in Neurolinguistics, Volume 4*. New York: Academic Press (1979).

ULATOWSKA, H.K., HILDEBRAND, B.H., and HAYNES, S.M., A comparison of written and spoken language in aphasia. In R.H. Brookshire (Ed.), *Clinical Aphasiology Conference Proceedings*. Minneapolis: BRK (1978).

ULATOWSKA, H.K., MACALUSO-HAYNES, S., and MENDEL-RICHARDSON, S., The assessment of communicative competence in aphasia. In R.H. Brookshire (Ed.), *Clinical Aphasiology Conference Proceedings*. Minneapolis: BRK (1976).

ULATOWSKA, H.K., and RICHARDSON, S.M., A longitudinal study of an adult with aphasia: Considerations for research and therapy. *Brain and Language*, 1, 151–166 (1974).

ULRICH, G., Interhemispheric functional relationships in auditory agnosia. An analysis of the preconditions and a conceptual model. *Brain and Language*, 5, 286–300 (1978).

VALENSTEIN, E., Age-related changes in the human central nervous system. In D.S. Beasley and G.A. Davis (Eds.), *Aging: Communication Processes and Disorders*. New York: Grune & Stratton (1981).

VAN ALLEN, M.W., BENTON, A.L., and GORDON, M.C., Temporal discrimination in brain-damaged patients. *Neuropsychologia*, 4, 159–167 (1966).

VAN BUREN, J.M., The question of thalamic participation in speech mechanisms. *Brain and Language*, 2, 31–44 (1975).

VAN DEMARK, A.A., Comment on PICA interpretation. *Journal of Speech and Hearing Disorders*, 39, 510–511 (1974).

VAN DEMARK, A.A., LEMMER, E.C.J., and DRAKE, M., Measuring reading comprehension in aphasia with the RCBA. Paper presented to the

American Speech and Hearing Association Convention, Detroit, November (1980).

VAN RIPER, C., *Speech Correction: Principles and Methods* (5th Ed.). Englewood Cliffs, N.J.: Prentice-Hall (1972).

VETTER, H.J. (Ed.), *Language Behavior in Schizophrenia.* Springfield, Ill.: Charles C. Thomas (1968).

VIGNOLO, L.A., Evolution of aphasia and language rehabilitation: A retrospective exploratory study. *Cortex,* 1, 344–367 (1964).

VON STOCKERT, T.R., Recognition of syntactic structure in aphasic patients. *Cortex,* 8, 323–334 (1972).

VON STOCKERT, T.R., and BADER, L., Some relations of grammar and lexicon in aphasia. *Cortex,* 12, 49–60 (1976).

WADA, J., and RASMUSSEN, T., Intracarotid injection of sodium amytal for the lateralization of cerebral speech dominance: Experimental and clinical observations. *Journal of Neurosurgery,* 17, 266–282 (1960).

WAGENAAR, E., SNOW, C.E., and PRINS, R.S., Spontaneous speech of aphasic patients: A psycholinguistic analysis. *Brain and Language,* 2, 281–303 (1975).

WAGNER, M.T., and HANNON, R., Hemispheric asymmetries in faculty and student musicians and nonmusicians during melody recognition tasks. *Brain and Language,* 13, 379–388 (1981).

WALLER, M.R., and DARLEY, F.L., The influence of context on the auditory comprehension of paragraphs by aphasic subjects. *Journal of Speech and Hearing Research,* 21, 732–745 (1978).

WAPNER, W., and GARDNER, H., A note on patterns of comprehension and recovery in global aphasia. *Journal of Speech and Hearing Research,* 22, 765–772 (1979a).

WAPNER, W., and GARDNER, H., A study of spelling in aphasia. *Brain and Language,* 7, 363–374 (1979b).

WAPNER, W., and GARDNER, H., Profiles of symbol-reading in organic patients. *Brain and Language,* 12, 303–312 (1981).

WAPNER, W., HAMBY, S., and GARDNER, H., The role of the right hemisphere in the apprehension of complex linguistic materials. *Brain and Language,* 14, 15–33 (1981).

WARREN, R.L., HUBBARD, D.J, and KNOX, A.W., Short-term memory scan in normal individuals and individuals with aphasia. *Journal of Speech and Hearing Research,* 20, 497–509 (1977).

WARRINGTON, E.K., and SHALLICE, T., The selective impairment of auditory verbal short-term memory. *Brain,* 92, 885–896 (1969).

WATAMORI, T.S., and SASANUMA, S., The recovery processes of two English-Japanese bilingual aphasics. *Brain and Language,* 6, 127–140 (1978).

WATSON, J.M., and RECORDS, L.E., The effectiveness of the Porch Index of Communicative Ability as a diagnostic tool in assessing specific behaviors of senile dementia. In R.H. Brookshire (Ed.), *Clinical Aphasiology Conference Proceedings.* Minneapolis: BRK (1978).

WATZLAWICK, P., *The Language of Change: Elements of Therapeutic Communication.* New York: Basic Books (1978).

WEBSTER, E.J., *Counseling with Parents of Handicapped Children: Guidelines for Improving Communication.* New York: Grune & Stratton (1977).

WEBSTER, E.J., and NEWHOFF, M., Intervention with families of communicatively impaired adults. In D.S. Beasley and G.A. Davis (Eds.), *Aging: Communication Processes and Disorders.* New York: Grune & Stratton (1981).

WEIDNER, W.E., and LASKY, E.Z., The interaction of rate and complexity of stimulus on the performance of adult aphasic subjects. *Brain and Language,* 3, 34–40 (1976).

WEIGL, E., and BIERWISCH, M., Neuropsychology and linguistics: Topics of common research. *Foundations of Language,* 6, 1–18 (1970).

WEIGL, E., and FRADIS, A., The transcoding process in patients with agraphia to dictation. *Brain and Language,* 4, 11–22 (1977).

WEINBERG, J., DILLER, L., GERSTMAN, L., and SCHULMAN, P., Digit span in right and left hemiplegics. *Journal of Clinical Psychology,* 28, 361 (1972).

WEINSTEIN, E.A., and KELLER, N.J.A., Linguistic patterns of misnaming in brain injury. *Neuropsychologia,* 1, 79–90 (1963).

WEISENBURG, T.H., A study of aphasia. *Archives of Neurology and Psychiatry,* 31, 1–33 (1934).

WEISENBURG, T.H., and MCBRIDE, K.E., *Aphasia.* New York: Commonwealth Fund (1935).

WEISS, H.D., Neoplasms. In M.A. Samuels (Ed.), *Manual of Neurologic Therapeutics with Essentials of Diagnosis.* Boston: Little, Brown (1978).

WEPMAN, J.M., The organization of therapy for aphasia: I. The in-patient treatment center. *Journal of Speech and Hearing Disorders,* 12, 405–409 (1947).

WEPMAN, J.M., *Recovery from Aphasia.* New York: Ronald Press (1951).

WEPMAN, J.M., A conceptual model for the processes involved in recovery from aphasia. *Journal of Speech and Hearing Disorders,* 18, 4–13 (1953).

WEPMAN, J.M., The relationship between self-correction and recovery from aphasia. *Journal of Speech and Hearing Disorders,* 23, 302–305 (1958).

WEPMAN, J.M., Aphasia therapy: Some "relative" comments and some purely personal prejudices.

In J.W. Black and E.G. Jancosek (Eds.), *Proceedings of the Conference on Language Retraining for Aphasics.* Columbus, Oh.: The Ohio State University (1968).

WEPMAN, J.M., Aphasia therapy: A new look. *Journal of Speech and Hearing Disorders, 37,* 203–214 (1972).

WEPMAN, J.M., Aphasia: Language without thought or thought without language. *Asha, 18,* 131–136 (1976).

WEPMAN, J.M., BOCK, R.D., JONES, L.V., and VAN PELT, D., Psycholinguistic study of aphasia: A revision of the concept of anomia. *Journal of Speech and Hearing Disorders, 21,* 468–477 (1956).

WEPMAN, J.M., and JONES, L.V., *Studies in Aphasia: An Approach to Testing.* Chicago: Education-Industry Service (1961).

WEPMAN, J.M., and JONES, L.V., Five aphasias: A commentary on aphasia as a regressive linguistic phenomenon. In D. Rioch and E. Weinstein (Eds.), *Disorders of Communication.* Baltimore: Williams and Wilkins (1964).

WEPMAN, J.M., and JONES, L.V., Studies in aphasia: Classification of aphasic speech by the noun-pronoun ratio. *British Journal of Disorders of Communication, 1,* 46–54 (1966).

WEPMAN, J.M., JONES, L.V., BOCK, R.D., and VAN PELT, D., Studies in aphasia: Background and theoretical formulations. *Journal of Speech and Hearing Disorders, 25,* 323–332 (1960).

WEPMAN, J.M., and VAN PELT, D.A., A theory of cerebral language disorders based on therapy. *Folia Phoniatrica, 7,* 223–235 (1955).

WERNICKE, C., The aphasia symptom complex: A psychological study on an anatomic basis. In G.H. Eggert (Trans.), *Wernicke's Works on Aphasia: A Sourcebook and Review.* The Hague, Netherlands: Mouton (1977).

WERTZ, R.T., Neuropathologies of speech and language: An introduction to patient management. In D.F. Johns (Ed.), *Clinical Management of Neurogenic Communicative Disorders.* Boston: Little, Brown (1978).

WERTZ, R.T., Word Fluency Measure (WF). In F.L. Darley (Ed.), *Evaluation of Appraisal Techniques in Speech and Language Pathology.* Reading, Mass.: Addison-Wesley (1979).

WERTZ, R.T., COLLINS, M.J., WEISS, D., et al., Veterans Administration cooperative study on aphasia: A comparison of individual and group treatment. *Journal of Speech and Hearing Research, 24,* 580–594 (1981).

WERTZ, R.T., DEAL, L.M., and DEAL, J.L., Prognosis in aphasia: Investigation of the High-Overall Prediction (HOAP) method and the Short-Direct or HOAP-Slope method to predict change in PICA performance. In R.H. Brook-shire (Ed.), *Clinical Aphasiology Conference Proceedings.* Minneapolis: BRK (1980).

WERTZ, R.T., DEAL, L.M., and DEAL, J.L., Clinical significance of the PICA high-low gap. In R.H. Brookshire (Ed.), *Clinical Aphasiology Conference Proceedings.* Minneapolis: BRK (1981).

WERTZ, R.T., KITSELMAN, K.P., and DEAL, L.A., Classifying the aphasias: Methods, prognostic implications, and efficacy of treatment. Miniseminar at the American Speech-Language-Hearing Association Convention, Los Angeles, November (1981).

WERTZ, R.T., ROSENBEK, J., and COLLINS, M.J., Identification of apraxia of speech from PICA verbal tests and selected oral-verbal apraxia tests. In R.H. Brookshire (Ed.), *Clinical Aphasiology: Collected Proceedings 1972–76.* Minneapolis: BRK (1978).

WEST, J.A., Auditory comprehension in aphasic adults: Improvement through training. *Archives of Physical Medicine and Rehabilitation, 54,* 78–86 (1973).

WEST, J.A., GELFER, C.E., and ROSEN, J.S., Processing true and false affirmative sentences by aphasic subjects. In R.H. Brookshire (Ed.), *Clinical Aphasiology Collected Proceedings 1972–1976.* Minneapolis: BRK (1978).

WEST, J.F., Imaging and aphasia. In R.H. Brookshire (Ed.), *Clinical Aphasiology Conference Proceedings.* Minneapolis: BRK (1977).

WEST, J.F., Heightening the action imagery of materials used in aphasia treatment. In R.H. Brookshire (Ed.), *Clinical Aphasiology Conference Proceedings.* Minneapolis: BRK (1978).

WHITAKER, H.A., Linguistic competence: Evidence from aphasia. *Glossa, 4,* 46–54 (1970).

WHITAKER, H.A., and NOLL, J.D., Some linguistic parameters of the Token Test. *Neuropsychologia, 10,* 395–404 (1972).

WHITAKER, H.A., and WHITAKER, H., Lexical, syntactic, and semantic aspects of the Token Test: A linguistic taxonomy. In F. Boller and M. Dennis (Eds.), *Auditory Comprehension: Clinical and Experimental Studies with the Token Test.* New York: Academic Press (1979).

WHITBOURNE, S.K., Test anxiety in elderly and young adults. *International Journal of Aging and Human Development, 7,* 201–210 (1976).

WHITE, N., and KINSBOURNE, M., Does speech output control lateralize over time? Evidence from verbal-manual time-sharing tasks. *Brain and Language, 10,* 215–223 (1980).

WHITEHOUSE, P., CARAMAZZA, A., and ZURIF, E.B., Naming in aphasia: Interacting effects of form and function. *Brain and Language, 6,* 63–74 (1978).

WIEGEL-CRUMP, C., Agrammatism and aphasia. In Y. Lebrun and R. Hoops (Eds.), *Recovery in Aphasics.* Amsterdam: Swets & Zeitlinger (1976).

WIEGEL-CRUMP, C., and KOENIGSKNECHT, R.A., Tapping the lexical store of the adult aphasic: Analysis of the improvement made in word retrieval skills. *Cortex,* 9, 411–418 (1973).

WILCOX, M.J., DAVIS, G.A., and LEONARD, L.L., Aphasics' comprehension of contextually conveyed meaning. *Brain and Language,* 6, 362–377 (1978).

WILLIAMS, M., *Brain Damage, Behaviour, and the Mind.* New York: John Wiley & Sons (1979).

WILSON, P., Application of the symbolic match-to-sample task in language training. In R.H. Brookshire (Ed.), *Clinical Aphasiology Collected Proceedings 1972-1976.* Minneapolis: BRK (1978).

WING, S.D., NORMAN, D., POLLOCK, J.A., and NEWTON, T.H., Contrast enhancement of cerebral infarcts in computed tomography. *Radiology,* 121, 89–92 (1976).

WINNER, E., and GARDNER, H., Comprehension of metaphor in brain damaged patients. *Brain,* 100, 717–729 (1977).

WITELSON, S.F., Hemispheric specialization for linguistic and nonlinguistic tactual perception using a dichotomous stimulation technique. *Cortex,* 10, 3–17 (1974).

WITELSON, S.F., Neuroanatomical asymmetry in left-handers: A review and implications for functional asymmetry. In J. Herron (Ed.), *Neuropsychology of Left-Handedness.* New York: Academic Press (1980).

WOLF, J.K., *Practical Clinical Neurology.* Garden City, N.Y.: Medical Examination Publishing Co. (1980).

WULF, H.H., *My World Alone.* Detroit: Wayne State University Press (1979).

WYKE, M., An experimental study of verbal associations in dysphasic patients: A qualitative analysis. *Brain,* 85, 679–686 (1962).

YARNELL, P.R., Crossed dextral aphasia: A clinical radiological correlation. *Brain and Language,* 12, 128–139 (1981).

YARNELL, P.R., MONROE, P., and SOBEL, L., Aphasia outcome in stroke: A clinical neuroradiological correlation. *Stroke,* 7, 516–522 (1976).

YORKSTON, K.M., and BEUKELMAN, D.R., A system for quantifying verbal output of high-level aphasic patients. In R.H. Brookshire (Ed.), *Clinical Aphasiology Conference Proceedings.* Minneapolis: BRK (1977).

YORKSTON, K.M., and BEUKELMAN, D.R., An analysis of connected speech samples of aphasic and normal speakers. *Journal of Speech and Hearing Disorders,* 45, 27–36 (1980).

YORKSTON, K.M., MARSHALL, R.C., and BUTLER, M., Imposed delay of response: Effects on aphasics' auditory comprehension of visually and nonvisually cued material. *Perceptual and Motor Skills,* 44, 647–655 (1977).

ZAIDEL, E., A technique for presenting lateralized visual input with prolonged exposure. *Vision Research,* 15, 283–289 (1975).

ZAIDEL, E., Auditory vocabulary of the right hemisphere following brain bisection or hemidecortication. *Cortex,* 12, 191–211 (1976).

ZAIDEL, E., Unilateral auditory language comprehension on the Token Test following cerebral commissurotomy and hemispherectomy. *Neuropsychologia,* 15, 1–17 (1977).

ZAIDEL, E., Concepts of cerebral dominance in the split brain. In P. Buser and A. Rougeul-Buser (Eds.), *Cerebral Correlates of Conscious Experience.* Amsterdam: Elsevier (1978a).

ZAIDEL, E., Lexical organization in the right hemisphere. In P. Buser and A. Rougeul-Buser (Eds.), *Cerebral Correlates of Conscious Experience.* Amsterdam: Elsevier (1978b).

ZAIDEL, E., Long-term stability of hemispheric scores on the Token Test following brain bisection and hemidecortication. In F. Boller and M. Dennis (Eds.), *Auditory Comprehension: Clinical and Experimental Studies with the Token Test.* New York: Academic Press (1979).

ZURIF, E.B., Language mechanisms: A neuropsychological perspective. *American Scientist,* 68, 305–311 (1980).

ZURIF, E.B., and CARAMAZZA, A., Psycholinguistic structures in aphasia: Studies in syntax and semantics. In H. Whitaker and H.A. Whitaker (Eds.), *Studies in Neurolinguistics, Volume I.* New York: Academic Press (1976).

ZURIF, E.B., and CARAMAZZA, A., Comprehension, memory and levels of representation: A perspective from aphasia. In J.F. Kavanagh and W. Strange (Eds.), *Speech and Language in the Laboratory, School and Clinic.* Cambridge, Mass.: MIT Press (1978).

ZURIF, E.B., CARAMAZZA, A., FOLDI, N.S., and GARDNER, H., Lexical semantics and memory for words in aphasia. *Journal of Speech and Hearing Research,* 22, 456–467 (1979).

ZURIF, E.B., CARAMAZZA, A., and MYERSON, R., Grammatical judgments of agrammatic patients. *Neuropsychologia,* 10, 405–417 (1972).

ZURIF, E.B., CARAMAZZA, A., MYERSON, R., and GALVIN, J., Semantic feature representations for normal and aphasic language. *Brain and Language,* 1, 167–188 (1974).

ZURIF, E.B., GREEN, E., CARAMAZZA, A., and GOODENOUGH, C., Grammatical intuitions of aphasic patients: Sensitivity to functors. *Cortex,* 12, 183–186 (1976).

Index

A

Acute care hospital, 22–23, 127, 128–129
Acute stage of recovery, 84–86
    ischemia, 35–36
Adaptive strategies (*see* Agrammatism)
Administration of aphasia tests, 132, 133–
    134, 169, 184
Age:
    content of treatment, 285
    differential diagnosis, 146
    hemisphere asymmetry, 65–66
    prognostic factor, 222, 228–229, 237
Aging:
    differential diagnosis, 137, 147, 205–206
    recovery, 228–229
Agnosias, 5, 7–8, 130, 147–148
    auditory, 7, 32, 68
    color, 7, 32, 68
    for faces (prosopagnosia), 7, 32, 54, 68
    tactile (astereognosis), 8, 31, 68, 181
    visual, 7
    visual object, 7, 32, 68, 151
Agrammatism, 12–13
    adaptive strategies, 108–109, 258, 262
    in Broca's aphasia, 20, 58–59, 151
    comprehension, 119–122
    economy of effort, 107–108
    research, 106–109
    treatment, 150–151, 239, 253, 258, 274–
    275
Agraphia, 15
Alajouanine, T., 3, 13, 14–15, 216

Albert, M. L., 6, 9, 64, 66, 111, 113, 115,
    136–138, 139, 170, 177, 213, 220, 271,
    272
Alexia, 17, 124–125
Alexia with agraphia, 59, 139
Alexia without agraphia, 8, 32, 139
Alpha suppression (*see* Electroencephalogra-
    phy)
Alternative communicative modes, 255–257,
    261, 299
Alzheimer's disease, 2, 137
American Indian Gestural Code
    (AMERIND), 3, 233, 257, 272
Amount of recovery, 210–211, 213–214,
    216–217, 224–225
Anger, 293–294, 297
Angiography, 45
Angular gyrus, 29, 32, 58, 59–60, 139
Anomia, 10
Anomic aphasia, 21, 22 (*see also* Circumlocu-
    tion; Mild aphasia)
    differential diagnosis, 144, 183
    language research, 97, 98, 100, 102, 118,
    121, 205
    recovery and prognosis, 215, 220, 224,
    236
    site of lesion, 59–60, 68
    treatment (mild aphasia), 255, 263, 272–
    274
Anosognosia, 17, 20–21
Answering questions:
    assessment, 131, 150
    recovery, 215, 226